Second Edition

LANGDON PARSONS, M. D.

*Clinical Professor of Gynecology
Emeritus, Harvard Medical School*

HOWARD ULFELDER, M. D.

*Joe V. Meigs Professor of Gynaecology, Harvard
Medical School; Chief of the Vincent
Memorial Hospital (Gynecological Division of the
Massachusetts General Hospital)*

An
Atlas
of
Pelvic Operations

Illustrated by

MILDRED B. CODDING, A.B., M.A.

*Surgical Artist, Department of Surgery, Harvard
Medical School and Peter Bent Brigham Hospital
Boston, Massachusetts*

W. B. Saunders Company   PHILADELPHIA·LONDON·TORONTO

W. B. Saunders Company: West Washington Square
Philadelphia, PA 19105

1 St. Anne's Road
Eastbourne, East Sussex BN21 3UN, England

1 Goldthorne Avenue
Toronto, Ontario M8Z 5T9, Canada

Listed here is the latest translated edition of this book together
with the language of the translation and the publisher.

Spanish (*2nd Edition*) — Elicien, Barcelona, Spain

Italian (*2nd Edition*) — Editrice Universo, Rome, Italy

An Atlas of Pelvic Operations   ISBN 0-7216-7096-2

Print No.: 9   8   7

Dedicated to

JOE V. MEIGS

GEORGE W. W. BREWSTER

ARTHUR W. ALLEN

These, our teachers, are no longer here to add encouragement to our efforts; but we shall never cease to feel a great debt of gratitude for their contributions to our personal and our professional lives. This Atlas is a product of the school of gynecologic surgery which they developed and in which we operate as grateful students.

Preface

This book has been treated with generous affection since it first appeared in 1953. Criticisms of it have been few and always appropriate, and we are convinced that it has filled a need because there are so many young men and women in our specialty who say they use it frequently for reference and because there is a steady volume of sales each year to those who are at the beginning of their careers in Gynecology.

We believe that a revision is now indicated, chiefly to include procedures which were not well established at the time of previous writing but also to drop one or two operations in each section because they appear now to be inappropriate or because they are no longer used.

Once we had made the decision to undertake a change in content, we included of necessity serious consideration of changes in format. This has resulted in a major revision primarily in response to criticism that the size and shape of the original Atlas made it awkward to manage. The major subdivisions have not been changed, although the introductory pages to each section have been eliminated and any appropriate comments previously included in that area have now been attached to the text which accompanies the illustrations. A reader familiar with the previous effort will perhaps immediately notice the inclusion of a bit of philosophy with the running text. We do not believe that this will alter the conciseness and the usefulness of our previous arrangement which was planned quite deliberately to offer the reader a guide to technique in the performance of selected operative procedures.

The section on malignant disease has been almost entirely rewritten, the emphasis now being on the presentation of major bloc operations which deal with genital tract carcinoma, and we have eliminated staged operations and procedures which attack carcinoma in nongenital pelvic organs.

It should be stressed that radical surgery for cancer in organs of the pelvic area differs markedly in both scope and magnitude from the operative procedures employed for benign disease within the same organs. The problems compound when one elects to perform one of the exenteration procedures.

The primary aim of operations designed to cure cancer in the organs of the female pelvis is to eradicate the disease both at the local site and in areas to which it may be expected to extend. To be successful an operation must be planned to conform to the extent of the pathologic involvement. This presupposes a thorough understanding on the part of the surgeon of the life history of the particular neoplasm he is dealing with and a working knowledge of the normal pathways of extension. The emphasis is on cure; to achieve it, all the potential tumor-bearing tissue must be removed. It is not enough to obtain a limited survival or palliation when a more extensive surgical procedure might produce permanent salvage.

To understand thoroughly the varied ramifications of malignant processes requires considerable experience. These radical surgical procedures should not be undertaken unless the surgeon can, in good conscience, feel that he can successfully deal with the presenting problems. Unfortunately, the training required to handle cancer in the pelvis is available to only a few men in the larger teaching hospitals where there is a greater concentration of malignant disease. It is also true, however, that malignancy in the pelvis does not respect geographical distribution and much of it will be encountered in hospitals remote from metropolitan cancer centers. The problem in many instances, then, must be solved by surgeons who have little specialized training in this field.

It is our hope that the surgeon who has had sufficient surgical training and finds himself confronted with the problem of having to deal with pelvic cancer will find the description of these procedures helpful in carrying out what we consider to be adequate surgery for the common pelvic neoplasms.

We would add a note of caution about the performance of the exenteration procedures. These are formidable operations which should not be undertaken lightly by even the more experienced surgeon unless he has been exposed to the problems inherent in the operation and has the necessary support from the resident, nursing and laboratory services of his hospital. Our reason for including the exenteration operations is simply that they are being widely performed. By providing a step-by-step description of each operation, stressing the danger points and the means of avoiding them, we hoped to provide some helpful hints to the surgeon who is faced with the problem of extensive malignant disease and feels that he is capable of dealing with it.

In general, the steps of other operative procedures recorded here are designed to keep the operator out of trouble by pointing out to him the exact area in the operation where danger is apt to be present and attempting to show how complications may be avoided.

There are obviously many ways of performing operative procedures for any given manifestation of disease or functional disturbance in the pelvic area. The operations described in this Atlas by no means represent the only methods of achieving a successful outcome. Rather than present a description of multiple procedures of comparable usefulness, we have selected the operative techniques employed in the institutions in which we work. The methods described and illustrated here have been carried out repeatedly by surgeons of varying degrees of proficiency and in varying stages of surgical training and have proved to be both safe and effective. Complications have usually been avoided and morbidity and mortality have been low. We have selected only operations which are in common use.

The reader will immediately note that we have not outlined the indications for or against a given operative procedure. These are subject to many variables and tend to change with the passage of time. Furthermore, an operation may be sound in principle and execution but the indication for its use open to question.

Once the surgeon has elected to perform a specific operation, however, we hope that this Atlas will provide a "road map" which will guide him through to a satisfactory conclusion with the greatest possible ease and safety.

We have not included any consideration of the physiological aspects of preoperative and postoperative management. This is a deliberate omission for we are not writing a general textbook of surgery, and both preoperative and postoperative management, in principle as well as in fact, are subject to constant change.

The title, "Atlas of Pelvic Operations," indicates the nature of the work. It is not restricted to gynecological procedures. It is our hope that the procedures outlined will be useful to surgeons with varying interests who find themselves operating in the pelvic area, and not simply to the physician who limits his practice to the specialty of gynecology. It is our feeling that the surgeon operating in the pelvis should be capable of dealing with any type of pathology he encounters. Because the preoperative diagnosis of pelvic conditions may not be accurate at all times, on occasion the surgeon will be confronted with tissue abnormalities he did not expect. For this reason the Atlas includes many general surgical operations outside the field of what is generally considered to be gynecological surgery. They are described to help the surgeon deal with these problems as they are encountered. Whether the surgeon feels that he is capable of performing any given procedure is a matter of judgment based on conscience and experience.

It is impossible to put together a work of this sort without the support of colleagues and the house staffs of the hospitals in which we work. We extend our thanks to the administrative staffs of the Massachusetts General Hospital, the Vincent Memorial Hospital, the University Hospital, and Massachusetts Department of Public Health Hospital for Cancer at Pondville, and the Palmer Memorial Hospital of the New England Deaconess Hospital. In particular we would also like to express our special thanks to the Peter Bent Brigham Hospital and Dr. Francis D. Moore for permission to use the services of our artist, Miss Mildred Codding.

The authors greatly appreciate the interest and cooperation of Celso Ramon-Garcia, who advised in the revision of the section on operations for infertility.

We are deeply indebted for the wholehearted cooperation of Miss Signe Windhol, who managed to keep smiling through the long, tedious secretarial work required in the final typing of the manuscript.

We reserve our most important expression of gratitude to Miss Mildred Codding, who created her fine drawings with loving care and devotion. Her talent in producing the illustrations is exceeded only by her patience in dealing with her two demanding and temperamental coauthors. Our admiration and respect for her are boundless.

Our final thanks are due our publishers, who have facilitated every phase in the preparation of this revision and done everything in their power to help produce another fine teaching text.

It may be as amazing to the reader as it is to us that after this revision of the Atlas the authors remain as good friends as we were at the completion of the first edition.

LANGDON PARSONS
HOWARD ULFELDER

Contents

Section I ABDOMINAL OPERATIONS

Section II VAGINAL AND PERINEAL OPERATIONS

Section III   OPERATIONS FOR MALIGNANT DISEASE

Section I

Abdominal Operations

CONSIDERATIONS PRELIMINARY TO ALL ABDOMINAL SURGERY

Before discussing the detailed steps involved in pelvic operations, it is appropriate to review some of the general considerations that have a bearing on the ease and success with which this type of surgery may be performed.

Preoperative Preparation

Preoperative and postoperative care are integral components in the success of modern surgery, but the limited scope of this Atlas will not permit a detailed discussion of them. Today, antibiotics, blood and fluid replacement, electrolyte balance and intestinal deflation are all major factors in preventing many of the unfortunate complications of surgery that once were commonplace. In general, the surgery is in itself superior to that of past decades, but the recent advances in preparation for operation and its aftercare have made surgery easier and have permitted a more thoroughgoing attack on disease than was hitherto possible. This is as true of operations in the pelvis as it is of those in other areas of the body.

In part, the difficulties of pelvic surgery are in inverse ratio to the accuracy of the preoperative diagnosis. With the increasing costs of hospitalization there is a tendency to rely on the presenting pathological signs and symptoms without sufficient preliminary study or even preparation for operation. Too frequently the patient enters the hospital one afternoon, and operation is scheduled for the following morning.

If the surgeon is prepared for the unexpected, his ability to cope with the problem is considerably improved. There is a too frequent tendency to belittle the problem when unsuspected disease is encountered in the pelvis. If the surgeon is presented with a history of bleeding in a patient with a large abdominal tumor, the surgical procedure seems obvious. Failure to consider the possibility that the small or large bowel may be involved or kidney function impaired through encroachment of the tumor may unduly complicate the actual operation, particularly if these findings are discovered for the first time after the abdomen has been opened.

Therefore, although we have important additions to our facilities for treatment, the increasing costs tend to restrict their use to dealing with complications after they have happened rather than in preventing their occurrence.

The preliminary use of a long intestinal tube whenever bowel disease is known to exist or has a reasonable chance of being present will materially aid the surgeon and patient.

Investigation of the urinary tract for possible involvement of the bladder or ureter may modify the planned surgical attack.

Unexpected infection or operative difficulty may result in hemorrhage beyond the expectations of the surgeon. Adequate preliminary evaluation of the blood picture is essential. It is also important to have adequate amounts of replacement blood available to cover unexpected loss. A train of unfortunate events frequently follows the attempt to replace blood under the stress of operative emergency.

When bowel disease may be present, it may be well to prepare the bowel with chemotherapeutic agents in anticipation of inadvertent damage. The same precaution should be taken if there is a possibility of trauma to the urinary tract.

Inasmuch as profound alterations in the electrolyte balance may occur in the postoperative period, it is advisable to obtain a preliminary evaluation of the nitrogen excretion, chlorides, blood sugar, serum protein, sodium and potassium. Facilities for obtaining all these values are not always available, but the surgeon should have such evaluations as can be determined. The preliminary tests may indicate a need for medical correction before operation is undertaken.

Appraisal of thyroid function in the presence of subjective symptoms may be indicated. Hypothyroid patients, for example, do not tolerate morphine well.

The choice of anesthesia may be altered by unexpected findings revealed in a chest roentgenogram.

An electrocardiogram made because of the presence of minimal symptoms may serve as a base line for comparison if complications arise in the postoperative period.

Even in the presence of obvious palpable lesions in the pelvic area, other abnormalities, organic or physiological, may be present and may bear on the successful outcome of the contemplated operation.

Anesthesia

In general, anesthesia should permit successful and easy access to any pathological state that may be encountered within the abdomen even though preoperative evaluation places the disease in the pelvis. For example, the surgeon who encounters extensive diverticulitis of the sigmoid colon in a patient whose preoperative diagnosis suggested only the presence of endometriosis should not be handicapped in performing a transverse colostomy because of the inadequacy of the level of anesthesia.

Preoperative evaluation of the patient is important. It is helpful to have the anesthetist consider the needs of the patient in relation to the contemplated operation. The history of an old back injury or of headache following previous spinal anesthesia may influence the surgeon or anesthetist in the choice of inhalation rather than spinal anesthesia.

The patient's history may give some indication of hypersensitivity to the common preoperative drug medications. Known sensitivity exists to both morphine and barbiturates. Since adverse drug reaction would affect both the immediate operation and the subsequent postoperative course these facts should be known in advance. Properly administered preoperative drug therapy will aid materially in smoothing the operative procedures. A high degree of cooperation between surgeon and anesthetist is essential to success.

It seems pertinent at this point to indicate certain preliminary steps which may help to eliminate some of the common errors associated with intra-abdominal surgery for pelvic pathology.

Examination and Curettage under Anesthesia

It is of utmost importance that all observations made in the clinic or office be rechecked at the time of operation. The urinary bladder must first be emptied completely. Thorough inspection of the external genitalia, vagina and cervix, as well as digital examination of the rectum and vagina, is definitely indicated. Too many abdominal explorations are performed on the basis of a diagnosis reached by digital examination alone.

Description of gynecological disease and the specific indications for pelvic surgery are not within the scope of this text. In general, removal of the uterus by the abdominal route is performed for such conditions as fibromyomata, pelvic inflammatory disease, endometriosis and abnormal uterine bleeding. It is imperative, however, to keep constantly in mind the possibility of the occurrence of both malignant growths and pregnancy within the uterus. Most of the tragedies in gynecological surgery involving removal of the uterus arise either because these entities were not suspected or because the preoperative investigation was inadequate. For example, in a patient with a history of abnormal intermenstrual spotting the cervix may reveal a focus of carcinoma within the endocervix.

Curettage will indicate the size and contour of the uterine cavity and will detect the vast majority of lesions within the uterus and cervix. Curettage itself is not 100 per cent accurate, and the frozen section interpretations of the curettings may be less so. It is of great importance that the laboratory receive every specimen removed at curettage, however small. If malignant disease is suspected from the history and the physical findings, but the pathological findings are doubtful on the basis of frozen section, definitive treatment should await the report of study of permanent specimen preparations.

If the operator will make it an invariable rule to perform a thorough examination when the patient has been anesthetized, together with a diagnostic curettage in every instance in which pelvic laparotomy is contemplated, many unfortunate mistakes will be avoided.

Exploration of the Upper Abdomen

When the peritoneal cavity has been entered and before any procedure is started on the pelvic viscera, the upper abdomen should be carefully explored with the examining hand to determine coexistent disease which may have a bearing on the immediate operation or the patient's subsequent convalescence. For example, ovarian tumors may represent metastases from the gastrointestinal tract. Concomitant primary neoplasms can exist in both bowel and genital organs. Pre-existing gallstones may precipitate an attack of acute cholecystitis during the period of convalescence from pelvic laparotomy. Knowledge of the concomitant disease would influence the type of operation in the first instance and would ensure a more accurate diagnosis and proper therapy in the second.

Mobilization of the Uterus and Adnexa

This phase of intra-abdominal surgery is difficult to illustrate pictorially, but represents an essential preliminary maneuver for any surgical procedure in the female pelvis.

In order to secure an adequate operating field, the intestine must be gently packed out of the pelvis with moist gauze. Frequently, however, the uterus and adnexa are fixed in the pelvis by previous surgery or by inflammatory disease. In such instances the bowel may be densely adherent to the uterus, adnexa or broad ligaments. It is

imperative that the bowel be freed from these structures and packed out of the field before the uterus is removed. The proper line of cleavage is best established by gentle, gloved finger manipulation. Where the bowel loops can be grasped, separation is often possible by gentle rolling of the tissue between the thumb and forefinger; only occasionally will help from a sharp instrument such as a knife or scissors be needed. The useful slogan, "stay on the uterine side," should be followed closely, for it is better to leave benign disease on the attached viscera than to remove a section of small bowel or sigmoid with the specimen.

The adnexa must be freed from the posterior leaves of the broad ligaments and sigmoid before any attempt is made to remove either the adnexa or the uterus, or both. Application of a tenaculum to the fundus or a clamp on the tubal angle and ovarian ligament for traction may be a helpful maneuver.

It is important to recognize that the fixation of tissues resulting from either endometriosis or malignant lesions differs materially from that encountered in pelvic inflammation from other causes. This observation has practical value. A line of cleavage can always be established between pelvic inflammatory disease involving tube and ovary and the attached viscera. For the most part, mobilization in pelvic inflammation should be begun from below upward. A suction apparatus should be available for ready use in the event an abscess is entered. Whenever firm bands of tissue are encountered, they should be brought under complete vision before clamps are applied. The presence of adhesive bands that will not separate suggests that either vessels are present or a false cleavage plane has been established.

The invasive tendency of endometriosis differs from that of pelvic inflammation. Ovarian endometriosis invades the posterior leaf of the broad ligament and cannot be separated without rupture of the adherent chocolate cysts. Great care must be taken that endometriosis has not invaded the small bowel or sigmoid adherent to the pelvic masses. The approach to this type of pathology is usually made from above downward rather than from below upward as in pelvic inflammation. It is extremely important to stay on the uterine side in the dissection.

When the surgeon encounters a large malignant ovarian cyst or pathologic state involving the side wall of the pelvis, it is important to ascertain the position of the ureter by exposing it at the pelvic brim through the posterior peritoneal covering.

The mobilization of the uterus and adnexa simply constitutes a preparation of an adequate operative field and represents a basic preliminary step for whatever type of pelvic surgery the surgeon elects to perform.

Positioning of the Operating Team

The diagram indicates the usual position of the surgeon and his assistants and nurses.

The surgeon (operator) stands to the left of the patient. This is the optimum position for a right-handed surgeon operating in the lower abdomen. By shifting his feet and turning his body toward the head he is in a satisfactory position to do any necessary exploration or operation in the upper abdomen as well. By and large, this position is maintained throughout the operative maneuvers described. Occasionally, the surgeon may shift to the opposite side of the table to have better access to the lateral structures deep in the left pelvis. When this is done, it will be indicated to the reader. Such a move is usually made when the over-

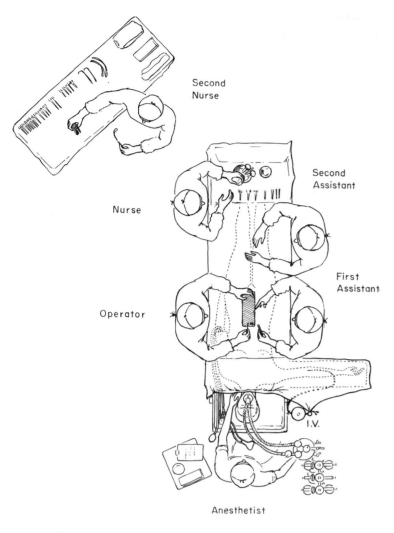

Diagrammatic Representation of Operating Room for
Pelvic Surgery.

second nurse, standing in front of the instrument table, anticipates the nurse's need for supplies not available on the Mayo stand, such as suture material, sponges or infrequently used instruments. If only one nurse is scrubbed, the larger instrument table is so placed that from her position to the left of the surgeon she may supply her own needs from it.

The first assistant stands directly opposite the surgeon just below the board carrying the patient's extended arm. He should be cautioned not to hyperextend the patient's shoulder by pushing too firmly against the board in his zeal to provide more effective assistance.

The second assistant, if available, usually takes his place to the right of the first assistant opposite the nurse. His job is to aid in exposure by retraction as directed.

Consistently throughout this Atlas the drawings have been made from the position which offers the most unobstructed view of the field, usually from just behind or beside the surgeon. Since the operator stands on the left side of the table, in most cases the reader may assume that the patient's feet are toward the top of the page. A special effort has been made to keep the relationships in all plates (except for the insets and close-ups) accurate on a scale approximately two-thirds of normal size.

Postoperative Management

This important phase of pelvic surgery strives for anatomic healing and physiological recovery in the shortest possible time and with minimum discomfort. Every decision made and every order written in the postoperative period must take these factors into account, perhaps favoring one at the expense of another in individual cases.

The orders which accompany the patient as she leaves the operating room should be concise and specific and should avoid the routine in favor of the individual need. Recording of the vital signs is essential and must be maintained throughout the recovery period. Periodic registering of pulse, respiration and blood pressure is also important during the period of returning consciousness after anesthesia. The patient should be constantly observed during this time, preferably in a special room or ward. She should be turned often enough to give each lung a chance to expand. The order sheet must include specific orders for administration of an opiate for relief of pain and discomfort.

Blood and fluid replacement are based on the calculated need. Both the volume and the electrolyte content will vary with circumstances. In general, a total fluid intake of approximately 2000 cc. daily should be maintained. Such quantities often cannot be taken by mouth in the immediate postoperative period, and intravenous supplement will be necessary. The actual amount, the rate of administration and the time the infusion is to be given should be clearly stated in the postoperative orders.

After the patient's recovery from anesthesia a different set of problems arises. Recordings of the pulse, temperature and respirations are continued, and the patient will need further opiates for pain and discomfort. A change of drug may be indicated if nausea and vomiting persist. The blood pressure readings are recorded as the individual case dictates.

Dysfunction of the urinary bladder after pelvic laparotomy is common but not routine. Although a variety of plans for management are in vogue, the basic precept should be the avoidance of overdistention; even one such episode may stretch the bladder to such an extent that the faculty

hanging edge of the abdominal wound interferes with exposure of the pelvic wall. Moreover, separate bilateral procedures, such as extraperitoneal lymph node resection, will be made easier if the surgeon changes his position to the side on which the operation is to be done.

The anesthetist occupies a position at the head of the patient. The anesthesia machine, if inhalation is the chosen method, will be set up to the right of the anesthetist. The work table with his supplies and charts will be on the left. He is protected from the operating field by linen drapes over a wire hoop which attaches to the table and is adjustable either forward or backward. The wire hoop permits him to have constant direct observation of the patient's face as well as an unobstructed working field. The patient's right arm is extended on a board (placed beneath the mattress) to permit intravenous infusion. The upright used to support the infusion bottle is placed to the right of the anesthetist behind the board supporting the arm. The entire pathway of the intravenous fluid is under the direct vision of the anesthetist, whose duty it is to regulate the speed and quantity of the flow.

A blood pressure cuff is in place on the patient's left arm, which is tucked beneath her body with the fingers extended. The surgeon's movements are thus unencumbered. The tubes from the sphygmomanometer lead toward the patient's head, allowing the anesthetist to make the necessary observations from behind the protective drapes.

The nurse, standing on the same side as the surgeon, is able from her position at the patient's feet to feed the instruments to him from a Mayo stand placed over the foot of the table. The main instrument table is on her left. A

of complete emptying is not recovered for days. An order for catheterization should be written to cover the immediate postoperative situation. When bladder difficulty can be expected from the kind of operation performed, an in-dwelling catheter may be inserted at the conclusion of the operation. Orders should then be left to cover the management of the catheter. Small prophylactic doses of nontoxic chemotherapeutic agents may be advisable if repeated catheterizations have been necessary or the nature of the surgery suggests bladder infection.

Ileus may be expected for one or two days after operation, and it will be advisable to restrict the intake by mouth to clear fluids in small amounts until normal peristalsis has been re-established. At times the ileus is severe enough to produce gastric dilatation. Simple gastric lavage may bring much relief. In severe cases a Levin tube in the stomach or a longer tube in the small intestine may be indicated. The large bowel is usually less prompt than the small intestine in its recovery of tone, but this delay is rarely the cause of serious difficulty. Enemas for relief should be ordered with due regard to the immediate findings and to the type of operation performed. They should not be given purely as a routine measure.

With a strong wound closure early ambulation is possible and should be encouraged as a means of minimizing postoperative tissue wasting. It may have some bearing on reducing the incidence of postoperative pulmonary emboli. To this end it is better to have the patient walk to the point of tolerance than to sit up in a chair for protracted periods.

Complications are infrequent, but should be anticipated and forestalled as far as possible. In general, they will develop least often when surgery is gentle and hemostasis is complete and when a happy balance between activity and comfort is maintained during the recovery period. Every available therapeutic regimen which has proved useful during convalescence should be understood and used as indications suggest. This applies particularly to antibiotics. The surgeon would do well to question exactly what he hopes to accomplish with any agent he uses. Routine use of any one or combination of drugs on the theory that they probably will not cause any harm and may do some good should be condemned.

Postoperative pain and discomfort vary enormously from patient to patient. The surgeon should therefore not fall back on standardized orders for opiates since some patients will require more, some less, medication for a similar discomfort. The wound itself is most painful immediately after the operation and the patient usually requires an opiate for relief. Within a day, however, physical comfort seems to improve as the patient resumes moderate activity, and it may be wise to change to medications with less depressant effects. As the convalescence progresses a great variety of causes for discomfort may develop; each should be treated in its own appropriate fashion and an attempt made to eliminate the cause as well as to stifle the pain.

Intangible factors play a role in the recovery phase after surgery. Most people abhor illness and disability and are anxious to return to the security of their daily routine. All are apprehensive to a greater or lesser degree, and attentiveness and sympathy on the part of the physician are very much in order and will help to sustain the patient through the trials of convalescence. The doctor who is wise and sincere cannot consider his job done until the patient is restored to full activity; he must be ready with explanations and advice at any point along the path to this goal. Each patient must be regarded as an individual problem.

HELPFUL HINTS FOR HYSTERECTOMY

For the sake of emphasis the measures used to avoid pitfalls inherent in the technique of abdominal hysterectomy will be outlined and discussed.

1. A preliminary examination under anesthesia should always be done. In this manner the office examination is checked.

2. The bladder should be emptied by catheter regardless of whether the patient has previously voided. A distended bladder can add enormously to the technical difficulties of hysterectomy.

3. The importance of curettage has already been stressed. This step should never be omitted.

4. When the peritoneum has been opened, the upper abdomen must be explored. It is well for the surgeon to have an established routine for such an examination. One might begin with palpation of the right kidney, liver, gallbladder, stomach, duodenum and pancreas, left kidney and spleen. The examining hand then passes rapidly over the colon from the cecum to the sigmoid. The aorta and adjacent nodal areas are then palpated, together with the base of the small bowel mesentery. It matters little how this is done as long as it follows a set pattern.

5. Mobilization of the uterus and adnexa must precede any attempt to remove the uterus.

6. The intestines must be kept out of the field of operation. Adequate anesthesia and the Trendelenburg position may suffice, but often moist gauze packs will also be necessary. It is important to minimize the pressure of the packs on the viscera, particularly the large vessels crossing the brim of the pelvis.

7. Whenever the history or physical findings suggest the likelihood of carcinoma within the uterus, Kelly clamps should be placed across the tubal isthmus and ovarian ligament on both sides. These clamps take the place of the tenaculum usually inserted on the fundus of the uterus. Adequate traction is thus maintained and spillage of viable cancer cells through the tubes prevented.

8. Development of the bladder flap as the initial step before dividing the ovarian vessels will greatly simplify the technique of hysterectomy. The bladder can be mobilized bloodlessly with the minimum expenditure of time, effort and risk. The anatomical relationship of the ureter to uterine artery and cervix is readily visualized. If the round ligament and ovarian vessels have been divided first, the lower portion of the broad ligament falls into accordian-like folds which make separation of the bladder, cervix and broad ligament much more difficult and bloody. For this reason the bladder flap should be developed as the initial step in the procedure.

9. To avoid injury to the dome of the bladder, the incision through the anterior sheath of peritoneum in the midline should be made with care. This thin peritoneal flap is then dissected off the bladder for 2 to 3 cm. At the conclusion of the operation this will serve to cover the raw areas completely and it will not be necessary to draw the bladder over the vaginal or cervical stump.

10. When the adnexa are to be left, it is important that the round and ovarian ligaments be divided and ligated separately. This is done in order that there be no tension on the ovarian vessel when the round ligament is resutured to the stump of the cervix or vagina in the reconstructive phase. Eliminating any tension on the ovarian pedicle ensures an adequate blood supply to the retained ovary.

11. When the ovaries are to be removed, it is of utmost importance that the relation of the ovarian vessel to the ureter be checked at the point where they cross the common iliac artery. This is one of the commonest sites of injury to the ureter and occurs largely because the proximity of the ureter is unsuspected. Injury may be avoided by tracing the course of the ureter as seen through the peritoneum and by elevating the vessels away from the ureter before applying the stitch ligature.

12. The second most common and the most unsuspected point at which the ureter may be damaged is the area of the uterosacral ligament where it is closer to the dissection than at any other time during the hysterectomy. The position of the ureter, bladder and uterine artery should be checked by palpating the base of the exposed broad ligament with thumb and forefinger. A characteristic snapping sensation is elicited as the ureter slips between the fingers.

The uterosacral ligaments are then clamped, divided and sutured close to the uterus well away from the ureter. By dividing the peritoneum between the sectioned uterosacral ligaments a bloodless plane of cleavage can be established which allows the peritoneum and uterosacral ligaments and ureters to be pushed downward away from the cervix and posterior vagina.

13. The maneuver just described is also useful in protecting the rectum against injury. Endometriosis of the rectovaginal septum frequently fixes the rectum to the posterior wall of the uterus between the uterosacral ligaments. It may be separated by sharply angulating the uterus toward the symphysis, producing a fracture through the peritoneum at a safe point. If the separation is not evident, it may be created by dividing the peritoneum between the ligaments with a long-handled knife.

14. There is another reason for separating the uterosacral ligaments in this manner. As soon as the surgeon has divided and secured the uterine vessels he approaches what is known as the "bloody angle" in total hysterectomy. This is a dangerous area. The operative steps in this region can be made bloodless. If the uterosacral ligaments are separated from the uterus, less tissue will be included in the clamp that must be applied to the cervical branches of the uterine vessels. It is also important to leave a cuff of tissue beyond the clamp to prevent retraction. Because of the cuff and primarily because less tissue is included there is less danger of tissue pulling out of the clamp and causing troublesome bleeding. Blind attempts to recapture the bleeding point further increase the likelihood of ureteral damage.

15. The majority of the vesicovaginal fistulae encountered in gynecology today come, not from poor obstetrics, but from injury to the bladder in the course of total hysterectomy. The initial development of the bladder flap is one important step in their prevention. The bladder may be gently stripped down from the cervix by the same pill-rolling motion used to separate the bowel from the uterus. As further protection the bladder should be separated from the uterine vessels. The bladder tends to be pulled up on the uterine vessels in a crescentic-shaped fold of tissue. This attachment may be gently freed with scissor dissection by staying in a plane superficial to the vessels. It is of the utmost importance that any tissue to be incised or sutured be under direct vision if injury to the bladder is to be avoided.

16. The mobilization of the bladder from the cervix is essential if the entire cervix is to be removed. Invariably, enough vagina is removed anteriorly and posteriorly, but some portion of the cervix may be left behind on the lateral vaginal fornix if insufficient attention is paid to these corners.

17. Because we recognize that the curettage is not infallible we have made it an invariable rule that every excised uterus and ovary should be opened at the operating table and their interior inspected before closure of the abdomen. If possible, the surgeon's observations should be checked by the resident pathologist.

ABDOMINAL HYSTERECTOMY

Total Hysterectomy

In the first sixteen plates the authors have chosen to carry the reader through an entire operation from the preliminary phases to the completed closure. Every pelvic laparotomy should be preceded by a preliminary examination and curettage under anesthesia. All too frequently the findings at operation are distinctly different from those noted in the office or on the ward. For example, the surgeon performing a laparotomy for a cystic adnexal tumor may find, if he has not checked his preoperative observations, that a physiological cyst has ruptured spontaneously and that the indications for surgery are no longer valid.

There are other reasons for performing this maneuver as a routine procedure. (1) The bladder is emptied. In rare instances the indications for the removal of centrally placed tumors may disappear as the bladder is deflated. The primary reason, however, is to be certain that the bladder is collapsed. A distended bladder can unnecessarily complicate the technical steps of an abdominal hysterectomy. (2) The cervix is inspected and the uterine cavity and the endocervical canal are evaluated. There are many explanations of abnormal uterine bleeding. The decision to preserve or remove the adnexa may depend on the findings at curettage. If performed as a routine step whenever hysterectomy is contemplated, the examination avoids the likelihood of discovering unsuspected disease after the uterus has been removed.

Figure 1. The patient should be lifted, not pulled, into the lithotomy position, with the buttocks at the end of the table. This is done to avoid skin abrasion which can produce a troublesome postoperative complication. Note the wide angled stirrups which permit the legs to lie easily without pressure on the medial calf. In this position the perineum is prepared with whatever antiseptic agent the surgeon elects to use. Placing of the linen drapes and, if the surgeon prefers, the application of the new adhesive drape completes the preparation of the operative field.

Figure 2. The lips of the labia are separated with the thumb and finger of the left hand, exposing the urethra. A lubricated catheter, either rubber, metal or glass, is inserted into the urethra and the bladder is emptied. To ensure complete evacuation the surgeon should apply pressure with his left hand on the abdominal wall above the symphysis.

Figure 3. A careful vaginal examination is carried out. Primarily we are concerned with the consistency of the cervix, the size, position, contour and mobility of the uterus and any abnormality, induration or fixation of the pelvic floor and adnexal areas. If there is any doubt, you may want to do a rectal examination. The complete relaxation of the patient under anesthesia may confirm or deny the preoperative observations.

Figure 4. The gross appearance of the cervix is evaluated. A biopsy should be made of any suspicious areas. Occasionally the anterior vaginal wall obscures the cervix. To simplify the placing of the tenaculum on the cervix the surgeon need only retract the bladder with the thumb of the left hand. Elevation and traction on the tenaculum expose the cervical os. A long probe is gently inserted in the cervical canal and advanced into the endometrial cavity. This enables you to determine the depth of the cavity. Care must be exercised and undue pressure avoided to prevent perforation of the uterine wall. This is particularly true of the small atrophic uterus in the older woman.

This description of the curettage is presented in abbreviated form. It will be described in greater detail in the section on vaginal procedures.

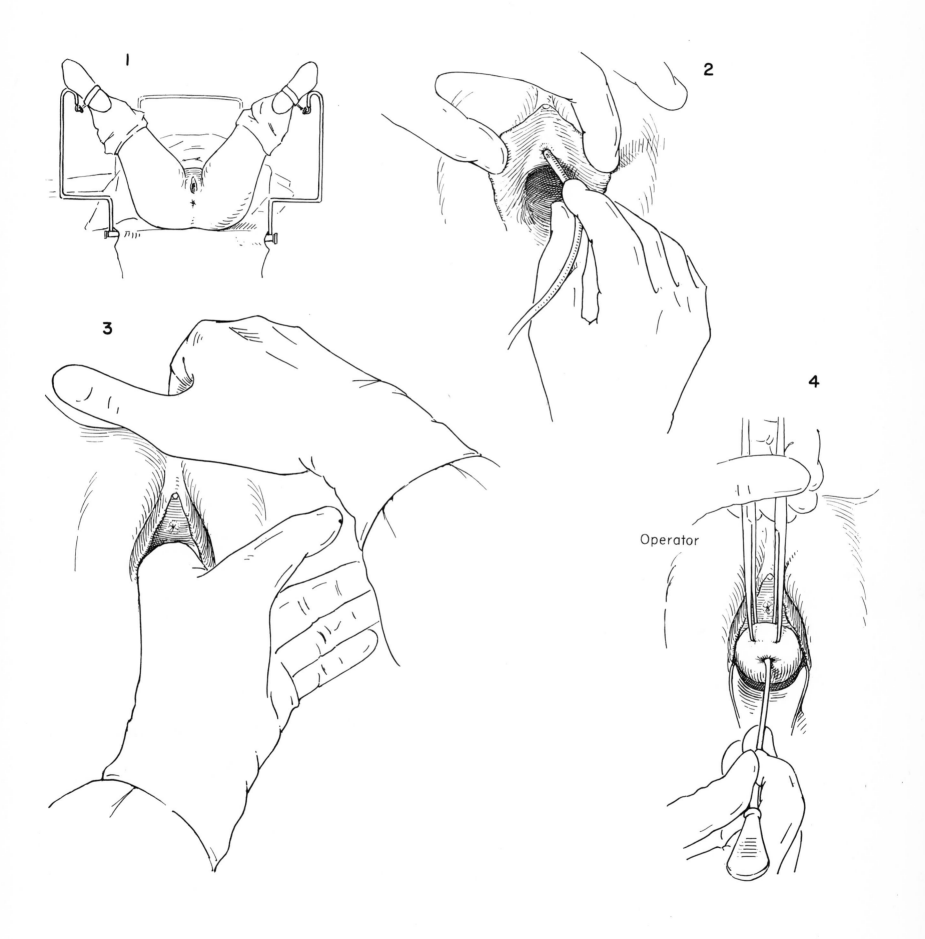

Figure 5. Before introducing a graduated type of Hank dilator into the cervical canal the surgeon has previously determined the depth of the endometrial cavity by inserting a probe.

The dilators must be used gently to avoid possible perforation. To increase his sense of touch the surgeon holds the tenaculum in his own left hand. If the assistant holds it he has no idea how much pressure he is exerting. The smallest of the series of dilators is followed serially by those of increasing diameter. In this manner the musculature of the cervix is stretched gradually. The so-called glove stretcher produces too much leverage and may split the cervix; for this reason it is no longer used.

In introducing the dilator the surgeon should avoid forcing it into the canal, for the plunger-like action can force endometrial tissue through the tube into the peritoneal cavity.

Figure 6. To ensure a complete diagnosis every piece of tissue, however small, must be saved and presented to the pathologist. This is the reason we insert fine meshed gauze or a sheet of rubber into the vagina beneath the cervix to aid in the collection of the uterine contents. The tissue is more likely to be lost if caught in the interstices of the usual coarse gauze.

In performing the curettage it is important to distinguish between the material taken from the endocervical canal and that scraped from the endometrial cavity. It is wise then to begin the curettage by concentrating on the endocervix. The scrapings should be inspected and set apart in their own container. The surgeon then directs his attention to the uterine cavity. Special attention should be given to the cornua of the uterus. This area is the "blind spot" in any curettage.

Each time the curette is introduced and withdrawn the material obtained should be inspected. The surgeon then has a better idea of the origin of the tissue. It is common procedure, but a poor idea, to scrape the cavity thoroughly before withdrawing the curette and to evaluate the endometrium grossly. If it has a shiny surface it is less likely to be malignant. On the other hand, if it has a granular yellowish appearance and breaks up easily when you run your finger over it, the suspicion of cancer arises. As we noted in the beginning, every piece of endometrium, however small, should be sent to the pathologist for careful examination.

Figure 7. Inasmuch as the curette may fail to dislodge a polyp which has a broad base or is suspended by a stalk which allows it to lie free in the cavity, another grasping type instrument should be used to explore the cavity.

INSET A. We have found that the forceps usually employed to explore the common duct at the time of cholecystectomy serves the purpose admirably. It is shown here being introduced into the uterine cavity.

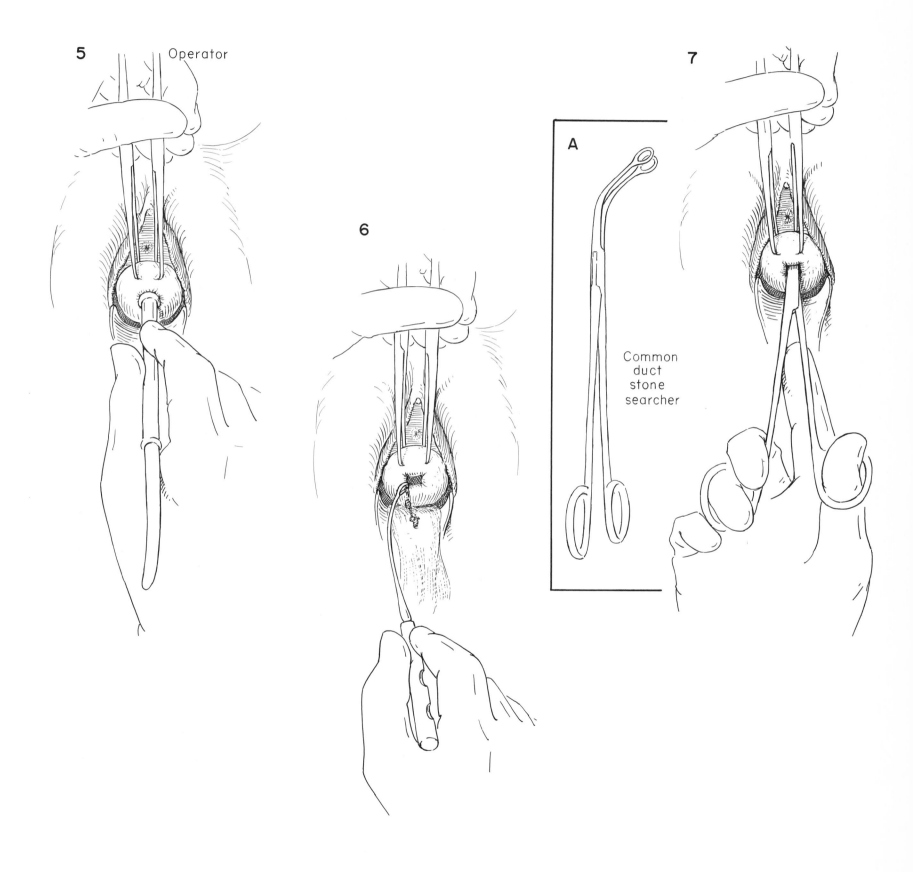

5 Operator

6

7

A

Common
duct
stone
searcher

Figure 8. Proper positioning of the patient on the operating table is important to the surgeon and to the patient during her subsequent convalescence. The patient is shown in the position generally preferred by surgeons operating in the pelvic region. The degree of depression of the head of the table should be enough to permit the intestines to fall back out of the pelvis naturally and easily. This reduces the amount of gauze packing required to maintain an operative field clear of any intestine that may tend to hamper the necessary surgical procedures. Forceful packing traumatizes the bowel, increases the likelihood of postoperative ileus and exerts so much pressure on the contents of the upper abdomen and diaphragm that the anesthetist has a more difficult time with the administration of anesthesia. The chances of postoperative atelectasis are also increased. An extreme Trendelenburg position will also complicate the problems of the anesthetist.

The patient is maintained in the moderate Trendelenburg position by breaking the foot piece of the table at the level of the popliteal space. Attention should be paid to this detail, for an improper break may create abnormal pressure on the calf and result in thrombosis of the popliteal veins and subsequent embolus. To further secure the position of the patient the feet are tied by a long, wide-tailed cotton strap that passes around the ankle and is fastened to the cross bar beneath the foot of the table. Note that no shoulder braces are used. There is, therefore, less danger of brachial stretching and subsequent paralysis.

The trunk of the body is supported by a straight table. This is an important detail that must be checked because angulation, either in extension or flexion, maintained during a long operation could produce troublesome backache in the convalescent period.

To permit intravenous infusion of an anesthetic agent, saline or blood, the arm is extended on a flat board that passes beneath the operating table mattress. To avoid obstructing the surgeon's movement the patient's extended arm should be on the opposite side of the table. Care must be taken that the shoulder is not abducted excessively and brachial stretching induced. With the patient in proper position an adjustable frame can be used to exclude the anesthetist from the operative field and still provide ample room for him to work at the head of the table.

The reader should note that the surgeon stands at the left of the patient with the first assistant directly opposite, while the nurse and the instrument table are on the side of the surgeon. The skin is now prepared. If the surgeon elects to use an adherent drape it should be placed in position at this time.

INSET A. After proper preparation of the skin and walling off with linen drapes a paramedian incision is made beginning at the symphysis and passing upward to curve slightly to the left if the surgeon elects to extend the incision above the umbilicus.

Figure 9. The incision extends through the skin and fat to the level of the fascia.

Figure 10. The assistant clamps each bleeding vessel as it is encountered.

Figure 11. The vessels so secured are ligated with fine suture material.

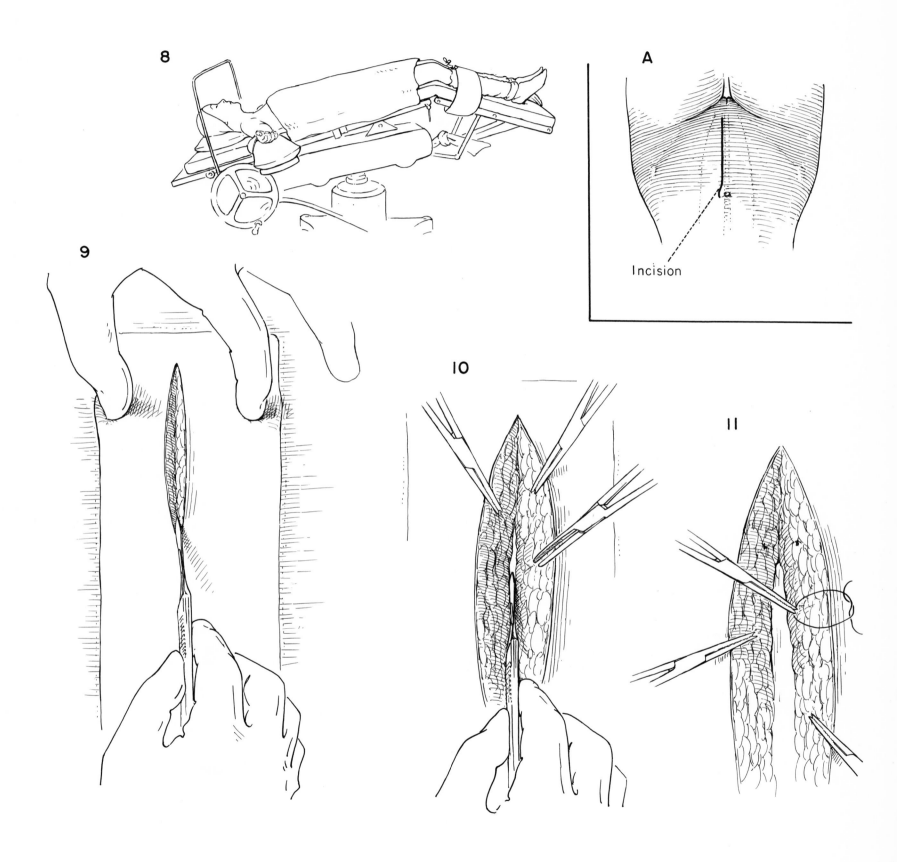

8

9

A

Incision

10

11

Figure 12. If an adherent drape is not used, the skin of the abdominal wall should be isolated from the wound created by the incision. This may be done in a variety of ways. Frequently towels are applied to the incised skin edges and held in place by clips. A refinement would be suturing the towels to the skin edge with a running type of suture. The surgeon may elect to fix the towels in place with dura clips. Another method often used employs large gauze squares or packs as skin edge covers and deep wound protectors. The leading edges are turned in facing each other and fixed to the skin with towel clips. The free, or turned in, edge then covers the fat of the abdominal wall and keeps it from contamination. Any of these methods will protect the operative field from the surrounding skin.

The incision is deepened to expose the underlying fascia as the surgeon and assistant apply counterpressure on the incised wound edges and the overlying fat. Individual vessels in the fat have been clamped and ligated as previously indicated.

The actual incision in the fascia is made slightly to the left of the midline, beginning at the symphysis and passing up and toward the umbilicus. The underlying rectus muscle on the left side is exposed.

Figure 13. To facilitate the separation of the edge of the left rectus muscle from the fascia the assistant applies clamps to the cut edge of the fascia on the medial side. The assistant then elevates the clamps and holds the fascial edge on tension as the surgeon retracts the muscle laterally with his left hand. Care must be taken not to damage the deep epigastric vein which lies on the undersurface of the muscle close to the free edge. If inadvertently damaged it must be secured and ligated to avoid the formation of a hematoma.

Retracting the muscle with his left hand the surgeon now dissects the muscle from its bed, exposing the peritoneum lying beneath. One may expect to find veins of varying caliber lying obliquely on the surface of the peritoneum. They must be individually isolated, divided and ligated.

Figure 14. To avoid the possibility of creating a hernia at the lower end of the incision the surgeon will be wise if he dissects out the pyramidalis muscle which crosses the lower end of the wound obliquely. With the leading edge identified, the muscle can be freed from its bed without dividing it. When the wound is closed the pyramidalis will lie obliquely across the rectus, thereby strengthening the lower abdominal wall.

Figure 15. As the surgeon separates the pyramidalis from the apposing rectus muscle he will invariably encounter vessels at the midportion of the muscle which can produce troublesome bleeding if they are inadvertently sectioned. These vessels should be identified, clamped and ligated with silk or cotton.

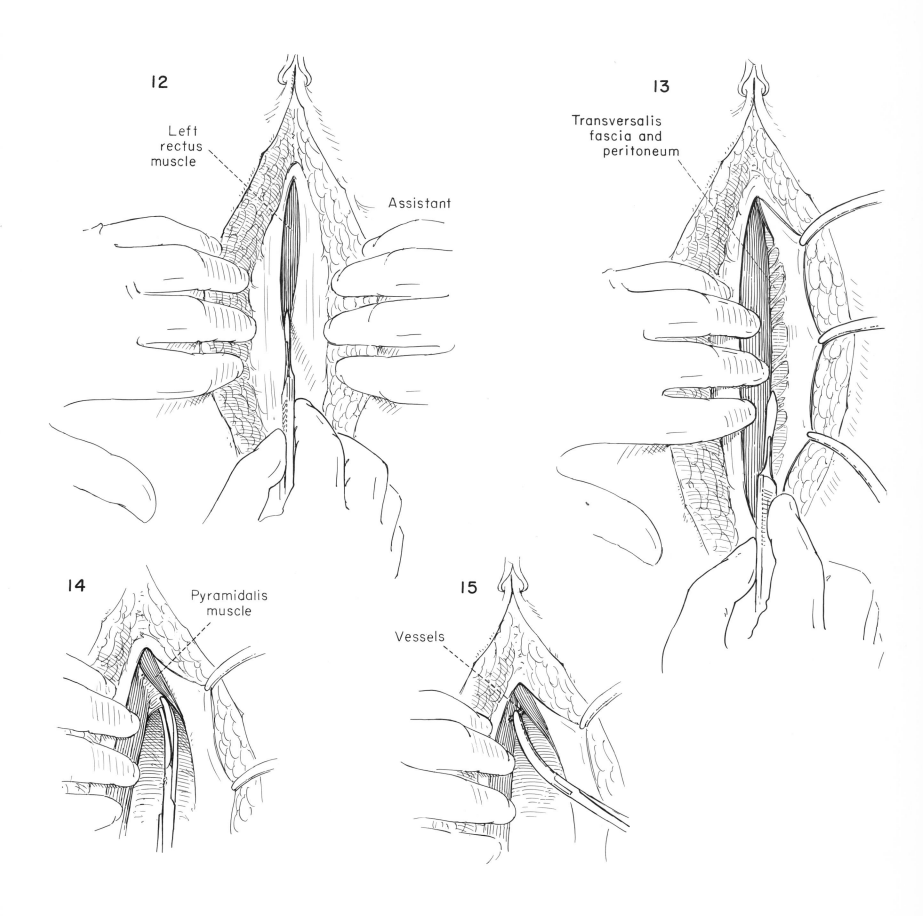

12

Left rectus muscle

Assistant

13

Transversalis fascia and peritoneum

14

Pyramidalis muscle

15

Vessels

Figure 16. The left rectus muscle is retracted laterally. The peritoneum presents through the whole extent of the wound. The surgeon and assistant grasp the peritoneum opposite one another with toothed forceps. The use of Kelly or Kocher clamps for this maneuver is to be condemned. Extreme care must be taken that bowel is not included in the forceps. Bowel may be adherent to the peritoneum. If there is any question, select another spot to enter the abdominal cavity. Should the peritoneum be taut because of incomplete anesthesia, wait until complete relaxation is acquired. The peritoneum is then elevated by forceps and an incision made through its full thickness to enter the abdominal cavity.

Figure 17. The opening is widened by lateral traction of the tissue forceps. After assuring himself that there is no bowel adherent to the peritoneum, the surgeon applies a Kelly clamp to the cut edge. The assistant carries out the same maneuver and clamps the opposite side.

Figure 18. The scalpel is now abandoned for curved scissors. After proper inspection of the undersurface of the peritoneum the incision is enlarged.

Figure 19. The surgeon then introduces the second and third fingers of the left hand into the opening of the peritoneum, extending them in the direction of the symphysis. This step protects the bowel from possible damage as the incision is enlarged. The extent of the incision downward is limited by the proximity of the bladder. The first observation of bleeding from the cut edge as the incision approaches the symphysis should give warning of the proximity of the bladder.

Figure 20. The same maneuver is carried out in an upward direction away from the symphysis.

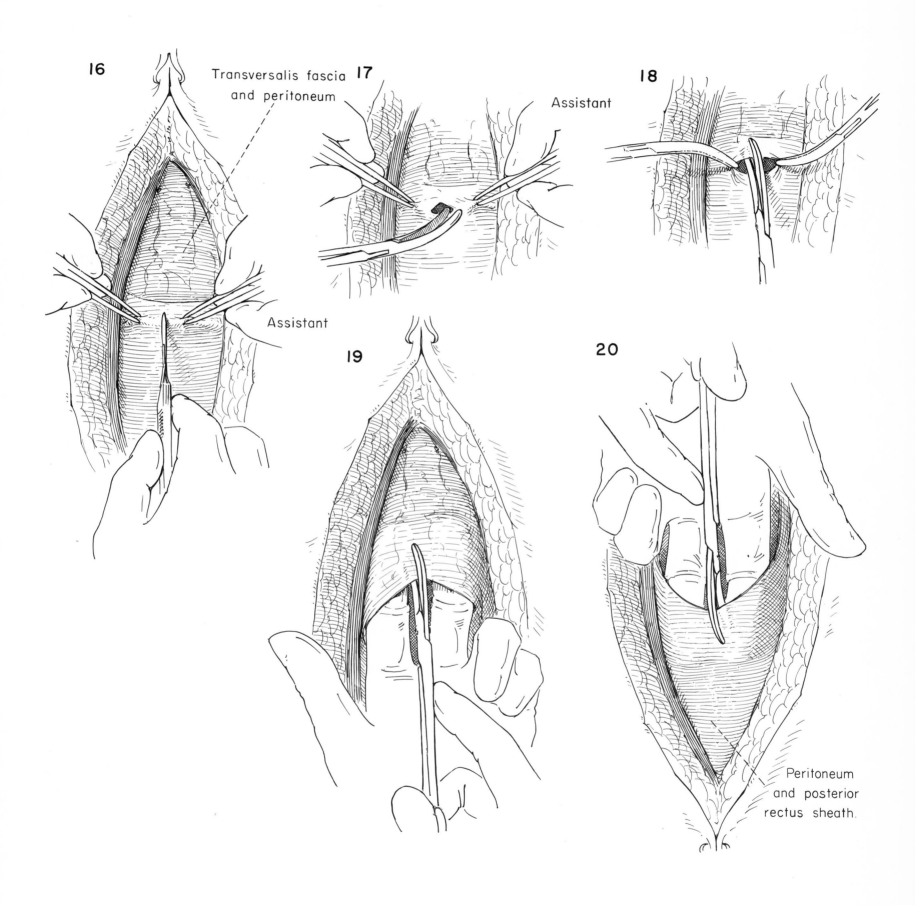

16 Transversalis fascia and peritoneum

17 Assistant

Assistant

18

19

20 Peritoneum and posterior rectus sheath.

Figure 21 (AND INSET A).   In this figure the surgeon standing on the left side of the patient inserts his left hand and begins the exploration of the abdominal cavity.

Unless the surgeon encounters an inflammatory process in the pelvis when he first enters the abdomen, he is obligated to explore the rest of the abdominal cavity despite the fact that his primary concern lies with the uterus and adnexa. (If there is an active inflammatory condition the risk of contaminating the upper abdomen is too great.) When no such condition exists the surgeon and patient have much to gain from a survey which includes palpation of the other organs in the abdomen. It can be done quickly and reasonably accurately if a systematic procedure is followed. There are many reasons for doing this. In the first place the preoperative interpretation of the cause of the symptomatology may be inaccurate even though the vaginal and rectal findings have been confirmed. The patient may have an asymptomatic Meckel's diverticulum or a retrocecal appendix. An unsuspected malignant lesion may be found in the stomach, small intestine or colon.

On exploration of the upper abdomen the surgeon frequently palpates asymptomatic gallstones. Although it is unwise to combine cholecystectomy with any pelvic operation other than appendectomy, it is of great importance to know that stones are present in the gallbladder. In the immediate postoperative period the patient may develop an attack of pain in the upper abdomen or lower right chest which may be incorrectly attributed to an embolus or infarct. Should the patient, several years later, have an attack of jaundice, the known presence of gallstones would immediately suggest the correct diagnosis.

If the problem is one of malignant disease in the uterus or the ovary, known to be present or suspected prior to exploration, the palpation of a metastasis in the liver may influence the surgeon to modify, or even abandon, the procedure previously planned. The same would hold true if the malignant process had spread to the nodes along the aorta.

Not to recognize the presence of coexistent disease may trap the surgeon into performing an inadequate or perhaps ill-advised pelvic operation. The time to explore comes immediately following the exposure of the peritoneal cavity. This maneuver is too often neglected by gynecologists concentrating on their particular province, the pelvis. The exploration should be systematic. With practice the exploration can be carried out very quickly and thoroughly.

Figure 22.   The greatest mistake the pelvic surgeon can make is to start removing organs before he has prepared his operative field. The lower pelvis must be cleaned of adherent bowel and omentum. The sigmoid should be dissected free of the left adnexa. If a low lying cecum projects into the operative field it can be displaced easily by incising the peritoneum lateral to and below it. Any adhesions, resulting from previous operative interference or existing infection such as pelvic inflammatory disease or endometriosis, should be dissected free from the uterus or adnexae. Once freed the intestine is then gently packed out of the pelvis with large, moist sponges or packs. Forceful packing should be avoided for it may interfere with the satisfactory administration of the anesthesia and can traumatize the organs in the upper abdomen, particularly the gallbladder.

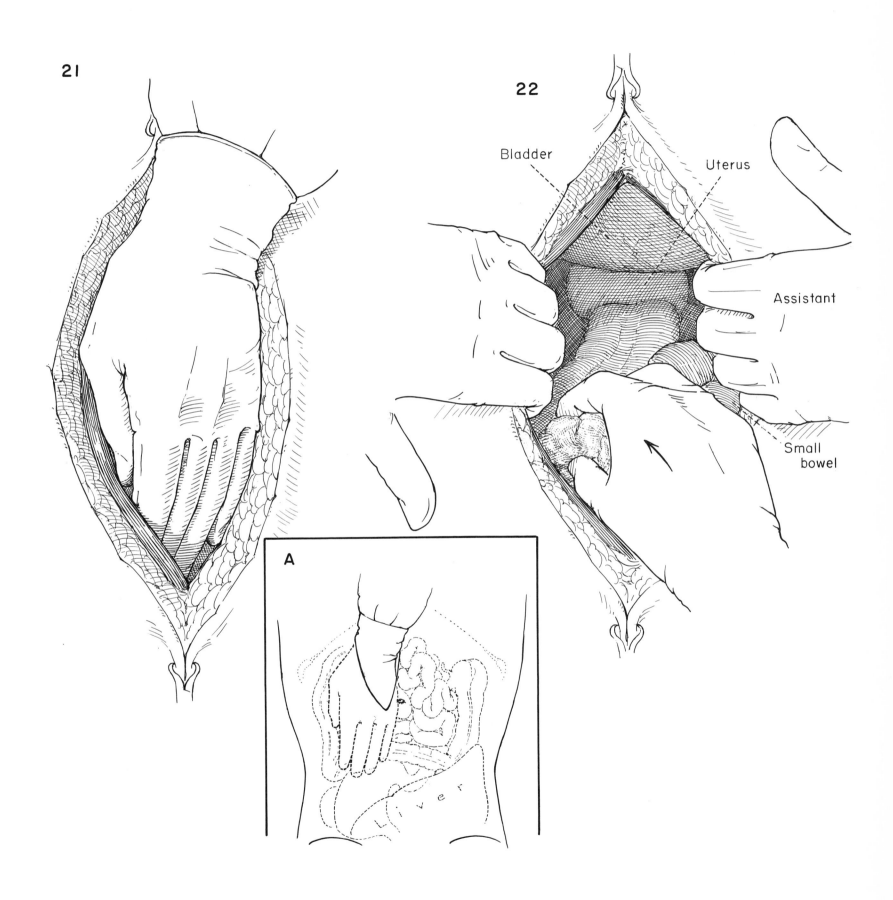

21

22

Bladder

Uterus

Assistant

Small
bowel

A

liver

Figure 23. After the operative field has been cleared by removal of any attachment of bowel or omentum to the uterus and adnexa, the wound edges are protected with moist gauze and the self-retaining retractor is introduced. It is our custom to insert the Balfour retractor with the crossbar toward the patient's head. We do this to avoid using the fixed lower curved retracting blade, preferring instead to employ the more mobile Deaver type retractor. In placing the self-retaining retractor the surgeon should exercise care to be sure that the blades do not compress the cecum, sigmoid, small bowel or iliac vessels.

Figure 24. The secret of all surgery in the pelvis, and particularly the operative procedures on the uterus or adnexa, is continued traction. This must be maintained throughout the operation.

The reasons this is so important are as follows:

1. The tissue cleavage planes are maintained. In picking up tissue you have less tendency to pick up structures or vessels that you do not want to incise.

2. Traction reduces the amount of bleeding. The individual vessels stand out more clearly and can be dealt with individually.

3. Injuries to the bladder and ureter are less likely to occur.

4. The course of the ureter is less tortuous and can frequently be seen when the structures are placed on tension.

5. The relationship of the bladder reflexion to the cervix and vagina is more clearly identified.

The traction is applied through an instrument placed on the fundus of the uterus. When there is no question of malignant disease of the endometrium, either from the history or the preliminary curettage or no obvious malignant tumor of the ovary is present, a tenaculum or double hook is applied to the uterine fundus. To aid in exposure the bladder is reflected by the Deaver retractor in the lower end of the wound. The uterus is fixed by holding it between the thumb and forefinger of the left hand while the surgeon applies the tenaculum to the fundus with the right. The tenaculum should include enough muscle tissue to keep it from pulling out and causing troublesome and unnecessary bleeding.

INSET A. When malignant disease of the endometrium is suspected or confirmed, it is unwise to traumatize the fundus with the tenaculum. As a substitute, a Kelly clamp is placed across the broad ligament close to the uterine body. This clamp includes the round and ovarian ligaments as well as the tube. In addition to avoiding trauma to the fundus, any leakage from the endometrium through the tube is prevented. Also, the peritoneal cavity is protected from accidental seeding.

INSET B. The broad ligament clamps are applied to both sides, and constant traction is maintained in this fashion in lieu of the uterine tenaculum.

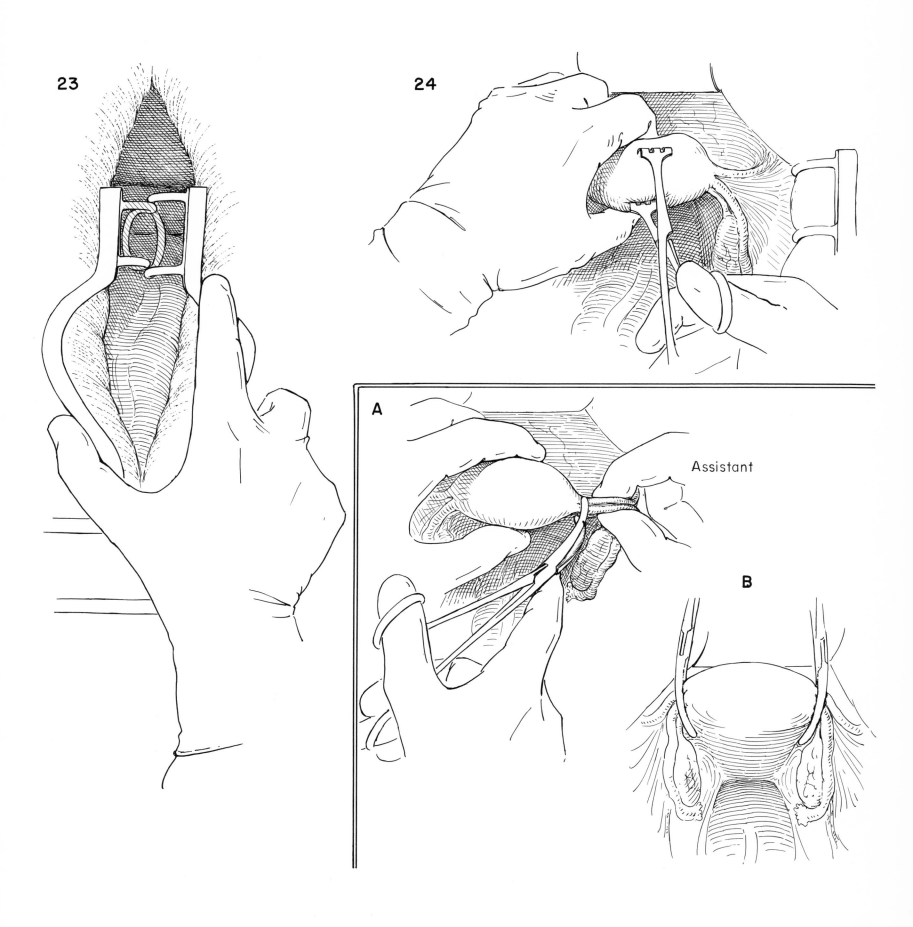

23

24

A

Assistant

B

The drawings on this page are designed to illustrate an important step which we feel helps to simplify the technique of total hysterectomy. It does so because it develops an operative field sufficiently large to enable the surgeon to identify the anatomy while at the same time providing him enough room to operate comfortably.

Figure 25. Because there is no suspicion of malignant disease in this patient the surgeon places a tenaculum on the uterine fundus. The assistant holds this on tension, drawing it upward and backward to expose the anterior surface of the peritoneum overlying the bladder and base of the broad ligament. The traction keeps the peritoneum from falling into folds and makes it easier for the surgeon and the assistant to pick it up. The point selected from the incision in the peritoneum should be lateral to the uterus and bladder below the round ligament at about the level of the cervix. The peritoneum between the forceps held by the surgeon and the assistant is then incised.

Figure 26. Traction on the Kelly clamps placed on the distal edge of the divided peritoneum exposes a relatively avascular area containing mostly areolar tissue. The anatomical landmarks immediately noted are the bladder lying medially and the external iliac vessels laterally.

The nurse and the assistant hold the clamps on tension while the surgeon inserts his index fingers back to back within the space. The two fingers move in opposing directions as the space is enlarged by separating the areolar tissue and pushing the posterior wall of the upper portion of the bladder away from the cervix.

When the space is completely developed the obliterated hypogastric and superior vesical artery, the uterine artery and the vein come into view. The external iliac artery and vein are seen laterally and below them the obturator nerve.

This maneuver, when done gently, can be performed quickly and bloodlessly.

Figure 27. The same step is repeated on the opposite side. The two Kelly clamps, medially placed on the incised peritoneal edge, are then held upward on tension. This permits the surgeon to divide the bridge of peritoneum between the two openings. This must be done with care to avoid damaging the dome of the bladder which is closely adherent to the posterior surface of the peritoneum.

Figure 28. Traction on the Kelly clamps exposes the fine tissue strands that hold the bladder to the surface of the peritoneum. They can be gently separated with blunt end scissors. When this step is completed and the bladder is pushed away from the peritoneum a free peritoneal flap is created. The importance of this step is apparent when the final peritonealization is done. It is then possible to pull the free edge of the peritoneum over the raw divided edge of the vaginal canal without disturbing the position of the bladder.

Inset A. The inset shows diagrammatically what has happened up to this point in the procedure.

Figure 29. The surgeon maintains traction on the uterus with the left hand while the right grasps the cervix between thumb and forefinger. Employing a gentle pill-rolling motion it is then possible to gently separate the lower attachment of the bladder to the anterior wall of the cervix and push it downward to the level of the vagina.

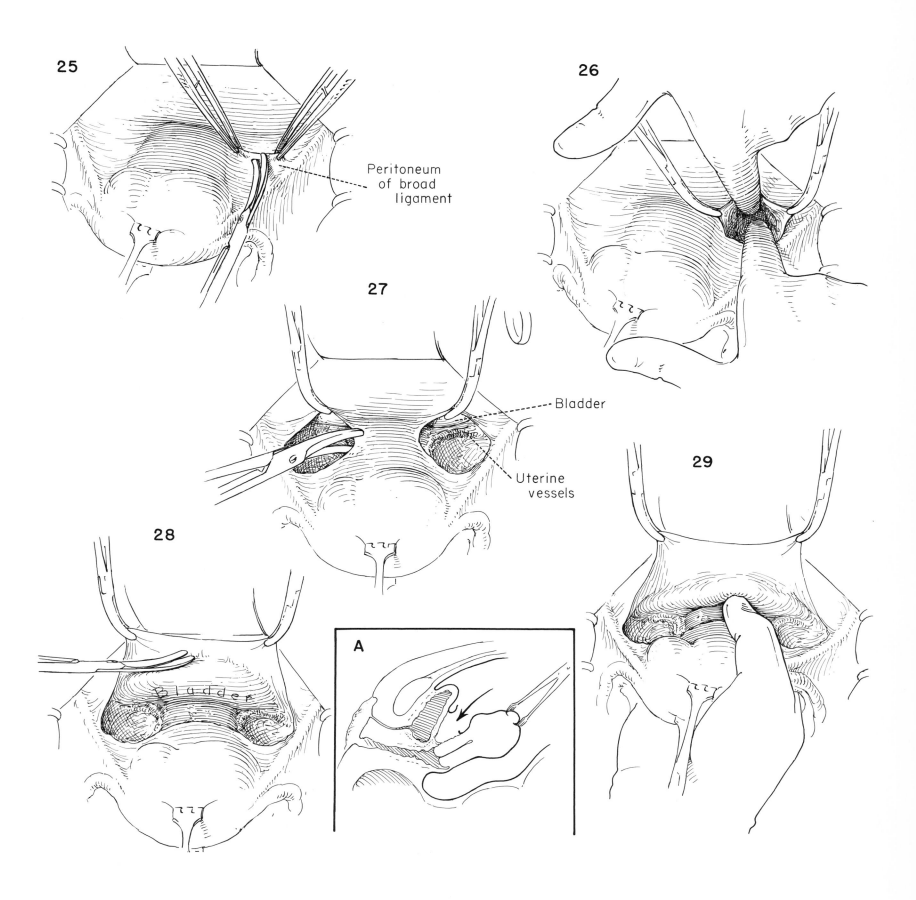

25

26

27

Peritoneum
of broad
ligament

Bladder

Uterine
vessels

28

A

29

The illustrations on this page demonstrate the technique of performing a hysterectomy when the surgeon elects to leave the tubes and ovaries intact.

Figure 30. The surgeon pulls the uterus toward him. This permits him to see the ovarian vessels and allows him to place the stitch ligature in the bloodless area between them and the round ligament. The location of this stitch, which includes the tube and ovarian ligament, is of great importance. The optimal position is approximately 1 inch lateral to the uterus. The round ligament will be sectioned closer to the uterus. In the reconstructive phase, after the uterus is removed, the round ligament will be approximated to the edge of the sectioned vagina. The tube and ovary will lie free without tension when this is done. It will materially reduce the possibility of retention cysts developing in the ovary. The suture is left long in anticipation of a reinforcing ligature.

Figure 31. After placing the initial suture the operator places a Kelly clamp on the uterine side of the ovarian ligament. The assistant holds the ligated suture on tension and prepares to apply a clamp on the stump of the ovarian vessels after the surgeon has divided them. The reason for this step is that it reduces the possibility of having the vessel retract out of the suture, which sometimes happens when two stitch ligatures are placed before the vessel is divided.

Figures 32 and 33. After dividing the vessels the surgeon places a second stitch ligature around the clamp on the vessel stump. The assistant now cuts the long ends of the initial tie. The second stitch ligature is now tied and cut.

Figure 34. With the uterus pulled toward him the surgeon removes the clamp previously placed on the uterine side of the infundibulopelvic ligament to prevent back bleeding. The clamp is then reapplied so that it includes all the structures arising at the cornu.

Figure 35. The surgeon now directs his attention to the round ligament. The uterus is drawn forward and the posterior leaf of the broad ligament is inspected to identify the location of the vessels. Once located the surgeon can now safely push the index finger of the right hand through the back of the broad ligament beneath the round ligament.

Figure 36. A stitch ligature is placed into the substance of the round ligament lateral to the clamp on the uterine side. The assistant then ties the suture. Note that the suture on the round ligament is about 1 inch closer to the uterus than those placed on the ovarian vessels.

Figure 37. The long end of the suture is clamped and held on tension by the assistant. The surgeon draws the uterus to his side and divides the round ligament. The long suture with the clamp is then allowed to hang outside the abdominal incision.

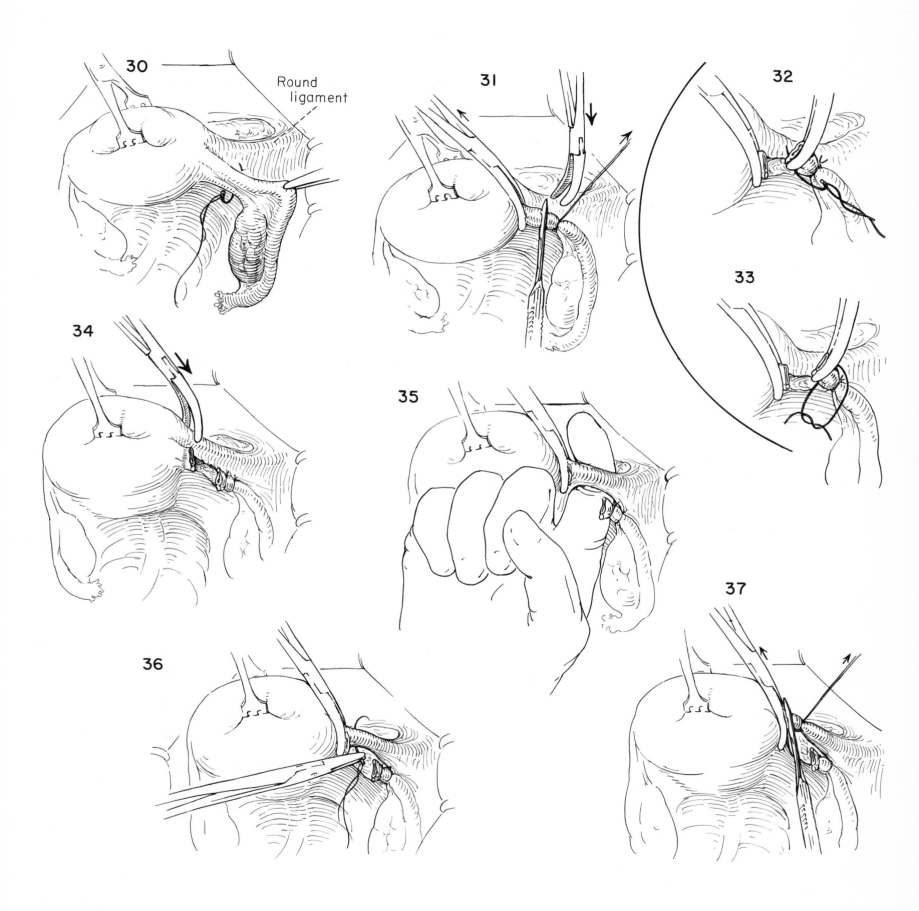

Round ligament

Figure 38.   The assistant now pulls upward on the suture placed on the round ligament while the surgeon retracts the uterus to the left side. With the broad ligament on tension the vessels within it are clearly outlined. The surgeon can now safely section the posterior leaf of the broad ligament with scissors without creating any troublesome venous bleeding. The incision is carried out under direct vision down to the level of the uterine vessels which can be seen crossing the base of the broad ligament.

The broad ligament on the opposite side is similarly treated.

Figure 39.   We are now concerned about the position of the ureter as the dissection is carried down toward the uterine vessels and bladder. If the surgeon will place his thumb and forefinger lateral to the uterus at the base of the broad ligament, the ureter can be felt to roll between the thumb and forefinger as a structure distinct from the uterine vessels.

Figure 40.   It is our basic concept that special instruments are not necessary in performing a hysterectomy. Only that amount of tissue that can safely be controlled should be included in the clamps used.

Before attacking the uterine vessels, then, we prefer to continue the mobilization of the uterus by isolating the uterosacral ligaments. It is important to note the position of the ureter in relation to them for they are very close to the line of dissection at this point and can easily be accidentally damaged.

The surgeon pulls the uterus upward and toward him and applies a Kelly clamp on the uterosacral ligaments close to the uterus. It is then divided.

Figure 41.   Because of the proximity of the ureter the surgeon must be very careful where he places the stitch ligature on the divided end of the uterosacral ligament. If there is any doubt he should dissect the area and locate the ureter before he ties his suture. The suture may now be ligated and divided.

Figure 42.   The same procedure is carried out on the patient's left side. The operator then connects the two areas by dividing the posterior peritoneum between the uterosacral ligaments.

INSET A.   The schematic sagittal section indicates that the uterus has now been circumcised and is free of all peritoneal attachments.

Figure 43.   With the uterus on tension the posterior peritoneal leaf between the ligaments is dissected downward. Not infrequently the rectum is pulled up on the back of the uterus between the uterosacral ligaments. The step outlined allows the rectum to be pushed back away from the posterior uterine and vaginal walls. In addition to the obvious advantage obtained by this maneuver in protecting the rectum and ureter from accidental trauma by letting them fall back out of the way, there is another important reason for carrying out this step. The dissection permits the Kelly clamps to be placed on the uterine vessels without having to include too much tissue in them. This reduces materially the hazard of having the vessel retract out of the clamp or suture. If it does, troublesome bleeding occurs which is difficult to arrest because the source of the bleeding is not readily located. If clamps are placed blindly to secure the retracted vessel there is a very real danger of including the ureter in the clamp.

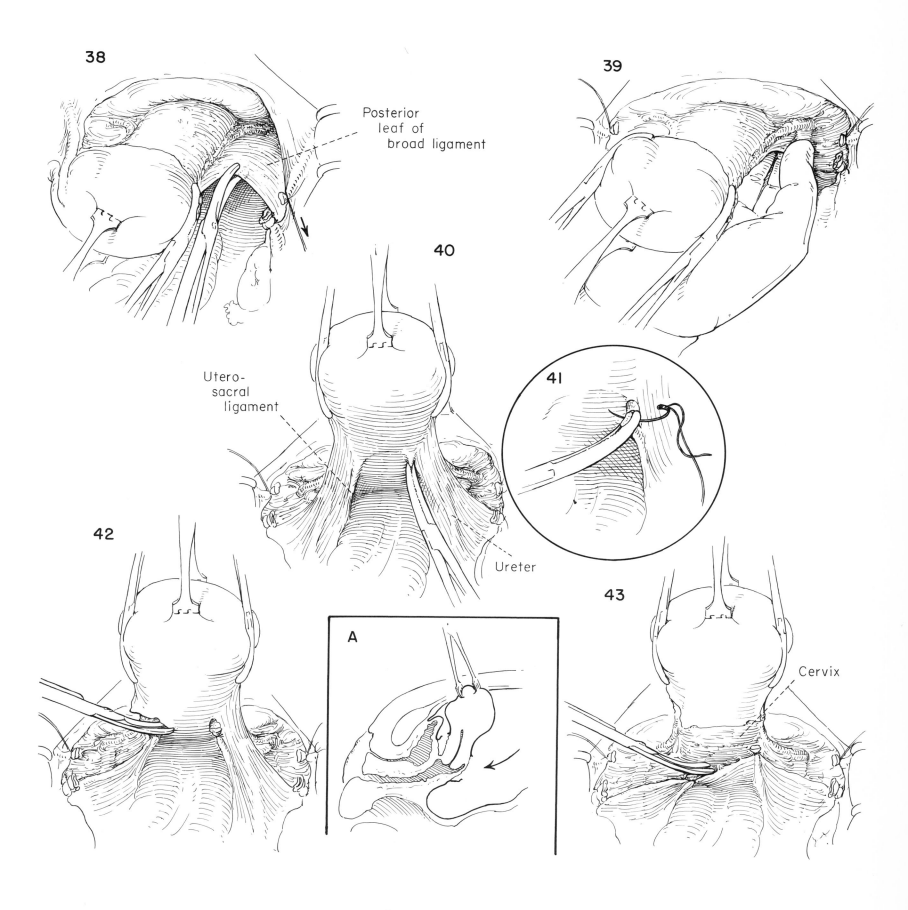

38

39

Posterior
leaf of
broad ligament

40

Utero-
sacral
ligament

41

Ureter

42

A

43

Cervix

The presentations on this page are concerned with an important phase in the technique of abdominal total hysterectomy, namely, the management of the uterine vessels. On the previous page we noted that it was important not to include in the clamps placed on the uterine vessels more tissue than the clamp could be expected to hold. To do so is to run the risk of having the vessel retract out of the clamp. In addition there are two other factors which will greatly facilitate and make safer the handling of vessels.

1. The vessels should be clearly identified and the clamps applied close to the uterus under direct vision.

2. The identification will become easier if the surgeon will keep the uterus under constant traction in the direction away from the side he is operating on. Isolating the individual vessel minimizes the danger of including other structures in the clamp.

Figure 44. The surgeon exposes the uterine vessels on the right by pulling the uterus toward him. He then applies a Kelly clamp on the vessels close to the uterus and above the level of the cervix. This clamp is placed to prevent back bleeding. It will be left in place throughout the removal of the uterus.

Figure 45. With the traction maintained to the left and with the vessels again under direct vision another Kelly clamp is applied below the so-called back clamp. It is placed in such a position that there will be enough tissue left to form a ¼ inch cuff as the vessels are divided between clamps.

Figure 46. Because there is always the chance that the vessel may pull out from under a single clamp or retract if the suture breaks in tying, a second clamp is placed on the cuff left protruding beyond the initial clip.

Figures 47 and 48. Throughout the operation we make a point of being able to see exactly where each suture is placed. Because the bladder has been advanced off the cervix (Fig. 29), the broad ligament kept on tension (Fig. 37), and the uterosacral ligaments dissected free from the cervix posteriorly (Fig. 43), the ureter has been displaced well lateral to the ligatures around the uterine vessels. The danger in the operation at this point is the proximity of the bladder. Extreme care must be taken not to damage it, thereby creating a vesicovaginal fistula.

It is important to identify the bladder edge before placing a stitch ligature around the vessels just below the most distal clamp. This step is facilitated by traction on the uterus.

Figure 49. The surgeon removes the most laterally placed clamp as the assistant ties the first ligature. The proximal clamp remains in place to prevent retraction of the vessel should the suture break in tying. It should be noted that from now on no stitch or clamp is placed lateral to the primary suture on the uterine vessels.

Figure 50. A second stitch ligature is now placed around the clamp previously applied to the cuff of uterine vessels. It is tied, the clamp removed and the suture cut.

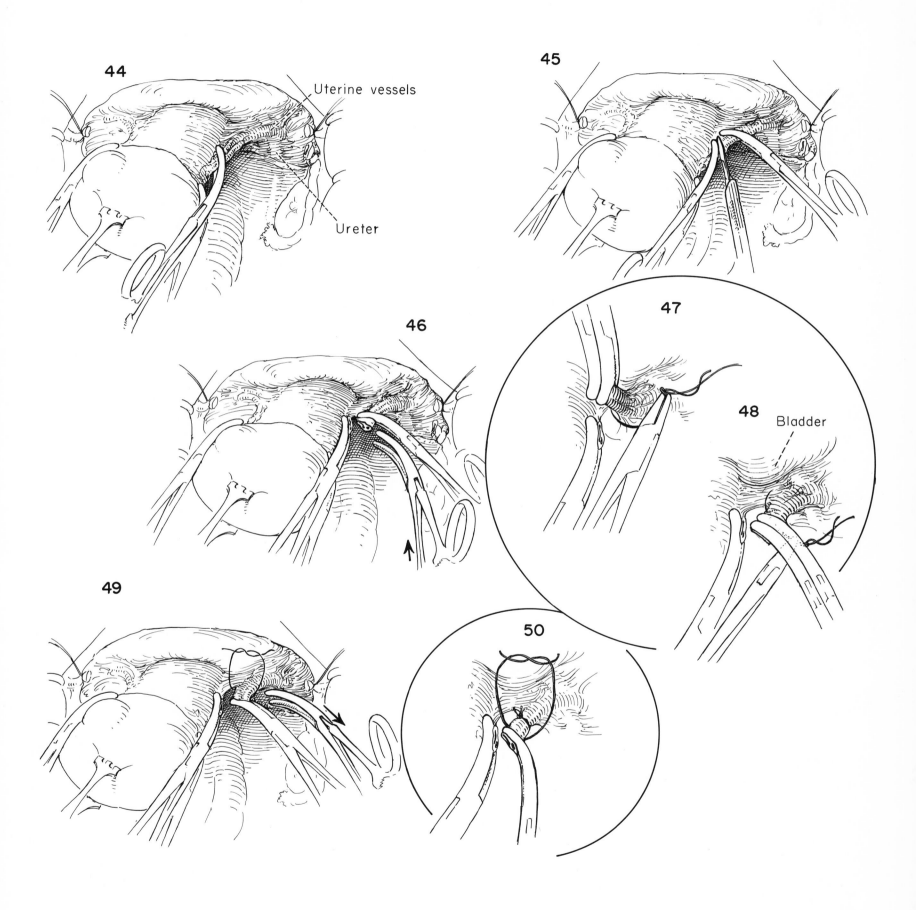

44   Uterine vessels   Ureter

45

46

47

48   Bladder

49

50

In performing a total removal of the uterus it is essential that all the cervix be removed. It is relatively easier to remove a portion of the anterior and posterior wall of the vagina, but it is much more difficult to circumcise the cervix on the lateral side. To accomplish the removal, without leaving a portion of the cervix on the vaginal wall at the lateral angle, it is necessary to mobilize the bladder well away from the vagina.

The steps depicted here indicate the simplest and safest method of separating the cervix from the bladder and exposing the lateral attachments of the bladder. This can best be done by developing a large enough operative field so that the bladder base can be visualized at all times. You are less likely to damage the bladder or ureter if you can see what you are doing. The greatest danger arises when you blindly attempt to apply a clamp to control bleeding vessels when you cannot identify them.

Figure 51. One of the factors that obscures the angle of the vagina is the lateral areolar attachments of the bladder which tend to pull the bladder up on the uterine vessels, forming a crescent-like fold. The surgeon must separate the areolar strands of these attachments by pulling the uterus to one side while the assistant picks up the bladder edge and retracts it. This is a very delicate maneuver. If the tissues are handled roughly, bleeding will certainly follow. To carry out the dissection in this area it is important to have a dry operative field.

Figure 52. When this is done on both sides the bladder is detached from the cervix. We are now at the point at which the previous dissection of the uterosacral ligaments from the posterior wall of the vagina proves so valuable.

The surgeon can now apply a Kelly clamp under direct vision without including a large amount of tissue. The placing of this clamp is important. The previous clamps on the uterine vessels were applied at right angles to the uterus. This clamp should be placed parallel to the cervix and medial to the sutures on the uterine vessels. It secures the cervical branches of the uterine vessels. It is not necessary to employ a back clamp.

Figures 53 and 54. After retracting the bladder the surgeon divides the tissue between the cervix and clamp, leaving a short cuff to prevent retraction. Again under direct vision a stitch ligature is placed and tied.

Figures 55 and 56. It is well to repeat the previous steps and cross the cardinal ligament in a series of small bites rather than include all the tissue in one large one. The need for clamps, and the number applied, will vary with each patient. The basic principle again is to include only as much tissue as can be safely controlled with the stitch. Note the position of the bladder. No clamp or suture is applied before identification of the position of the adjacent viscera.

Figure 57. By palpating the cervix between the thumb and fingers the extent of dissection is checked before proceeding further.

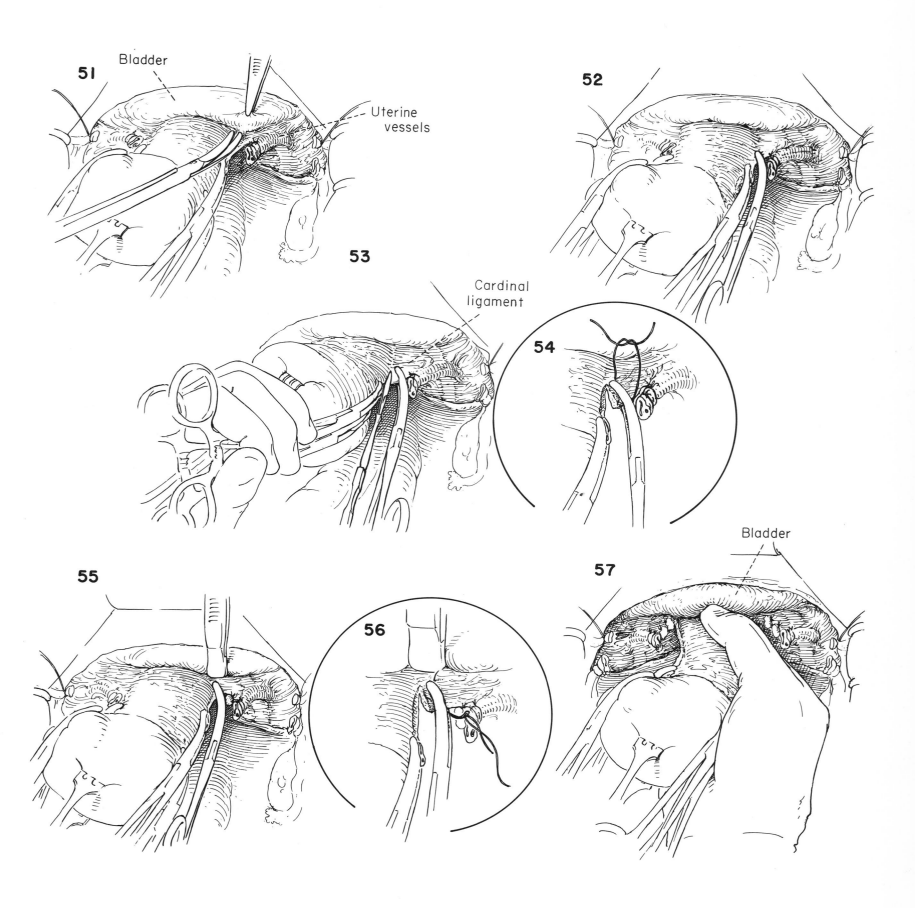

51 Bladder

Uterine vessels

52

53

Cardinal ligament

54

55

56

57 Bladder

The dissection to this point has completely freed the uterus on all sides. The bladder has been cleared from the anterior wall of the vagina. The uterosacral ligaments have been stripped from the posterior vaginal wall. The lateral angles have been freed of bladder attachments and the side walls of the vagina have been cleared. All the dissection has been carried out medial to the original clamp placed on the uterine vessels. It has been done anatomically with the important structures always in view.

Figure 58. Before pulling the uterus forward toward the symphysis the bladder edge has been retracted to avoid having it involved in the clamp the surgeon will place on the vaginal wall at the angle. To be certain that no part of the cervix is left behind the cervix is palpated and its relation to the vaginal wall determined. The clamp is now placed approximately ½ inch below the lateral edge of the cervix. The same procedure is carried out on the opposite side. The vagina is then entered by incising the tissue above the clamps.

Figure 59. The anterior vaginal wall has a tendency to retract beneath the bladder wall after it has been excised. To avoid the problem of having to search blindly for it later the assistant is alert to grasp the vaginal wall with a Kocher clamp when it can easily be seen. He must be certain that the bladder edge is retracted so that it is not included in the clamp he will apply. The surgeon has now transected the vaginal wall with the scissors, and the clamps are being placed on the anterior vaginal wall.

Figure 60. A Kocher clamp is placed on the posterior vaginal wall for two reasons. Primarily it will be used to maintain traction, for the uterus is about to be removed. It will also help to keep the vaginal canal open and will allow the surgeon freedom to place the running suture on the cut edge of the vagina.

Figures 61 and 62. With the bladder again held back a stitch ligature is placed around the clamp at the lateral angle of the vagina. This stitch is tied by the surgeon on his side and by the assistant on the other. The sutures are clamped and kept long to provide continued traction on the vagina, lost when the uterus was removed.

Figure 63. The vaginal canal is to be left open. There is a tendency for the vaginal epithelium to retract from the musculature carrying thrombosed, but unsutured, vessels with it. This may result in postoperative bleeding from the vaginal cuff. The cut edge of the vagina is therefore sutured with a running lock stitch around the entire circumference. Leaving the vagina open permits drainage and results in a less conical-shaped vagina. If the anterior wall is approximated to the posterior wall a pyramidal type of vagina is created which results in foreshortening of the canal, which is undesirable.

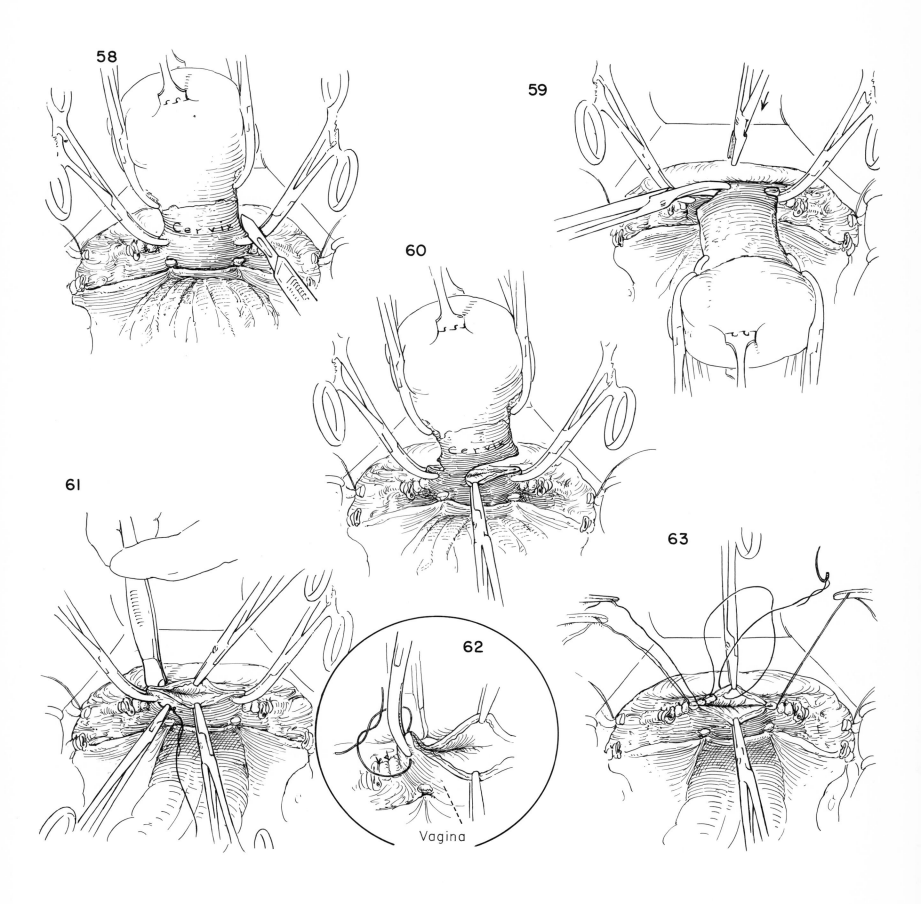

The removal of the uterus completes one phase of the total abdominal hysterectomy. The reconstructive portion is yet to be done. The steps to accomplish it are now outlined.

Figure 64. The traction sutures placed on the angles of the vagina have taken over the traction role following the removal of the uterus. The sutures are held on tension by the assistants as the surgeon grasps the uterosacral ligaments. A stitch ligature is placed through the ligament and the posterior vaginal wall. After completing the tie the same thing is done on the opposite side.

The approximation of the uterosacral ligaments to the posterior wall of the vagina accomplishes two things: it facilitates reperitonealization, and the reapposition of the uterosacral ligaments helps not only to support the vagina but also to keep the upper portion of the canal patent.

Figures 65, 66 and 67. In many of the techniques described for total hysterectomy no attempt is made to employ the round ligament in the reconstructive phase of the operation. The round and infundibulopelvic ligaments are allowed to hang free. Suturing of the cardinal ligaments to the angle of the vagina is considered sufficient support for the vagina. Although we also utilize the cardinal ligaments, we prefer to suture the round ligaments to the vaginal stump.

The round ligament, therefore, is brought back into the operative field as the surgeon draws the long suture toward him and places a mattress type of stitch ligature through the substance of the ligament. The stitch continues through the wall at the lateral angle of the open vagina. When completed and tied, the long suture originally placed on the round ligament is cut. The same maneuver is carried out on the opposite side.

The reason such pains are taken to divide the round ligament closer to the uterus than the infundibulopelvic ligament is now evident.

The drawing demonstrates how the ovary and tube hang freely without tension after the round ligament is approximated to the vagina. There is now no chance of interfering with the remaining blood supply to the ovary by narrowing the lumen through traction.

The reconstructive phase designed to maintain support of the vagina has been completed. The remaining figures on this page are concerned with reperitonealization of the raw areas on the pelvic floor created by the dissection. These must be covered to prevent bowel from becoming adherent to the operative site.

Figures 68, 69, and 70. There is a tendency for the surgeon to relax his concentration at this point but he must not forget that it is possible to include the ureter in his peritoneal stitch.

To be sure that this does not happen the assistant retracts the ovary to expose the raw cut edges of the pelvic peritoneum lying behind it. When the surgeon is certain that the ureter is out of the way be begins the running atraumatic peritonealizing suture at the lateral corner of the defect. When it has been tied, the peritoneal edges are approximated by the running stitch until the opposite side is reached and the defect closed.

Figure 71. The value of the initial step in freeing the bladder from the anterior peritoneum now becomes apparent. The bladder flap is brought down to cover the vaginal canal. The bladder remains undisturbed in its normal bed.

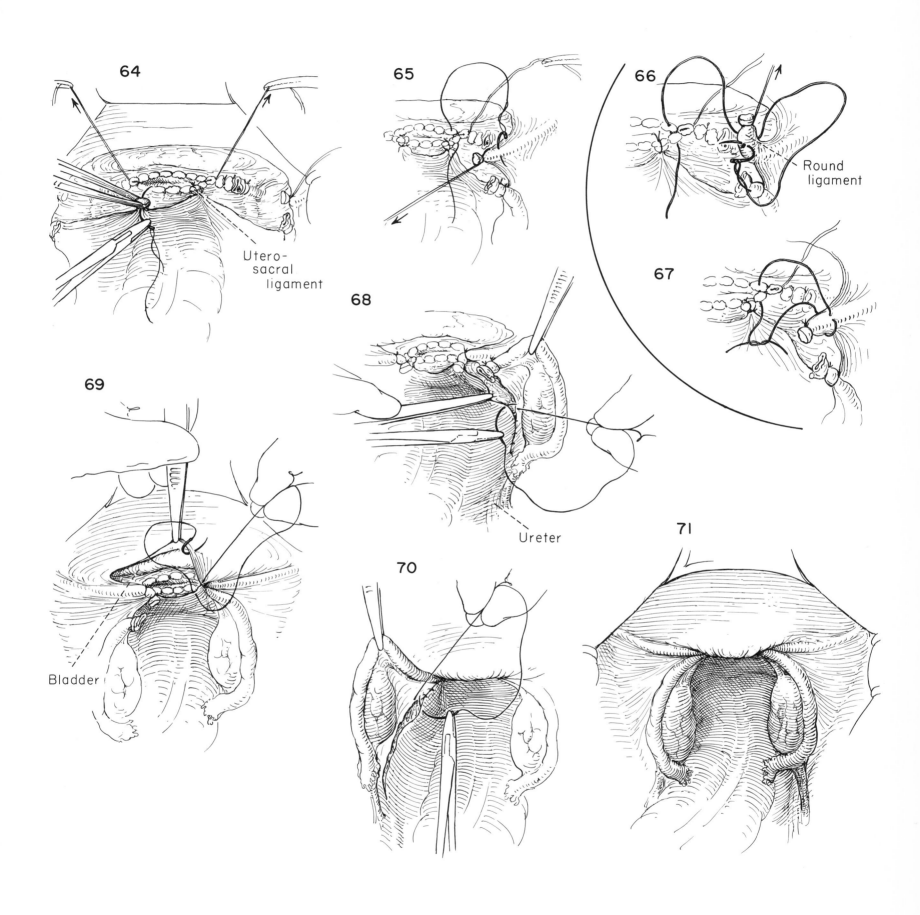

64

65

66

Round ligament

Utero-sacral ligament

67

68

Ureter

69

Bladder

70

71

Figure 72. The description of the technique of total abdominal hysterectomy as portrayed in this series of plates called for leaving the ovaries and tubes in place.

Unless the uterus is opened before the abdomen is closed the surgeon may have the unhappy experience of being told later by the pathologist that a totally unsuspected lesion is present and could compromise the ovaries that have not been removed. Even though a curettage has been performed routinely before every hysterectomy we must still remember that the results are not always 100 per cent accurate. This is particularly true of the cornua of the endometrial cavity. For example, the patient may have a submucous fibroid with carcinoma hiding behind it. A widely based polyp may contain malignant disease.

For this reason we recommend the routine opening of the uterus and inspection of the endometrial cavity at the operating table while the patient is still under anesthesia. If there is a pathologist in attendance he should inspect it. If none is available, the anesthetist or operating room attendant should be asked to open it. The surgeon then makes his own inspection.

In most instances nothing of consequence will be found, but if the examination is performed routinely the occasional lesion will be detected at a time when something can be done about it.

Figure 73. With the assurance that all the surgery within the abdomen is complete and that the surgeon has accomplished what he set out to do he may then prepare to close the abdomen. All packs are removed from the upper abdomen and given to the circulating nurse for counting. The same thing is done for the small sponges used in the operation. If the nurse has an incomplete count of small sponges and they cannot be located within the abdominal cavity, the surgeon should remember that it is possible that he may have left one in the deeper recesses of the wound and peritonealized over it. Should the count continue to be incorrect, the peritonealizing suture should be divided and this area inspected.

Figure 74. Although all raw edges have been covered with peritoneum, the small bowel sometimes descends into the cul de sac and becomes adherent to the operative incision in the pelvis. To prevent this and to keep the small intestine away from the cul de sac and the recent operative site the surgeon should grasp the redundant sigmoid and carefully place it so that it fills the lower portion of the pelvis.

Figure 75. As further precaution in prevention of the small intestine's adhering to the abdominal wall incision the surgeon should retrieve the omentum from the upper abdomen where the gauze packs have pushed it. The omentum should be inspected to be sure that it is intact and does not contain bleeding points. If they are present the defects should be closed and any bleeding vessel ligated with silk or catgut sutures.

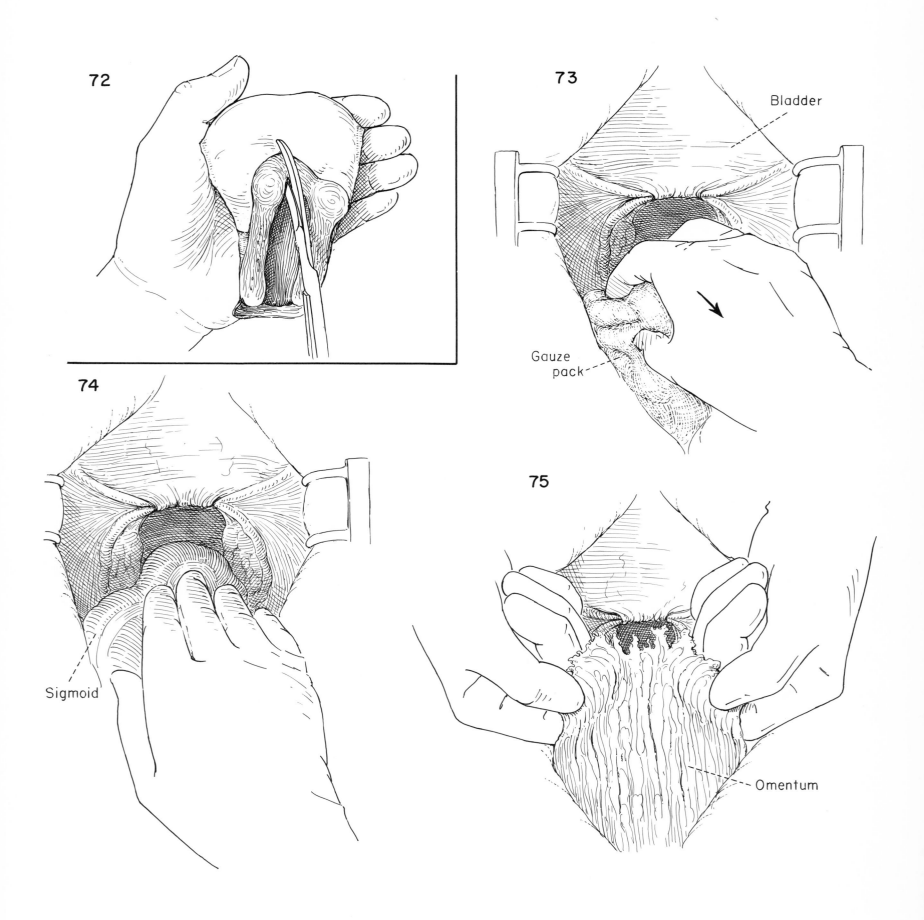

72

73 Bladder

Gauze
pack

74

Sigmoid

75

Omentum

With the operation completed and the sponge count reported correct, the patient is now ready for closure of the abdominal wall.

Figure 76. The omentum is so placed that the small intestine is completely covered. The self-retaining retractor is then removed.

Figure 77. The assistant exposes the upper end of the wound so that the surgeon may place the first suture through the peritoneum and posterior rectus sheath. This suture is continued as a running stitch from above downward. It approximates peritoneum to peritoneum.

Figure 78. The operator prepares to close the fascia. The assistant exposes it by retracting the fat of the skin edges. Interrupted silk or cotton sutures are placed and individually tied by the assistant. Exposure is helped by holding each suture on tension as the next one is laid in.

Figure 79. The skin towels are now removed. Interrupted sutures are placed at intervals in the subcutaneous fat to close the dead space.

Figure 80. The surgeon then closes the skin edges with evenly spaced, interrupted silk or cotton stitches. Care should be taken that each one enters at a right angle to the skin. This insures better approximation. The dressing is then applied.

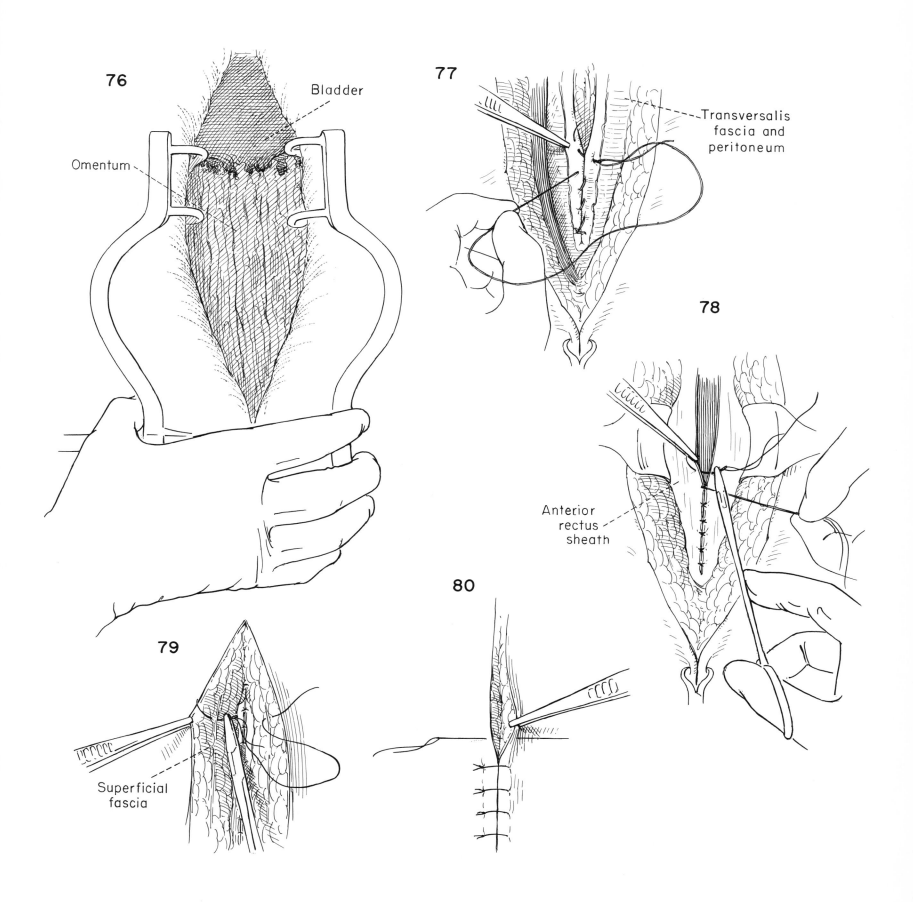

76   Bladder

Omentum

77   Transversalis fascia and peritoneum

78

Anterior rectus sheath

79

Superficial fascia

80

Modifications of Hysterectomy

REMOVAL OF OVARY AND TUBE

There are many occasions when removal of one or both ovaries will be indicated as an accompaniment of a hysterectomy. The main problem is to avoid damage to the ureter. It is not generally appreciated that the ovarian vessels and the ureter are in close apposition as they cross the common iliac vessels. This is the point at which clamps or stitch ligatures are commonly applied. Careless handling of tissue in this area, without first identifying the course of the ureter, increases the danger of including the ureter in clamp or stitch when troublesome bleeding is encountered.

When removal of the tube and ovary is indicated in the course of performing a hysterectomy the entire operation will proceed more easily and with greater safety if the surgeon will defer sectioning the ovarian vessels until after the bladder flap has been developed.

Figure 1. The broad ligament has been entered through the anterior peritoneal leaf on both sides of the cervix. The bladder has been reflected medially by finger dissection in a bloodless area. The peritoneal bridge is now being divided. The surgeon proceeds carefully, for the bladder is closely adherent to the flap.

Figure 2. A Kelly clamp is placed on the right tube and ovary. The tenaculum and the Kelly clamp are held together in the left hand, and the uterus and adnexa are pulled toward the operator. This places the right infundibulopelvic ligament with the ovarian vessels on stretch. Before placing the first stitch ligature, determine the position of the ureter in relation to the vessels. This is one of the commonest areas in which the ureter may be damaged. The ureter normally crosses the common iliac artery in close proximity to the ovarian vessels. Careless application of the first stitch ligature may include the ureter.

Figure 3. The stitch is tied by the assistant and kept on tension as the surgeon applies a Kelly clamp on the uterine side to prevent back bleeding. The surgeon then divides the vessel between clamps and cuts the initial suture as the assistant applies a clamp to the cut end of the ovarian vessels. A second stitch ligature placed around the clamped vessel provides a double ligation of the ovarian vessels.

Figure 4. The right adnexa and uterus are again pulled to the left, thereby placing the peritoneum on tension. The attachment is then divided in the bloodless area in the direction of the uterine cornu and up to the point of round ligament attachment.

Figure 5. The uterus is now pulled upward and forward toward the symphysis to expose the posterior sheath of the right broad ligament. Noting the position of the uterine vessels, the surgeon gently forces the index finger of the right hand through the broad ligament just below the round ligament. A Kelly clamp has been placed on the uterine end of the round ligament to prevent back bleeding.

MODIFICATIONS OF TOTAL HYSTERECTOMY
REMOVAL OF OVARY AND TUBE

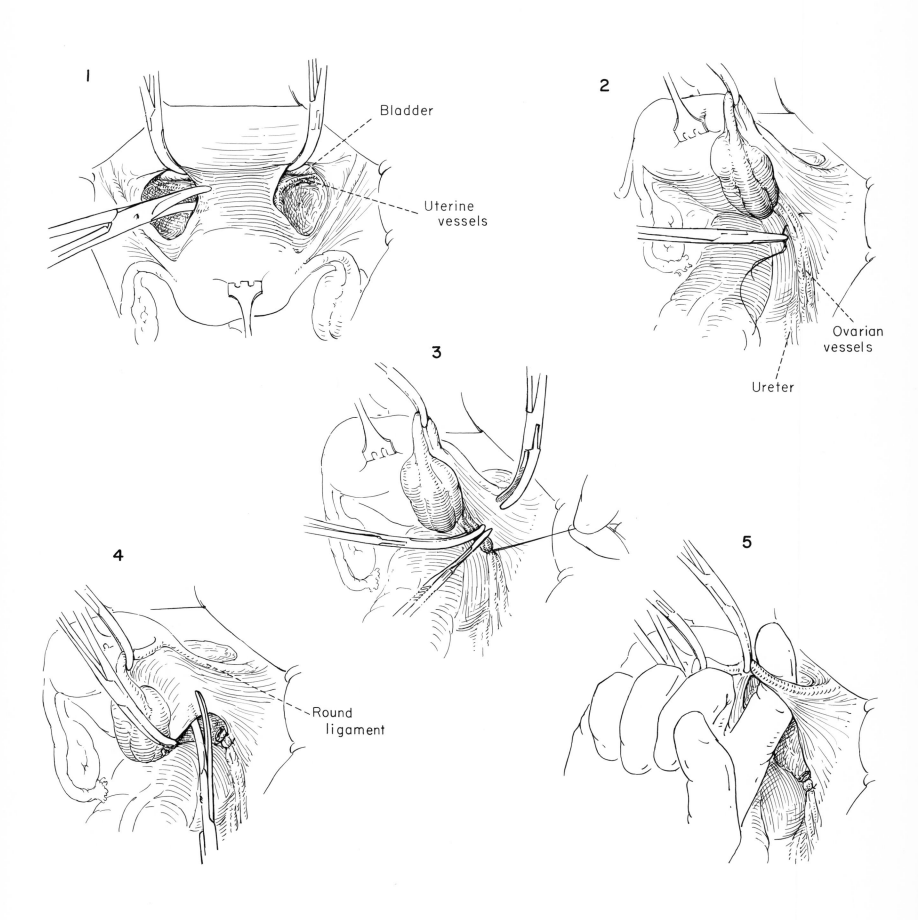

1

Bladder

Uterine vessels

2

Ovarian vessels

Ureter

3

4

Round ligament

5

Figure 6. The surgeon elevates the uterus and draws it toward him by applying light traction on the tenaculum and the clamps placed on the round ligament, tube and ovarian pedicle. This maneuver facilitates the passage of a stitch ligature through the substance of the round ligament.

Figure 7. The assistant ties the suture and leaves it long, with a clamp on the end to hang outside the abdominal cavity so that it will not be in the operative field. He then holds it on tension as the surgeon divides the round ligament between the clamp and the suture.

Figure 8. To further the exposure of the vessels within the broad ligament the surgeon holds the uterus on tension to the left while the assistant applies traction on the round ligament. When this is done there is less tendency for the broad ligament to fall into accordion-like pleats which may contain broad ligament veins. The posterior leaf of the broad ligament is then divided.

The surgeon then proceeds with the regular steps of the total hysterectomy.

PERITONEALIZATION

The problem of peritonealization after removal of both uterus and adnexa is quite different from the description given for the operation when the ovaries are left in place.

Figure 9. Note that the uterosacral ligaments have been sutured to the posterior vaginal wall in a previous step. There are two reasons for this maneuver: the patency of the vaginal wall at its apex is kept open, and the raw posterior peritoneal defect is eliminated.

Similarly, the raw defect in the broad ligament left after the tube and ovary have been removed is closed when the round ligaments are sutured to the corners of the vagina by a stitch ligature. This is the primary reason for this maneuver. The broad and uterosacral ligaments have a very limited role in providing support to the vagina. This is produced chiefly by the cardinal ligaments which have previously been sutured to the corners of the vagina.

Figure 10. An atraumatic suture picks up the peritoneum above and below the stump of ovarian vessels on the right. The suture is so placed that peritoneal surface approximates peritoneal surface. In this manner the cut end of the ovarian vessels is buried beneath the peritoneum. The opposite or left ovary lies freely without tension after the round ligament is sutured to the vagina.

Figure 11. A continuous over-and-over running suture closes the defect in the peritoneum. The free peritoneal edge overlying the bladder is included in the peritoneal covering over the vagina. Note that the free edge pulls down easily without disturbing the position of the bladder.

The peritonealization is now complete. The left ovary and tube remain. The right adnexa have been removed. If there is any doubt about the presence of disease in the ovary that is to be left, the surgeon should split the ovary in its long axis and inspect the inner surfaces. If it proves to be negative, the ovary is then closed with interrupted sutures.

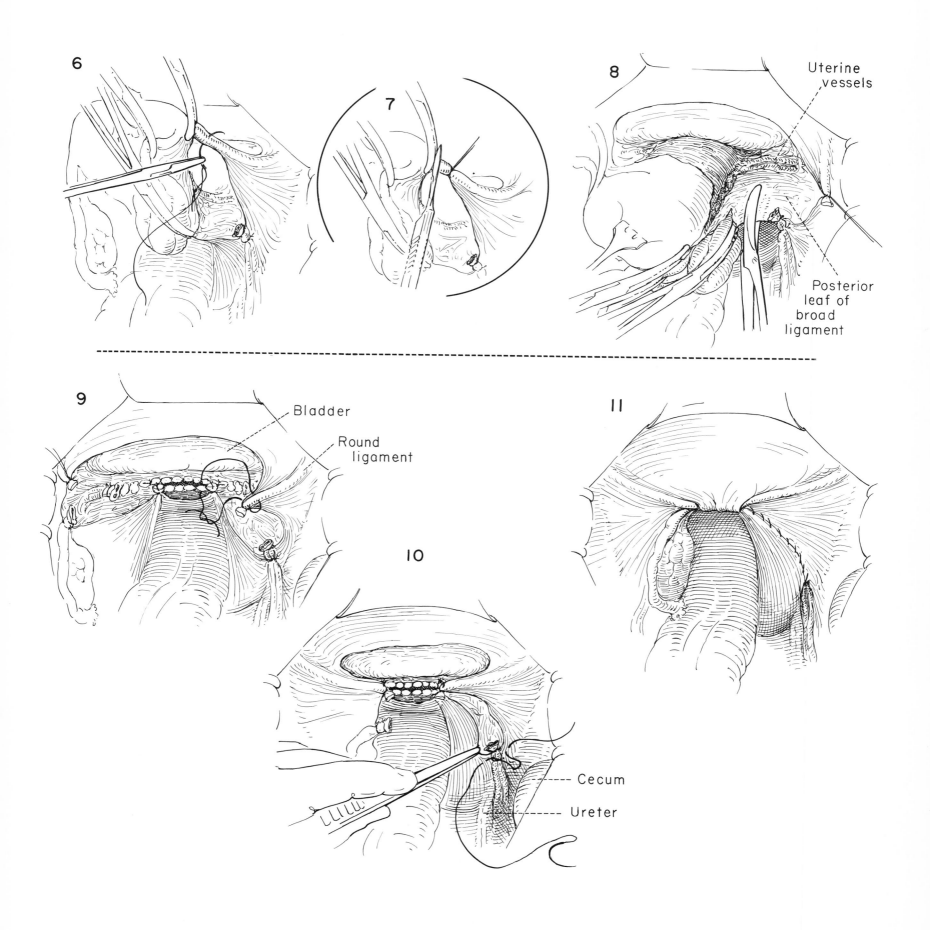

SUPRACERVICAL HYSTERECTOMY

There will be very few times when indications call for removal of the uterus that the surgeon will elect to perform a supravaginal or supracervical hysterectomy. This was once a common operation, but today the method has largely been superseded by total hysterectomy. A supracervical hysterectomy should never be performed if there is any suspicion of malignant disease in either the cervix or the endometrium. The operation of choice for cancer of the adnexa, either tube or ovary, would be bilateral salpingo-oophorectomy combined with total removal of the uterus.

At times, however, there may be such adherence of rectosigmoid or bladder to the cervix or posterior wall of the uterus that total removal of the uterus would create the hazard of entering either the bowel or the bladder. The same situation might exist in the presence of extensive benign disease such as pelvic inflammation or endometriosis.

It is conceivable that some unforeseen situation might arise in the course of a planned removal of the total uterus when it might be necessary to terminate the operation because of the patient's deteriorating condition. It would then be logical to remove only the intra-abdominal portion of the uterus.

The preliminary steps are identical with those for total hysterectomy and will not be repeated. The bladder flap has been developed, the adnexa left in situ, the round ligament divided and the broad ligament opened. The uterine vessels have been severed and doubly ligated. The bladder has been mobilized just enough to permit incision through the cervix and subsequent closure without endangering the bladder base.

INSET A.   Diagrammatic representation showing the uterus free of peritoneal cover with the line of incision indicated in the lateral view. The relationship of the cervix to the vaginal canal and posterior vaginal wall is outlined.

Figure 1.   The uterus is placed on tension by grasping all the clamps, including the tenaculum, in the left hand. The surgeon then incises the anterior wall of the cervix above the bladder reflexion and stump of the uterine vessels.

Figure 2.   The uterus is drawn sharply forward and upward toward the symphysis as the surgeon incises the posterior wall of the cervix above the uterosacral ligaments and the ligated uterine vessels.

Figure 3.   So that the traction will be continued on the cervical stump after the uterus has been removed, a Kocher clamp is placed on the anterior incised edge. Upward traction is applied by the surgeon on the tenaculum and by the assistant on the Kocher. In order that the endocervical lining be removed from the stump, the surgeon bevels the knife blade to bring about a conical excision of the cervical musculature with included endocervical epithelium.

Figure 4.   The uterus is again drawn forward against the symphysis to expose the posterior cervical wall. A Kocher clamp is placed on the posterior edge to aid in maintaining traction. The conical removal of the lower cervical segment is completed.

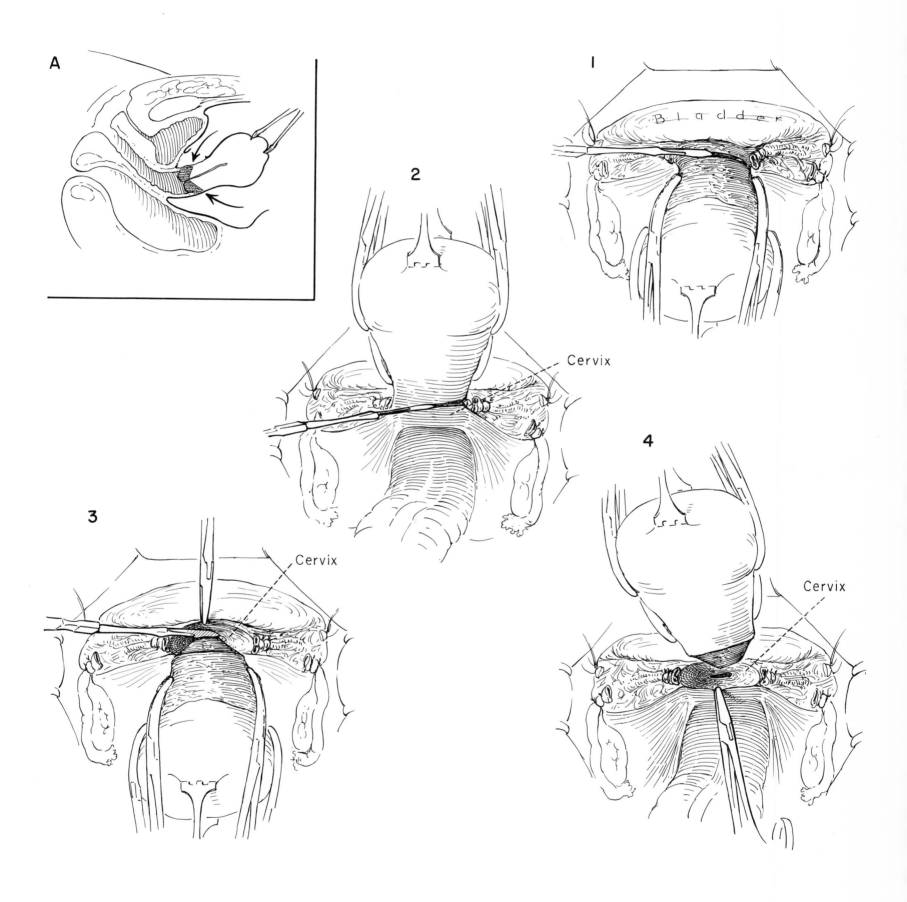

Figure 5. The bladder reflection in its relation to the cervix is determined before another Kocher clamp is placed on the anterior lip of the divided cervix.

The two lips of the cervix must be approximated to control bleeding. This is done by placing a series of interrupted sutures in the cervical stump. To facilitate these steps traction is made on the Kocher clamps as the surgeon places the first stitch ligature into the right angle of the cervix just medial to the point where the uterine arteries were doubly ligated. Because the cervical musculature is so dense and tough a smooth-pointed needle, however large, cannot easily traverse it. The procedure is made much easier if a cutting edge needle is used.

The sutures are placed through the posterior peritoneal reflection and deep into the muscle of both lips at the level of the apex of the cone. In this manner the vessels in the cervical stump are controlled.

Figure 6. A similar stitch is introduced in the muscle of the cervix on the opposite side. After the sutures have been placed in the cervical stump they are tied but not cut. It is necessary to continue traction but not essential to maintain it with a Kocher. If the surgeon will leave the ends of the suture long he can apply traction in this fashion while he leaves the operative site unencumbered by clamps. They may then be discarded. The rest of the closure is accomplished by applying traction on the clamps and placing interrupted catgut sutures across the entire body of the cervix. In this fashion the posterior surface of the cervical stump is peritonealized, eliminating the raw surfaces.

Figure 7. Although the uterine vessels have been divided, the cardinal ligaments which contain the cervical branches of the uterine artery have not been detached from the cervical stump. There is little chance then for the cervix to prolapse. Nevertheless, it is customary to attach the round ligaments to the stump.

You will note that the round ligament and the ovarian vessels have been ligated separately. There is an important reason for the individual ligations. If the round and infundibulopelvic ligaments are sutured together and brought to the cervical stump, tension is placed on the ovarian vessels. This tends to constrict the lumen and limits the blood supply to the ovary which has already lost some supply when the uterine branches to the ovary were resected. The tendency for the ovary to develop follicular or retention cysts is materially reduced when the ovaries are allowed to hang loosely.

Figure 8. The round ligament on the right is then approximated to the closed cervical stump with a mattress suture which passes through the substance of both. The same procedure is carried out on the left side.

Figure 9. Peritonealization is begun in the raw area beneath the right adnexa. Exposure of the incised peritoneal edges is provided by the assistant, who elevates the adnexa with smooth forceps. The anterior peritoneal edge of the bladder flap is best brought into view by a retractor placed in the lower end of the wound. A running suture approximates the cut edges of pelvic peritoneum from right to left.

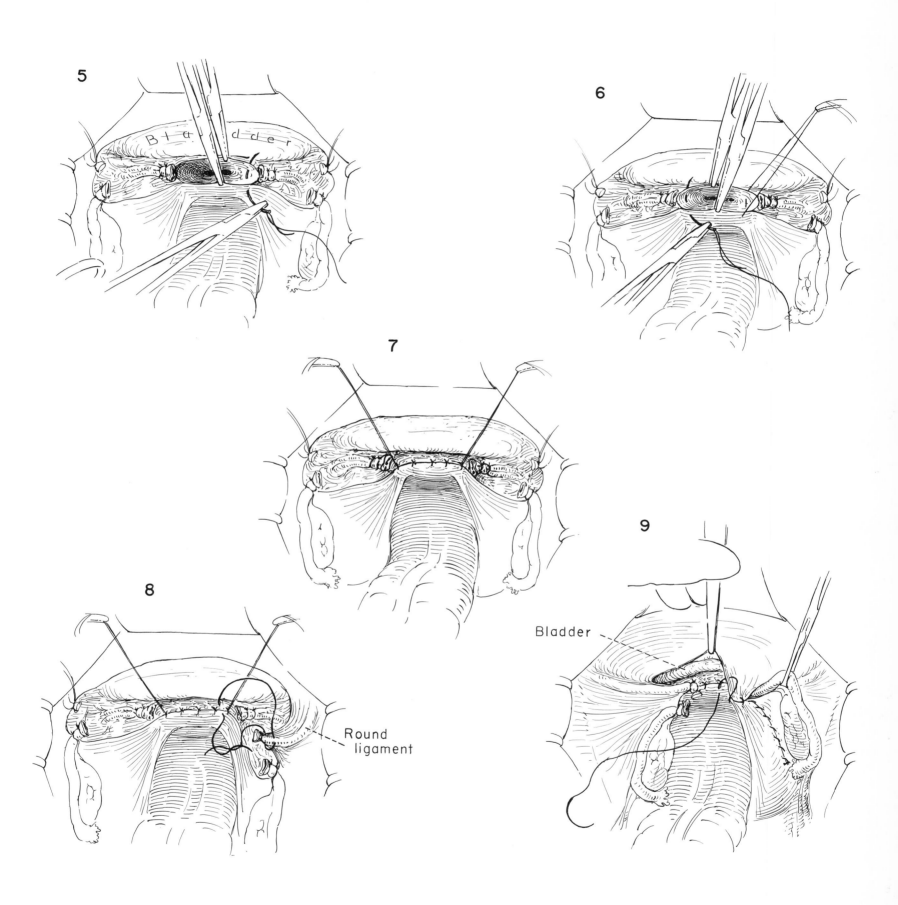

Round ligament

Bladder

MARSHALL-MARCHETTI OPERATION FOR STRESS INCONTINENCE OF URINE

There are many operations devised for the correction of stress incontinence. They are not always effective. For the majority of patients the authors prefer to concentrate on repairing the anatomical defect at the bladder neck, employing the vaginal approach.

The urethrovesical suspension operation designed by Marshall and Marchetti is performed as an abdominal operation. For the most part it is done as a definitive procedure on patients who have not been cured by a vaginal operation or who have been shown by test to have disruption of the dorsal urethral attachment to the symphysis when they strain down.

It has a logical place, however, when hysterectomy is called for. Many of these patients will have varying degrees of stress incontinence. If it is not corrected the symptoms will become worse after the uterus is removed. The Marshall-Marchetti can rightly be classified in the list of modifications of total hysterectomy.

The operation described here, however, depicts the steps employed when it is done as a definitive procedure in a patient with an intact uterus.

Figure 1. A midline incision has been made in the skin down to the symphysis, and the peritoneum has been opened. Wide retractors are placed in the wound to aid in the displacement of the rectus muscle. To assist in the separation of the muscle from the peritoneum beneath it a Kelly clamp is placed on the peritoneal edge while the surgeon gently teases the muscle away from the peritoneum. This is done on both sides. When traction is applied to the clamps on the peritoneum in an upward direction, the prevesical space lying between the symphysis and the lower peritoneum comes into view.

Figure 2. The surgeon inserts his right hand into the space and gently applies pressure, pulling the underlying bladder upward. This maneuver exposes the urethra at the point where it enters the bladder.

Inset A. This is a diagrammatic representation showing an inlying catheter in the bladder and the assistant's finger in the vaginal canal. The assistant applies traction on the catheter while he at the same time exerts upward pressure on the base of the bladder at its neck.

Figures 3 and 4. After the assistant has delineated the bladder neck the surgeon pulls up on the bladder and places a catgut suture in the para-urethral tissue and leads it out through the cartilaginous portion of the symphysis in the midline. The suture is left long and clamped. This is done on both sides.

Figure 5. The first two sutures are tied, approximating the para-urethral tissue to the symphysis. A second series of sutures are placed in the para-ureteral tissue and again into the cartilage of the symphysis proximal to the initial sutures.

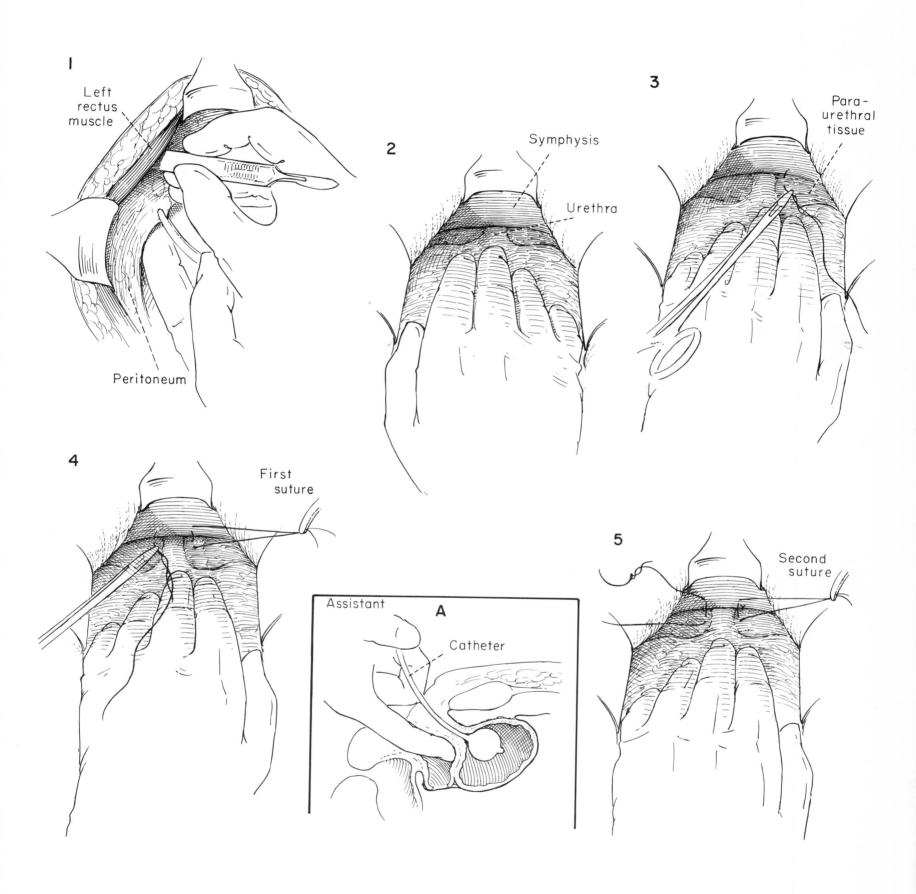

1 Left rectus muscle

Peritoneum

2 Symphysis

Urethra

3 Para-urethral tissue

4 First suture

Assistant A Catheter

5 Second suture

Figure 6. The assistant continues to elevate the bladder base by pushing upward on the bladder neck. The surgeon pulls the bladder upward by exerting pressure with the extended fingers of the left hand. A third series of interrupted catgut sutures are placed in the para-urethral tissue and the cartilage in the midline of the symphysis. After both have been properly placed they are individually tied and cut.

Figure 7. The series of three sutures so placed will have approximated the para-urethral tissue to the symphysis without tension. When this is accomplished the normal posterior vesicourethral angle is restored.

To provide additional support, interrupted sutures are placed in the anterior bladder wall and in the periosteum of the symphysis. These must be carefully introduced into the cartilage to avoid entering the cavity of the bladder on the one hand or stripping the periosteum from the underlying bone on the other. If the latter is done, there is danger that the patient may subsequently develop osteitis pubis. The necessary number of interrupted sutures are placed, ligated and divided.

Prevention of Enterocele

This procedure inevitably dislocates the vaginal apex forward in the pelvis and enterocele may then develop. If hysterectomy has been performed the suspension of the vaginal vault and peritoneal closure must correct for this.

In cases where the uterus is not removed, special steps to shorten the uterosacral ligaments and obliterate the deep cul-de-sac are indicated.

Figure 8. The peritoneal cavity has been opened, the uterus delivered and a stay suture placed at the fundus. The long suture is clamped and placed on constant traction. With the uterus on tension and the ovary held out of the way with forceps, the uterosacral ligaments come into view. The surgeon is seen grasping the ligament between thumb and forefinger. When this is done the ureter can be felt to roll beneath the finger.

Figure 9. After the location of the ureter has been ascertained, a suture is placed in the right uterosacral ligament and carried through the one on the opposite side as the assistant holds the tube and ovary out of the operative field. The surgeon draws the uterosacral ligament medially with forceps as he places the suture. This minimizes the danger of including the ureter in the stitch.

Figure 10. The suture is tied and divided. Several others are similarly placed. The approximation of the two ligaments tends to foreshorten them and restores the normal anatomical situation, thereby reducing the likelihood of development of an enterocele.

Figure 11. The peritoneum is being closed. Drains are placed on both sides into the prevesical space. They are brought out through stab incisions in muscle and fascia, permitting solid closure of the wound and avoiding the chance of hernia.

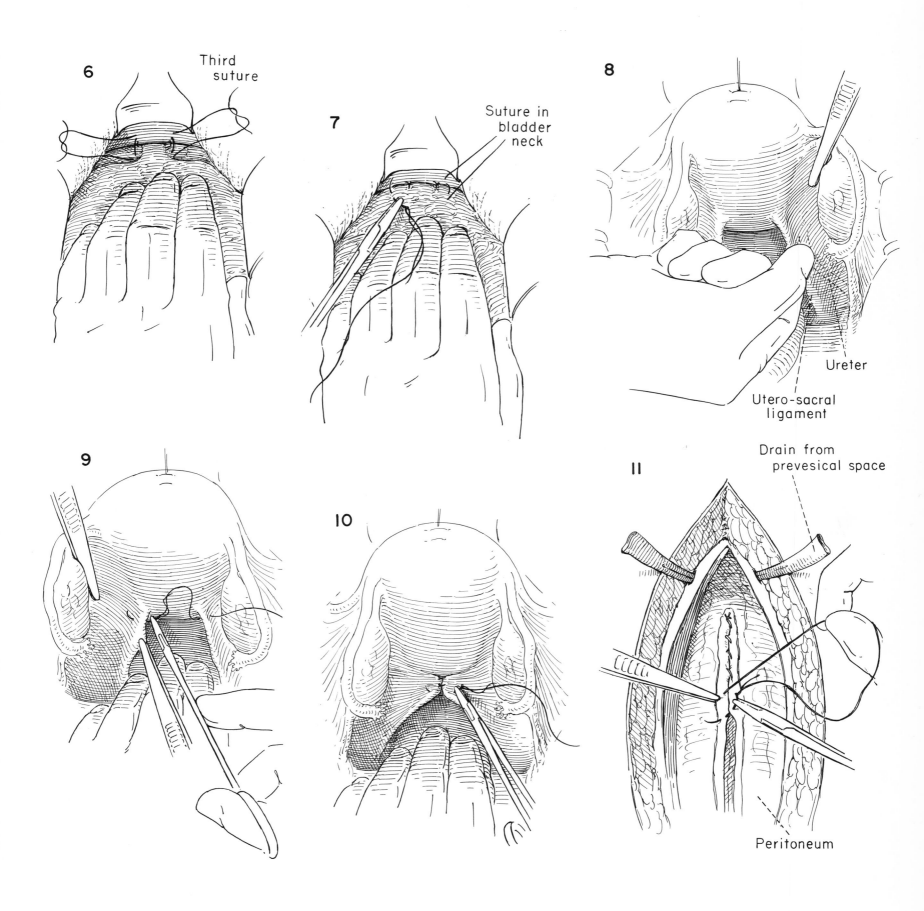

6 Third suture

7 Suture in bladder neck

8 Ureter

Utero-sacral ligament

9

10

11 Drain from prevesical space

Peritoneum

HYSTERECTOMY IN THE PRESENCE OF A LARGE LEIOMYOMA IN THE CERVICAL REGION

A fibroid tumor arising from the cervical portion of the uterus and extending into the leaves of the broad ligament below the pelvic floor may add to technical difficulties in performing the routine steps of a total hysterectomy.

The chief problems are hemorrhage and possible damage to the ureter or bladder. If certain precautions are observed, these potential elements of danger may be minimized.

To avoid damage to the ureter, its course in the pelvis should be checked. The ureter can always be seen beneath the peritoneum as it crosses the common iliac artery. To keep it constantly in view throughout the operation the surgeon should place stay sutures on the incised edge of the medial edge of the peritoneum.

Damage to the bladder as well as excessive bleeding from the plexus of veins in the region of the bladder floor may be avoided if the surgeon will take advantage of the fact that the fibroid tumor is normally encapsulated. The blood supply to the tumor lies within this capsule. An incision through it extending down to the superior surface of the tumor will permit its being shelled out of its bed, leaving the vessels, ureters and bladder on the capsule. With the tumor delivered, the operation proceeds in routine fashion.

Figure 1. Trauma to the ureter may be minimized by full exposure. The nurse pulls the uterus to the left while the assistant retracts the adnexa. The ureter can be seen beneath the peritoneum at the point where it crosses the common iliac artery. The surgeon and assistant grasp the peritoneum lateral to the ureter. The peritoneum is then incised.

Figure 2. Stay sutures of silk are placed on the medial peritoneal leaf and held long. This keeps the operative field open. The ureter can now be followed in its course overlying the fibroid.

Figure 3. The bladder flap has been developed, the tube and ovary ligated and sectioned, and the round ligament detached as in the routine steps of total hysterectomy. The ureter is gently retracted by grasping the supporting tissue rather than the ureter itself. The surgeon then dissects the ureter from the surface of the fibroid to the level of the crossing uterine vessels.

Figure 4. The routine steps of total hysterectomy are carried out on the left side. The uterus is held on traction, and the posterior peritoneum is divided transversely in such a manner that the right and left sides are connected. Exposure is increased by widening the operative field. The rectum is removed from danger.

Figure 5. The uterine vessels as they cross the surface of the fibroid and ureter are then doubly clamped under direct vision, divided and ligated.

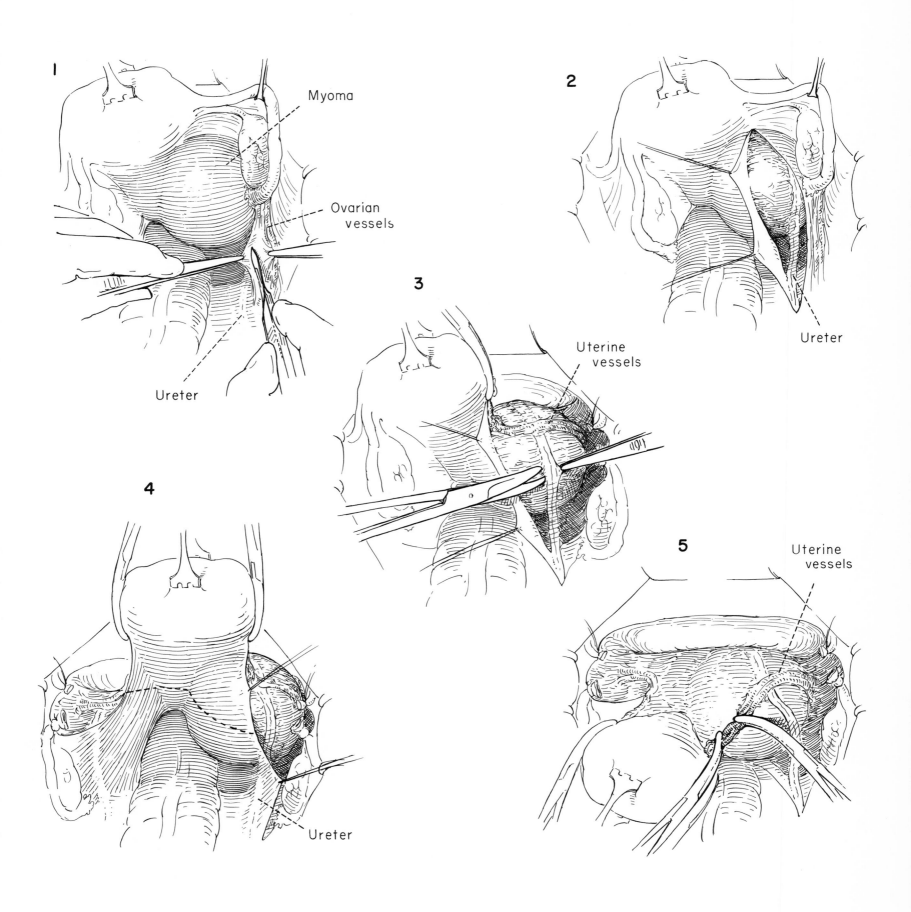

1

Myoma

Ovarian vessels

Ureter

2

Ureter

3

Uterine vessels

4

Ureter

5

Uterine vessels

Figure 6. To maintain tissue planes the uterus is held on tension and drawn to the left side by the surgeon. Note that a wide operative field has been created and that (1) the adnexal vessels and the round ligaments have been ligated and sectioned on both sides; (2) the bladder has been dissected from the cervix on the left side, opposite that of the tumor; (3) the posterior peritoneum has been dissected from the posterior wall of the cervix carrying the rectum out of the field of dissection; and (4) the uterine vessels have been doubly ligated and can be seen lying on the surface of the tumor in close relation to the ureter running lateral to them.

With the anatomy established and the operative field developed, the surgeon then incises the capsule overyling the superior surface of the leiomyoma.

Figure 7. The surgeon keeps traction on the uterus to the left while the assistant picks up the lateral edge of the incised capsule. This permits the surgeon to begin to develop a cleavage plane between the capsule and the fibroid tumor. This is done gently, employing the handle of the knife. Note that the ureter and the vessels lie on the lateral surface of the capsule away from the area being dissected.

The chief blood supply to the tumor lies within the thinned-out muscle layers or capsule of the tumor. When the dissection is done carefully very little bleeding will be encountered. Obvious bleeding vessels should be clamped and ligated.

Figure 8. Again the uterus is maintained on traction by the surgeon in the direction away from the side of the tumor. After defining the plane of cleavage between the tumor and the overlying capsule with the knife handle the surgeon may gently insert the fingers of his right hand into this cleavage plane. By gentle manipulation of the fingers it is possible for the surgeon to complete the separation of the fibroid from the capsule. Once the cleavage plane has been developed it is usually possible to gently elevate the tumor out of its bed without creating any appreciable loss of blood. Any obvious bleeding points must be secured and ligated.

Figure 9. With the tumor freed from the overlying capsule it is rolled out of its bed by rotating it toward the uterine side in an upward medial direction. Traction on the uterus is essential.

When the tumor has been delivered the uterus is held upward on traction in the midline and the fibroid is rolled upward. This permits the surgeon to see the posterior lateral corners of the vagina below the level of the inferior border of the tumor. Kelly clamps are then placed on both corners of the vagina.

Figure 10. Maintaining traction on both uterus and fibroid for purposes of exposure, the surgeon now transects the vaginal wall between the Kelly clamps. The bladder edge is under direct vision. The reconstructive steps of the total hysterectomy then proceed in the usual manner.

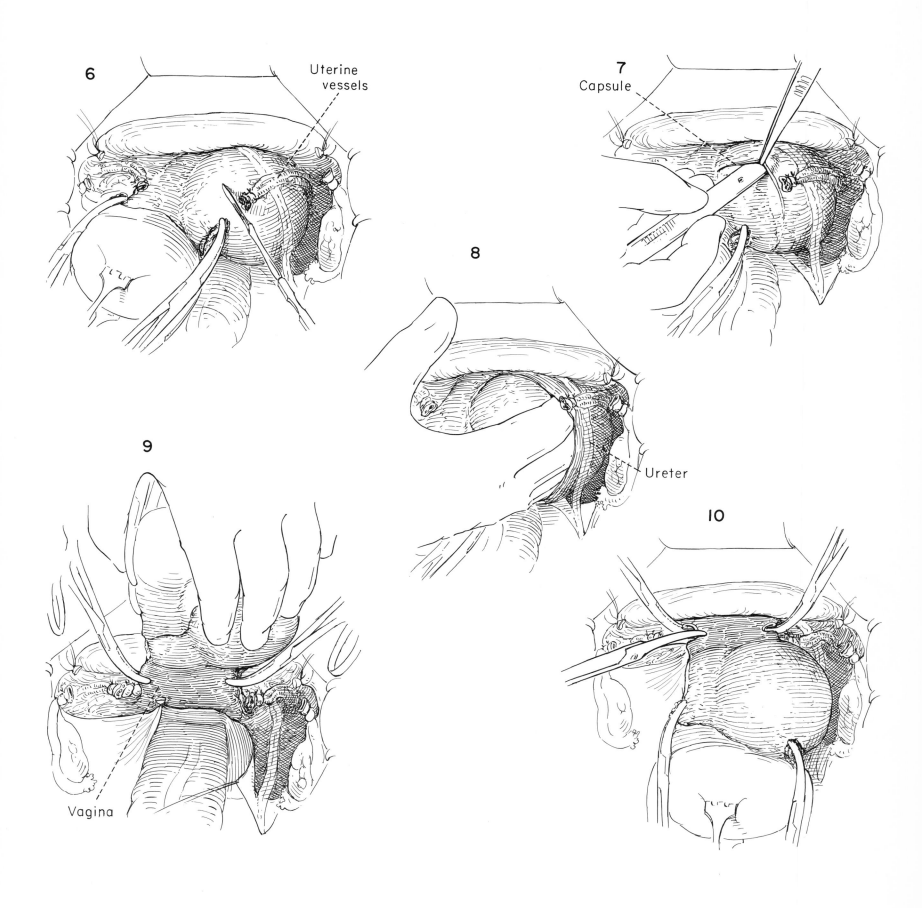

MOBILIZATION OF THE UTERUS AND ADNEXA

In performing surgery in the pelvis it is of prime importance to prepare an unencumbered operative field. It is a common error to attempt to remove the uterus, tube or ovary before it has been mobilized. One frequently finds small intestine adherent to the fundus, ovary or posterior leaf of the broad ligament. It must be freed before proceeding with the removal of any of the pelvic organs.

In sectioning adhesions which bind the intestine to the uterus it is important to stay on the uterine side of the dissection to minimize the risk of injury to the bowel. Immediate repair is indicated if damage occurs.

Similarly, the adnexa must be freed from the posterior leaf of the broad ligament. Once a plane of cleavage is established, pelvic inflammation separates readily, but endometriosis, because of its tendency to invade, can be freed only after rupture and spillage of the contents of the chocolate cyst.

Figure 1. The surgeon grasps the tenaculum on the fundus as he holds the small bowel in the fingers of the right hand. A gentle rolling of the bowel between the thumb and forefinger will either establish a plane of cleavage or will expose adhesions that may safely be divided by scissor dissection. If there is any question about the point of division, "stay on the uterine side." Leave a segment of uterus or ovary on the bowel, not bowel on the uterus.

Figure 2. The tube and ovary are often found densely adherent to the posterior surface of the broad ligament. With traction maintained on the fundus of the uterus, the palmar surfaces of the fingers of the right hand are placed against the posterior surface of the broad ligament below the ovary. By elevating the fingers in a "peeling motion," a cleavage plane is established and the tube and ovary dislodged from the adherent bed. Extensive pyosalpinx may be displaced intact. Chocolate cysts will invariably rupture. In either case, a suction tip should be held in readiness to aspirate inadvertent spillage.

Figure 3. The cecum may have become attached to the right adnexa as a result of previous pelvic inflammation or surgery. The uterus, the bowel and the tube and ovary are held on tension while the adhesive bands are divided.

Figure 4. The rectum is often fixed to the posterior vagina or cervix for one of various reasons. This area is thrown into sharp relief by upward traction on the fundus. The surgeon exerts counterpressure on the sigmoid by the flattened fingers of the left hand. The cleavage plane is exposed and the sigmoid stripped from the back wall of the uterus.

INSETS A AND B. These drawings indicate in a sagittal plane the situation before and after this dissection.

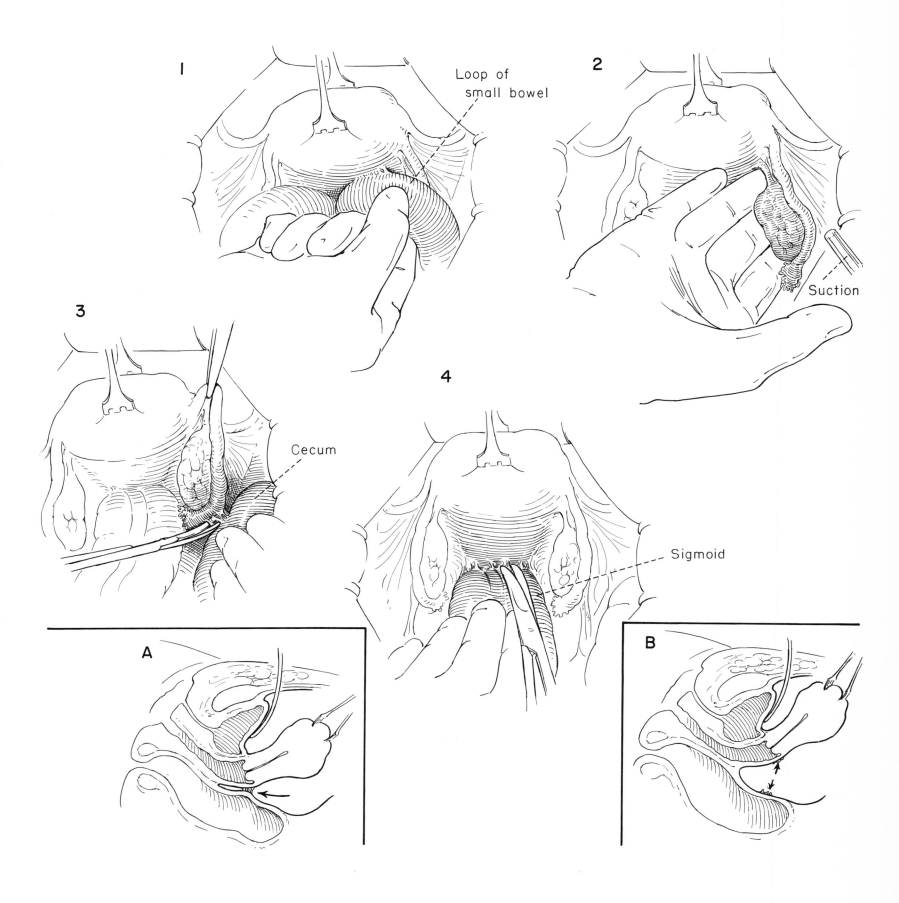

Figure 5. The rectum, in endometriosis of the rectovaginal septum, may be adherent to the posterior wall of the uterus between the attachments of the uterosacral ligaments. Separation does not occur in the usual fashion because of the invasive tendency of the disease. Separation is possible by two methods. The surgeon may apply traction to the tenaculum on the fundus. Sudden flexion in the direction of the symphysis cracks the peritoneal surface on the posterior wall of the uterus above the point of bowel attachment. If such separation does not occur, the surgeon lightly divides this peritoneal cover transversely above the area of bowel fixation. A plane of cleavage is created which will permit dissection of the rectum from the uterus without the danger of entering bowel.

Inset A. Diagram showing in sagittal section the result when peritoneum of the posterior cervix or vagina has been left on the bowel in order to achieve satisfactory mobilization.

REPERITONEALIZATION OF SIZEABLE DEFECTS ON THE PELVIC FLOOR

Figure 1. It is imperative in any pelvic procedure to ensure adequate peritoneal closure to prevent the possibility of intestine becoming adherent to any raw area. At times the surgeon may be confronted with the problem of not having enough normal peritoneum to provide complete peritonealization. This is particularly apt to occur when the surgeon finds it necessary to remove wide areas of the pelvic peritoneum in order that extensive implants of endometriosis can be completely excised. Similarly, much of the peritoneal cover may have to be sacrificed when extensive pathology of the adnexa has fixed it to the posterior leaves of the broad ligament. Although the defect may be too extensive to permit closure by mobilization of the existing peritoneum, complete peritonealization can be accomplished easily by utilizing the adjacent sigmoid colon. This can be done without materially altering the course of the bowel or creating the possibility of subsequent disturbance in function.

Figure 2. To ensure this the bowel must be brought to the defect in such fashion that it lies comfortably in position without distortion or tension. There is usually enough redundancy in the sigmoid colon to accomplish this with ease.

The properly selected area of the bowel is then grasped with Allis forceps which are placed in the tenia of the colon.

Figure 3. The sigmoid is then rotated to cover the defect. A series of interrupted atraumatic sutures approximates the cut edge of the peritoneum overlying the bladder flap to the longitudinal band of the sigmoid. The assistant aids by keeping the bowel in position with the Allis clamps. Interrupted sutures are used to avoid any puckering effect from a running suture.

Figure 4. This line of sutures is continued far enough laterally to obliterate openings or pockets into which small bowel might later descend.

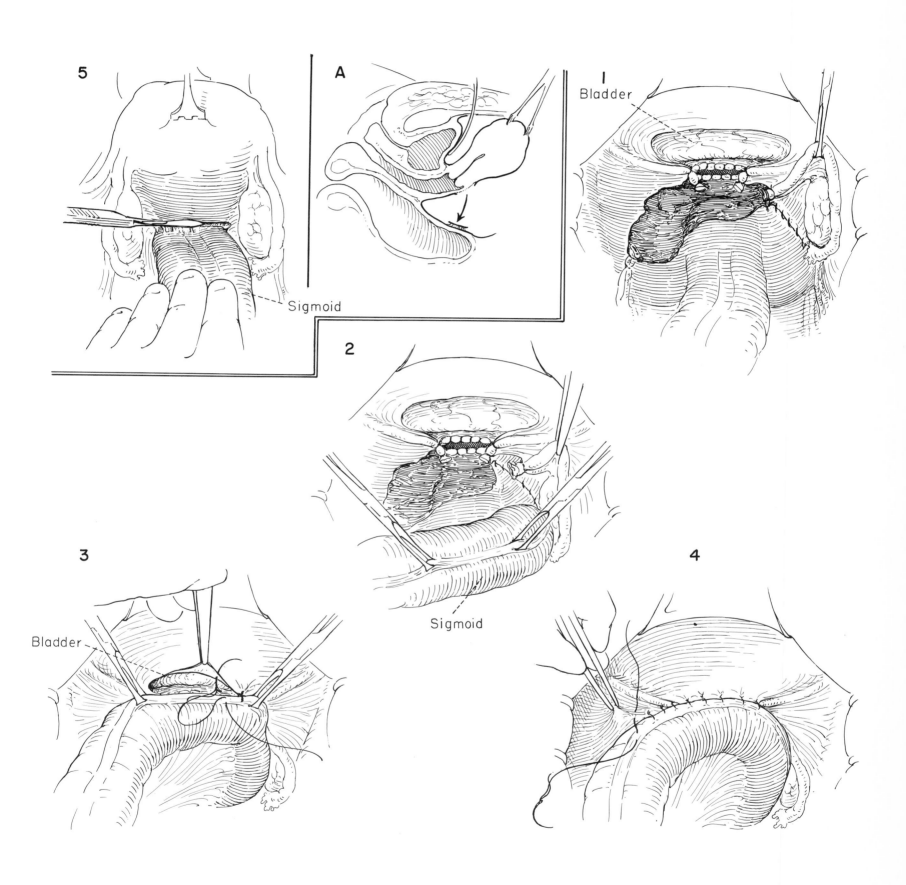

RESECTION OF THE ANTERIOR VAGINAL WALL FOR CORRECTION OF A SMALL CYSTOCELE

Normally we prefer to leave the vaginal canal open and whip over the cut edges with a running lock stitch. On rare occasions in the presence of a small cystocele, insufficient to require a vaginal plastic procedure from below, it is possible to correct the anatomical defect by removing a wedged V-shaped section of the anterior vaginal wall in its long axis along with the uterus and closing the vagina in a transverse direction with interrupted catgut sutures.

The foreshortening of the anterior vaginal wall that results will correct a small cystocele. Because of the shortening of the vaginal canal the procedure is not recommended for a bladder prolapse of any great degree.

Figure 1. The prime requisite for successful performance is adequate retraction of the bladder floor from the vaginal wall. The surgeon applies upward traction on the uterus while the assistant retracts the bladder floor. The vagina is entered laterally on both sides. Kelly clamps grasp the vaginal wall at the angles. The surgeon then removes a V-shaped segment of the anterior vaginal wall. The assistant prepares to grasp the leading cut edge of the vagina with a clamp.

Figure 2. The clamps at the angles are individually ligated with stitch ligatures. These are left long for traction. The surgeon then closes the open vagina with interrupted sutures which include the full thickness of both walls.

Figure 3. The vagina is now completely closed with interrupted sutures. Reconstruction and peritonealization then follow the procedure outlined in the technique of total hysterectomy.

THE INTRAFASCIAL TYPE OF HYSTERECTOMY

This type of hysterectomy differs from that previously described only in the steps with which the cervical portion of the hysterectomy is handled.

In the majority of instances these steps will not be necessary, but occasionally the surgeon is faced with pathological conditions which tend to fix the bladder floor to the cervix and anterior vaginal wall. The majority of vesicovaginal fistulae seen today follow damage to the bladder during total removal of the uterus. If there appears to be any danger of damaging the bladder floor the surgeon had best split the fascia overlying the cervix. There is always a plane of cleavage beneath it. It can be identified by introducing a Kelly clamp into the elliptical defect that appears in the fascial sheath after dividing the uterine vessels.

After dividing the fascia between the two openings the surgeon may then apply the lateral clamps so that the upper blade is below the fascia. No possible damage can occur to the bladder floor because it is above the clamp.

Figure 4. After doubly ligating the uterine vessels and applying traction to the uterus, the surgeon incises the fascia over the anterior wall of the cervix above the ligated vessels.

Figure 5. The fascia can then be gently stripped from the cervix with a minimum of bleeding. The assistant elevates the cut fascial edge as the surgeon dissects the cervix from the fascia with scissors or the handle of the knife.

Figure 6. After elevation of the fascia, the Kelly clamp on the cervical branches of the uterine artery may be placed beneath the fascial edge without risk of damage to the bladder, which lies superior to the fascial flap.

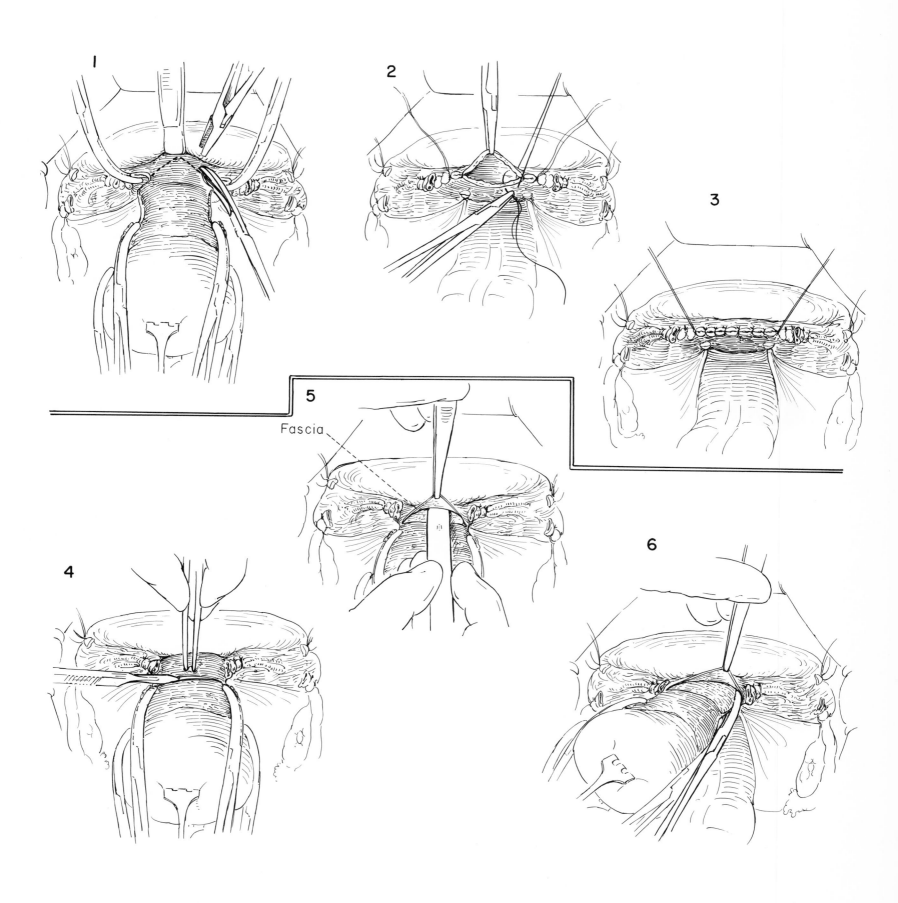

Fascia

Conservative Operations

There can be little doubt that the present trend in gynecology in the field of benign disease and anatomical derangement is away from the policy of performing hysterectomy as a routine procedure. The thoughtful approach to the problem of endometriosis is an excellent example of this trend toward conservatism.

EXCISION OF ENDOMETRIAL IMPLANT

Within the scope of the concept of conservative management of endometriosis, in which the primary aim is to preserve menstrual and ovarian function, there is logic in removing peritoneal implants which are prone to occur on the peritoneal floor, uterosacral ligaments and serosal surface of the bowel, provided the surgeon exercises reasonable care in so doing. The implant is more likely to produce severe dysmenorrhea and dyspareunia than far more extensive endometriosis within the ovary.

Some surgeons like to cauterize these areas. We prefer to excise them. The stellate scar surrounding the endometrial implant frequently involves only the peritoneum or serosal surface. The individual implants thus lend themselves to excision.

Figure 1. Exposure is provided by traction on a figure-of-eight suture placed in the fundus while the assistant retracts the sigmoid and elevates tube and ovary with a Babcock clamp. The Allis clamp often used may cause tissue damage.

Figure 2. The surgeon elevates the peritoneal flap and carefully dissects beneath it.

Figure 3. The peritoneum is then closed with interrupted atraumatic catgut sutures.

EXTENSIVE ENDOMETRIOSIS

Despite massive invasion of the ovary, uterus and sigmoid, the surgeon may elect to be conservative in order to preserve the childbearing function in the young, and ovarian function in the older patient.

The rectosigmoid, for example, may be separated from the area of attachment between the uterosacral ligaments in the manner previously described (page 58). Multiple implants on the pelvic peritoneum and uterosacral ligaments may be excised en masse by careful dissection of the peritoneum from the underlying structures.

Though the ovary may appear to be hopelessly compromised by endometrial cysts, a plane of cleavage can invariably be established between the cyst and normal ovarian tissue. Endometriosis, although it has invasive properties in other areas, is less likely to demonstrate this in the ovary. It is thus possible to preserve an ovary that might otherwise have been sacrificed. Many patients previously infertile have become pregnant following this procedure.

When the sigmoid is fixed to the back of the uterus, two methods are available to establish a proper cleavage plane: (1) if the uterus is drawn sharply toward the symphysis, the serosal surface may crack in the proper plane; (b) if not, a light stroke of the knife above the point of sigmoid attachment will create it.

Figure 1. Before undertaking any dissection of the endometriosis, the tube and ovary must be freed from the back of the broad ligament and the sigmoid from the posterior wall of the uterus. The ovary invariably ruptures. This figure shows a chocolate cyst involving the left ovary, the sigmoid adherent to the posterior wall of the uterus, small implants in the right ovary and a stellate scar on the serosal sigmoid surface.

Figure 2. The rupture of the chocolate cyst in the left ovary is evident. The sigmoid has been separated from the posterior wall of the uterus, exposing the uterosacral ligaments. The surgeon elevates the peritoneum beyond the obvious involvement by endometriosis and gently dissects it from any underlying structures.

Figure 3. The dissection is carried up on the back of the uterus. Firm traction on the flap with Allis forceps and upward traction on the uterus will facilitate this maneuver. The scar of endometriosis on the sigmoid is left undisturbed.

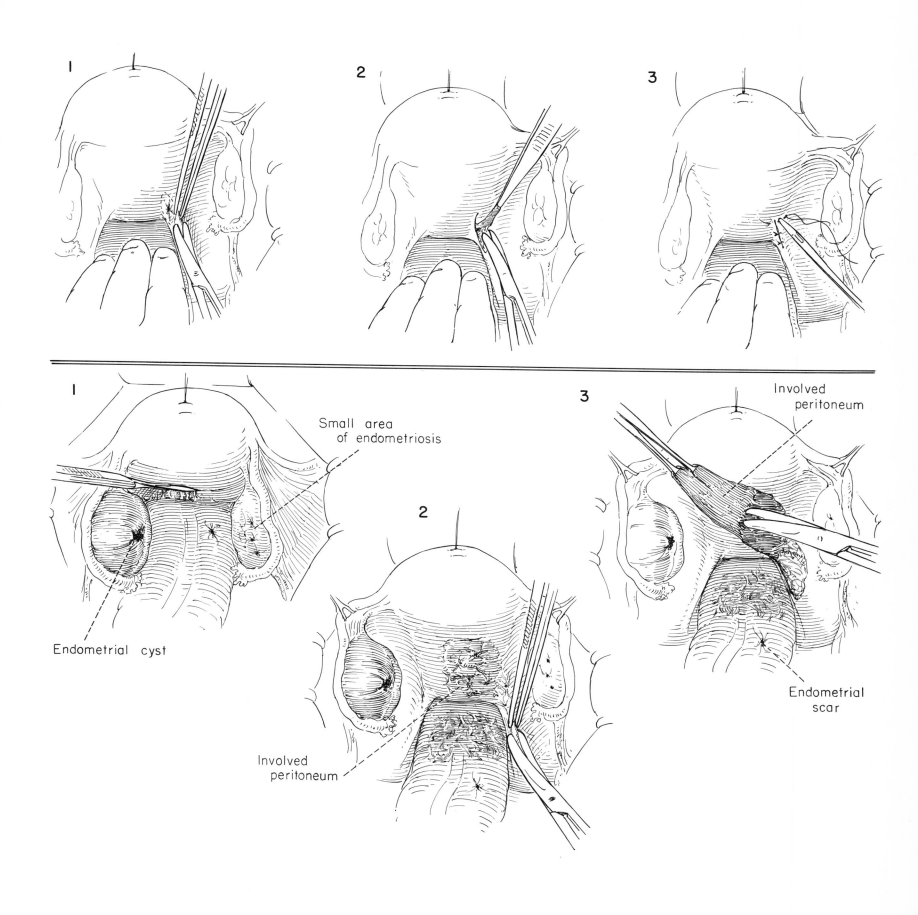

Small area
of endometriosis

Endometrial cyst

Involved
peritoneum

Involved
peritoneum

Endometrial
scar

Figure 4. Regardless of the extent of endometriosis within the ovarian substance, chocolate cysts can invariably be excised so that some ovarian tissue is left. A definite cleavage plane is usually present. Although there is a chance that the endometriosis may recur, the procedure is warranted when the primary aim is to enhance fertility and preserve ovarian function.

The uterus is held on traction by a figure-of-eight suture placed in the musculature of the uterine fundus. Since the uterus is to be preserved, this is less traumatic than applying a tenaculum, which tends to tear the muscle.

The surgeon then applies a Babcock clamp to the medial edge of the ovarian ligament in order to steady it. Recognizing the fact that normal ovarian tissue tends to thin out over the surface of the cyst wall, the surgeon selects a suitable area and incises the serosal peritoneal cover. The assistant places an Allis clamp to the incised edge and holds it on traction to aid in exposing the plane of cleavage between the cyst and the normal ovarian tissue.

The surgeon grasps the cyst, using gauze to facilitate easier traction, and gently separates the cyst with the handle of the knife as a blunt dissecting instrument. The cyst is then shelled out of the ovary. The resulting defect is closed and the ovary reconstructed with a running lock type catgut suture which begins at the pole and returns to the point of origin.

Figure 5. The chocolate cyst has been excised from the substance of the left ovary and the defect closed with a continuous catgut suture.

Small individual and coalescent cysts have been excised in a wedge-shaped segment from the right ovary. The ovary is then reconstructed with a running suture. The raw area on the pelvic floor and posterior uterine wall is too extensive to permit peritoneal closing either by approximation of the peritoneal edges or by uterine suspension.

REPERITONEALIZATION BY OMENTAL GRAFT

In many instances the raw area on the pelvic floor and posterior uterine wall is so great following an extensive conservative operation for endometriosis that it is impossible to provide a peritoneal closure either by approximation of the peritoneal edges, a Baldy-Webster type suspension or by use of the sigmoid. If the sigmoid does not readily cover the defect, a free omental graft can be utilized to provide effective closure.

Figure 6. The omental graft is applied as a patch and is a free graft. It must, therefore, be detached from the main omental body. The surgeon and the assistant place the free edge of the omentum on tension. The individual vessels within the omentum are clamped with Kelly clamps. The tissue is divided and the clamps individually ligated.

Figure 7. The free omental graft is then sutured to the peritoneum of the posterior uterine wall and pelvic floor by interrupted catgut sutures.

Figure 8. The defect is now covered by the omental graft, thus preventing adhesion of small or large bowel to the area denuded of peritoneum.

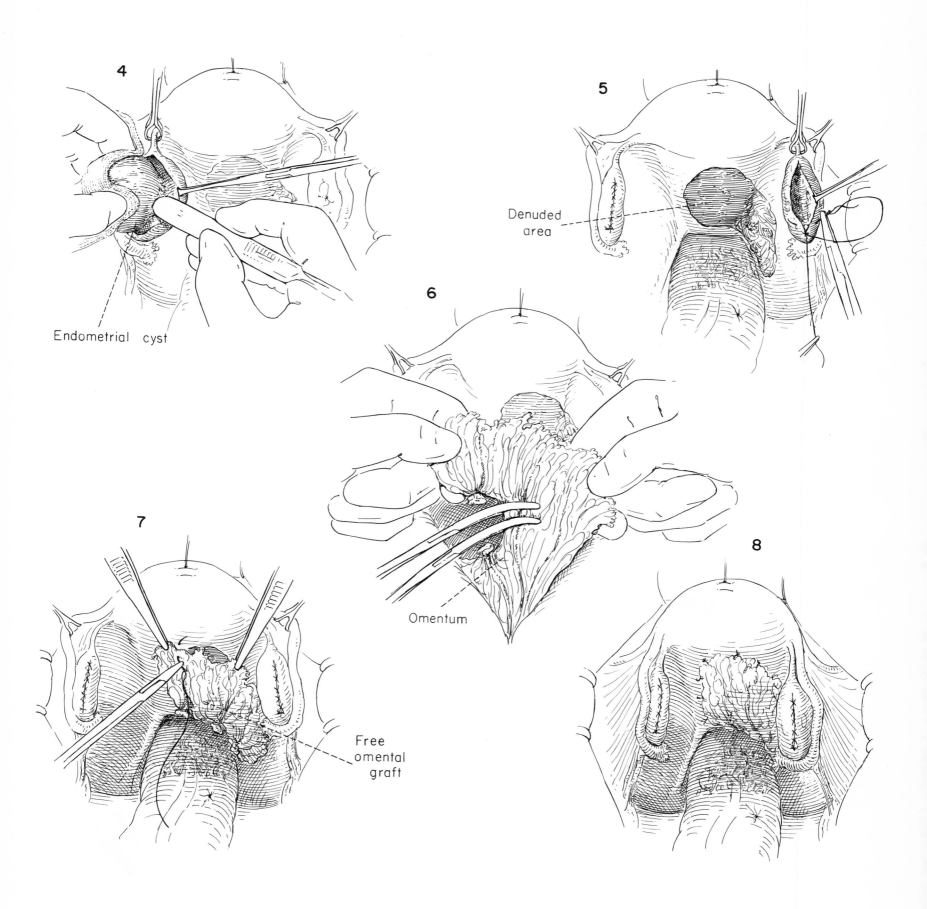

4

Endometrial cyst

5

Denuded area

6

Omentum

7

Free omental graft

8

OLSHAUSEN SUSPENSION

In the past, suspension of the uterus in retroverted position was a common operation. Although it is rarely used today as a definitive procedure, it still has a recognized place in gynecological surgery, particularly when the operation is performed in conjunction with other procedures designed to improve fertility. It is important that the uterus be suspended in such fashion that it will not break down under the stress of the enlarging fetus and that it not interfere with a successful delivery.

The Olshausen type of suspension has fulfilled these obligations over a long period of time and has the advantage of being a simple operative procedure.

Figure 1. The abdomen has been opened through a paramedian incision in the usual manner. The surgeon grasps the uterus with thumb and forefinger and draws the uterus up out of the pelvis to the position on the anterior abdominal wall where it lies without undue tension. This is important.

The assistant maintains the position of the uterus as the surgeon picks up the round ligament about 1/2 inch lateral to its point of insertion in the uterine wall. If placed too far out on the round ligament, an opening may be left to the lateral side through which small bowel might herniate.

The surgeon then places a cutting point stitch at this point, carrying two strands of heavy braided silk beneath the round ligament.

Figure 2. Kelly clamps are placed on the edge of the peritoneum and the anterior rectus fascia at the level selected for fixation. The assistant holds back the subcutaneous fat and skin with a retractor. The surgeon exposes the undersurface of the peritoneum by elevating the two Kelly clamps in the left hand while he introduces the stitch into the peritoneum, muscle and fascia.

Figure 3. The clamps are then drawn firmly to the midline, thus exposing the point of exit of the suture on the anterior rectus sheath.

Figure 4. The surgeon maintains traction on the left rectus fascia and peritoneum toward the midline while he returns the suture again through the fascia muscle and peritoneum. The point of exit on the peritoneal side should be approximately 1/2 inch from the point of the initial introduction. This suture is thus a mattress suture passing through all the structures noted.

Figure 5. The peritoneum and fascia are again elevated to the left by the Kelly clamps held in the left hand of the surgeon. The area of peritoneum between the two double strands of silk is then scarified with a knife blade.

Figure 6. The double strands of silk are drawn taut, pulling the round ligament and with it the uterus up to the scarified area on the abdominal wall. The process is repeated on the opposite side.

Figure 7. This shows the round ligament in relation to the abdominal wall after the suture has been tied.

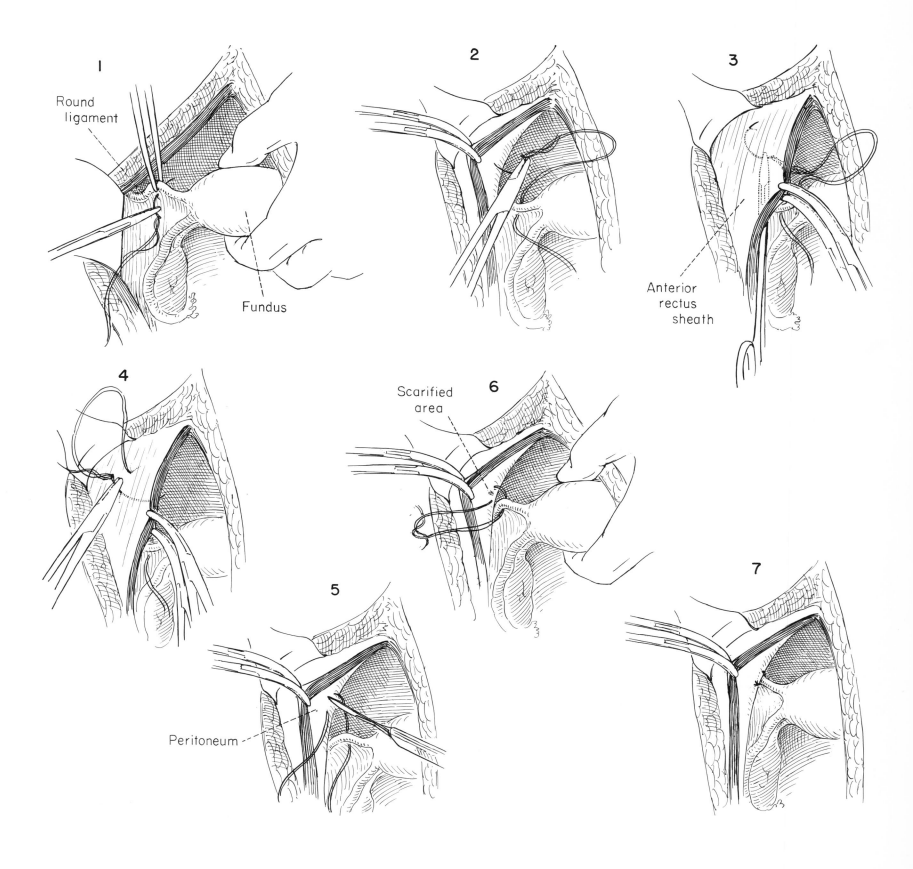

1

Round ligament

Fundus

2

3

Anterior rectus sheath

4

5

Peritoneum

Scarified area

6

7

BALDY-WEBSTER SUSPENSION

Although the surgeon would in all probability not select the Baldy-Webster type of uterine suspension as a sole definitive procedure in the rare instances when such a suspension might be indicated, nevertheless it does have a useful place in pelvic surgery.

The procedure is most useful when in the course of a conservative operation for endometriosis or pelvic inflammation the peritoneum of the broad ligament or posterior serosal surface of the uterus has been either sacrificed or traumatized. In this situation it is often difficult to mobilize enough peritoneum to cover the defect. It is also of value to cover the suture line of a posterior uterine wall myomectomy.

When the original disorder has been endometriosis the surgeon may want to maintain the uterus in forward position and may not be enthusiastic about peritonealizing the defect with either the sigmoid or a free omental graft. It is a relatively easy operation to bring the round ligaments through the posterior leaf of the broad ligament and suture this to the back wall of the uterus. The round ligaments can then be covered by mobilizing peritoneum. This is the Baldy-Webster suspension.

Figure 1. The uterus is placed on forward traction to expose the posterior leaf of the broad ligament. A bloodless area beneath the ovarian ligament is thus exposed. The assistant aids in the exposure by retracting the tube and ovary with a Babcock forceps. The surgeon picks up the peritoneum and incises it in the bloodless area with curved scissors.

Figure 2. The assistant retracts the adnexa while the surgeon inserts a Kelly clamp through the opening in the posterior leaf of the broad ligament and incises the anterior surface of the broad ligament between the open jaws of the clamp.

Figure 3. The opening in the posterior broad ligament is enlarged with curved scissors.

Figure 4. The assistant continues to hold back the tube and ovary while the surgeon pulls the uterus to the left. The surgeon inserts an Allis forceps through the opening in the broad ligament and grasps the round ligament at a point well away from the uterus.

Figure 5. A loop of the round ligament is pulled through the opening in the two leaves of the broad ligament onto the posterior wall of the uterus.

Figure 6. The assistant retracts the adnexa and uterus as the round ligament is approximated to the posterior uterine wall with interrupted sutures. A point midway between the fundus and cervix just lateral to the midline is the ideal position.

Figure 7. The same procedure is carried out on the left side. The defect in the posterior wall of the broad ligament must be closed to prevent herniation of small bowel through the opening. The surgeon places interrupted catgut sutures through the peritoneum lateral to the cut edge and secures it to the peritoneal surface of the uterus.

Figure 8. This shows the completed suspension and peritonealization. The uterus should lie easily, without angulation.

CONSERVATIVE OPERATIONS
BALDY-WEBSTER SUSPENSION

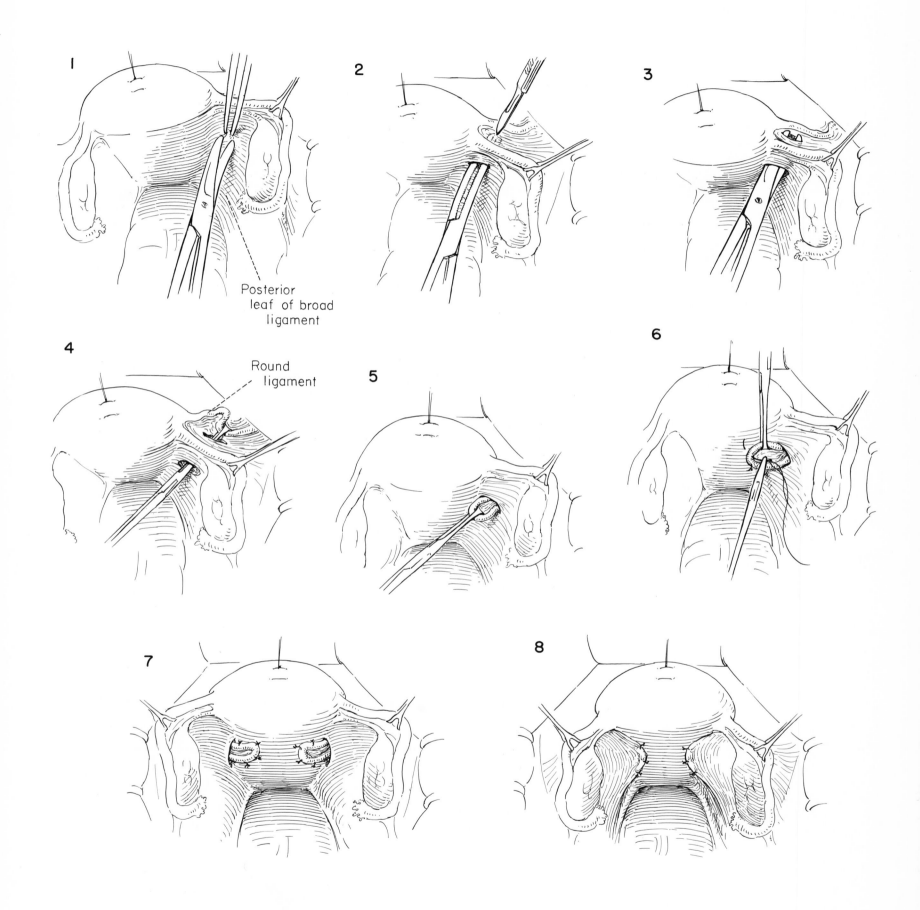

1

Posterior
leaf of broad
ligament

2

3

4

Round
ligament

5

6

7

8

MYOMECTOMY

Myomectomy, the term used for enucleation of leiomyomata from the uterus, has a logical and useful place in gynecological practice when the surgeon either discovers the tumor when he is operating in the pelvis for some other reason or when he feels that removal of the tumor will enhance the patient's chance of being able to become pregnant and deliver a normal child.

In the older patient, when a careful survey of the symptoms and physical findings indicates that surgery for the fibroid tumor, or tumors, should be performed, it is probably better to plan total removal of the uterus, particularly if the woman has completed her family or is at an age when pregnancy is no longer desired or advisable.

In the younger patient who either has symptoms attributable to the presence of benign tumors or has a fibroid tumor which is increasing in size or is located in a position within the uterus which would lessen her chances of producing a living child, it is far better to remove the tumors from the uterus. It is amazing how normal and functional a uterus can be after large or multiple leiomyomata have been excised.

The basic fact to remember in performing a successful myomectomy is that leiomyomata tend to displace rather than invade the uterine musculature. The main blood supply lies in the thinned out layer of muscle which resembles a capsule. When the surgeon incises this outer layer and satisfactorily establishes a plane of cleavage between the tumor and the capsule, the tumor can be enucleated with a minimal amount of blood loss. The surgeon need not be concerned that leaving the so-called capsule will increase the chance of recurrence, nor should the encroachment of the tumor on the endometrial cavity be a deterrent.

Figure 1. A figure-of-eight suture is placed through the muscle wall of the top of the fundus and held on traction away from the symphysis. A fibroid on the anterior wall of the uterus is thus exposed. The surgeon makes a transverse incision through the serosal surface of the uterus down through the capsule of the fibroid. There is always a plane of cleavage between the fibroid and the surrounding musculature.

Figure 2. The divided edges of the serosa and musculature are held on traction with Allis forceps by the surgeon and the assistant as a stitch ligature is laid in the substance of the tumor.

Figure 3. The assistant keeps the divided anterior musculoserosal layer on tension with an Allis forceps while the surgeon applies traction to the stitch through the fibroid and begins to separate the tumor from its bed.

Figure 4. The stitch ligature is then held sharply forward to expose the posterior wall of the fibroid. Allis forceps on the seromuscular coat increase the ease of the dissection by providing a wide field. The blood vessels lie in the connective tissue of the capsule. Individual bleeding vessels are clamped.

Figure 5. The tumor is enucleated, and the assistant ties any clamped vessel.

Figure 6. Closure is accomplished by placing a cutting point stitch through the serosa and muscle to include the depths of the cavity.

Figure 7. Obliteration of the dead space and closure are continued by a series of interrupted sutures similar to those in Figure 6. To complete the serosal approximation, fine interrupted sutures may be placed where needed between the deeper sutures.

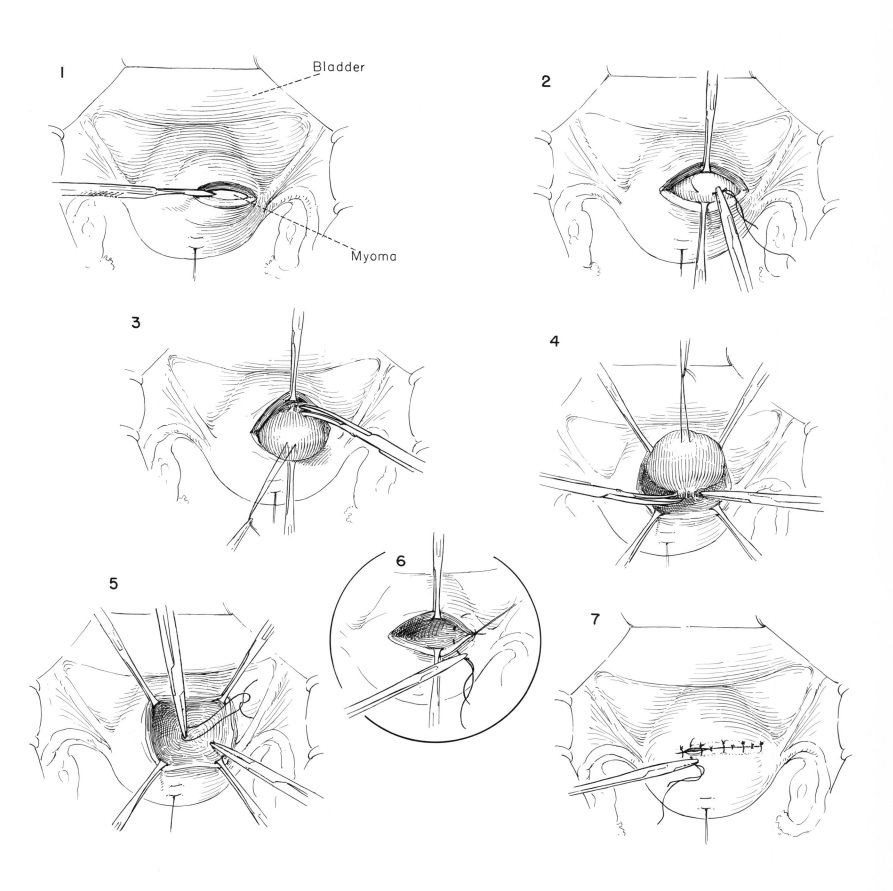

PRESACRAL NEURECTOMY

Section of the presacral nerve is an effective means of dealing with severe intractable pain localized to the midline when the patient has primary dysmenorrhea which cannot be controlled by other means or when she has increasingly severe menstrual cramps secondary to endometriosis that requires a conservative abdominal operation.

It is the authors' opinion that the mere removal of a segment of nerve at the bifurcation of the iliac vessels constitutes inadequate resection. The conception of the presacral nerve as a single trunk we regard as erroneous. The nerve bundle has so many ramifying pathways that a complete resection calls for a wide dissection of all the ramifications of the nerve, beginning above the bifurcation of the aorta and extending down along the iliac vessels over the promontory of the sacrum. The field must be kept meticulously dry. Great care must be taken to avoid possible damage to the midsacral veins which empty into the left common iliac vein.

Figure 1. The abdomen is opened through a paramedian incision and the bowel packed out of the pelvis. The patient is placed in the Trendelenburg position. The sigmoid is retracted to the left. The dotted line indicates the direction and the extent of the proposed incision in the posterior peritoneum.

The surgeon and the assistant elevate the posterior peritoneum from the underlying sacrum as the surgeon divides it with a knife. The incision is then extended down over the promontory and up over the bifurcation of the aorta.

Figure 2. Silk stay sutures are placed on the divided edges of the peritoneum and clamped long to hang outside the abdominal cavity. This provides a wide open operative field. The surgeon then sweeps the areolar attachments toward the midline from the undersurface of the right peritoneal flap with curved scissors.

Figure 3. The right ureter comes into view, lying adherent to the undersurface of the peritoneum. It must be identified and left undisturbed.

Figure 4. The dissection should be directed toward the right common iliac artery, and all the ramifying nerve trunks incised, leaving the adventitia of the vessel clean and glistening. The tissue is mobilized toward the midline as the dissection continues down along the internal iliac (hypogastric) artery. This vessel forms the lateral limits of the dissection.

Figure 5. The common iliac artery has been stripped clean of all nerve branches, and the bare, bony surface of the promontory of the sacrum is seen. The left common iliac vein runs almost transversely across the operative field to disappear beneath the right common iliac, where it joins the right common iliac vein to form the inferior vena cava. The nerve is elevated by forceps and gently dissected free of the superior surface of the vein. Small branching veins must be gently isolated, clamped and tied. The entire nerve bundle has been mobilized toward the midline.

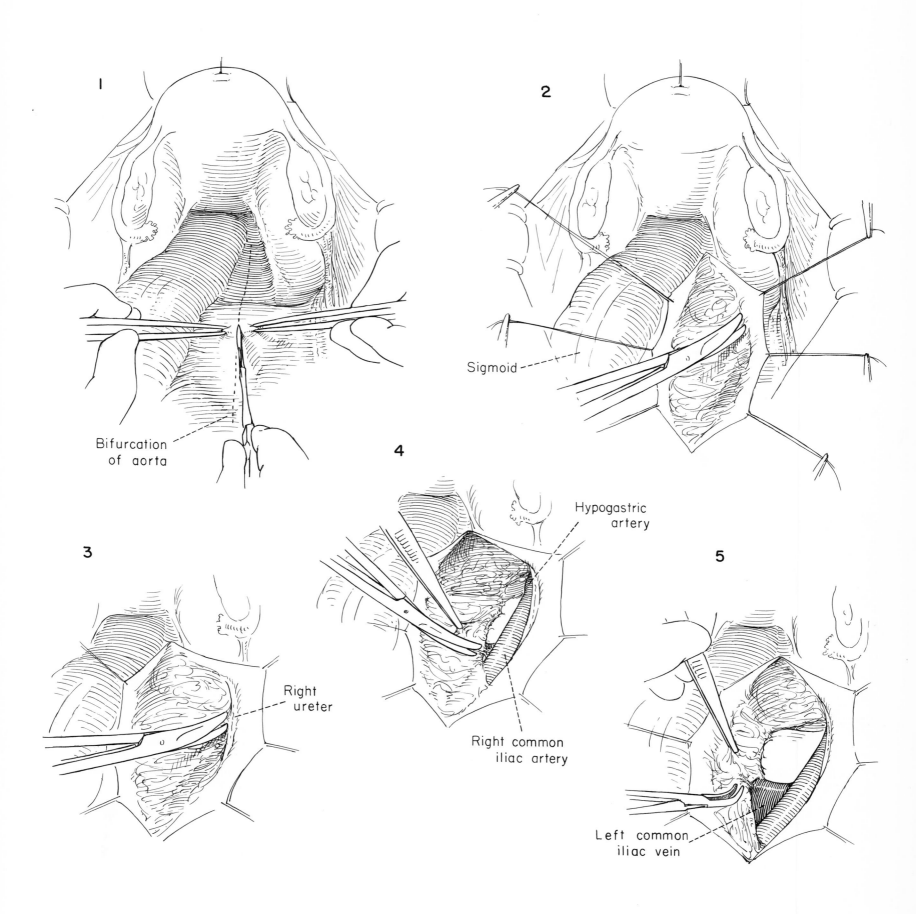

1

2

Sigmoid

Bifurcation
of aorta

4

3

Right
ureter

Hypogastric
artery

Right common
iliac artery

5

Left common
iliac vein

Figure 6. While the dissection of the right side proceeds readily with all anatomical structures easily identified, the resection of the nerve on the left can be a bit more complicated because the sigmoid colon must be reflected to expose the nerve.

To facilitate the exposure the left peritoneal flap is placed on traction by the assistant as the surgeon draws the nerve toward the midline and dissects the areolar attachments of the nerve from the undersurface of the left peritoneal flap.

The chief problem is identifying the sigmoidal vessels and distinguishing the main branch of the artery from the left ureter. When isolated and identified, the artery is left on the peritoneum as the dissection proceeds downward.

Figure 7. When the sigmoidal vessels have been identified, further medial traction on the nerve bundle exposes the left ureter. The exposure is materially improved when traction is placed on the peritoneal stay sutures. The dissection then continues as it did on the right side.

Figure 8. With traction maintained on the stay sutures on the peritoneum, the surgeon and assistant draw the bulk of the nerve mass medially as the dissection proceeds along the superior surface of the left internal iliac vein and the left iliac arterial trunks. Note the position of the left midsacral vein as it lies on the promontory of the sacrum prior to joining the left common iliac vein.

Figure 9. The nerve has now been freed of its lateral and inferior attachments to all vessels. It is still continuous with the main body of the trunk above and with the ramifications of the nerve in the lower pelvis. The main body of the nerve is then elevated and Kelly clamps are placed across its substance at about the level where it crosses the left common iliac vein.

The level for the division of the nerve is arbitrarily selected simply to make the dissection easier. Nothing will be gained by trying to resect it at a higher level for the sole purpose of keeping the nerve trunk in continuity. When the clamps have been placed the nerve is divided.

Figure 10. The surgeon then turns his attention to the distal end of the nerve, rotating it toward the symphysis and dissecting the undersurface of the nerve mass from the anterior surface of the sacrum for a distance of about 1 inch. Care must be taken not to damage the midsacral veins which, although no larger than the lead in a pencil, nevertheless may, when traumatized, cause formidable bleeding that is difficult to control. The surgeon will be happy to have dura clips available on the operating table in the event of damage. The best advice is to have the vessels in sight and avoid injuring them.

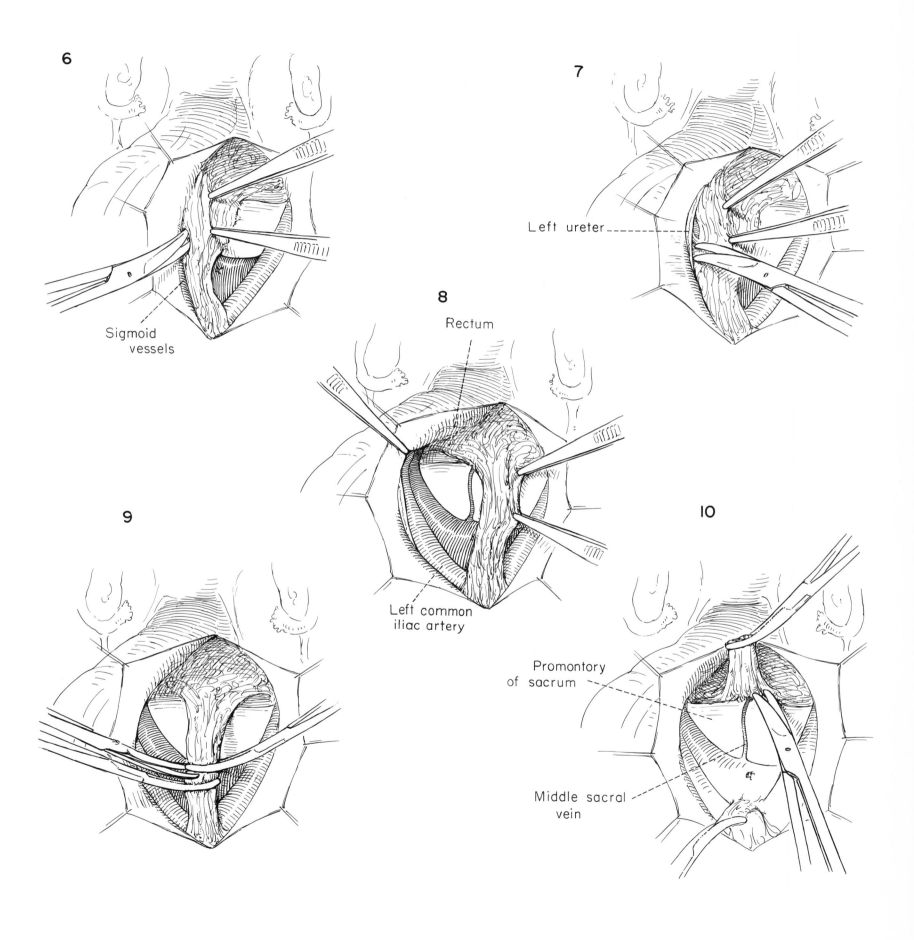

6

7

Left ureter

Sigmoid
vessels

8

Rectum

Left common
iliac artery

9

10

Promontory
of sacrum

Middle sacral
vein

Figure 11. The lateral dissection of the pelvic ramifications of the nerve have carried downward along the hypogastric vessels to the nerve plexus centering around the isthmus of the uterine cervix. Despite the extensive dissection in this area one rarely encounters a patient who has difficulty in emptying her bladder.

The nerve fibers have been freed from the overlying peritoneum in the midline at the level of the cervix. The surgeon then elevates the nerve and under direct vision applies Kelly clamps to the lateral extension of the nerve plexus on both sides. This is necessary since small blood vessels are present and it is of the utmost importance that the operative field be completely dry before the peritoneum is closed. After the clamps have been applied the lower extensions of the nerve are sectioned and removed, and the clamps are left in place.

Figure 12. Stitch ligatures are then placed to include the tissue in the Kelly clamps. The sutures are tied and divided.

Figure 13. With the lower dissection completed the surgeon now concentrates on the removal of the upper segment of the nerve. Light traction is applied to the clamp previously left on the upper portions of the nerve. The surgeon does this himself for it requires gentle handling since it lies directly over the aorta and vena cava. Holding the clamp in his left hand the surgeon rotates the nerve upward to expose the fine areolar attachments which bind the undersurface of the nerve to the wall of the aorta at its bifurcation. Under direct vision the attachments are gently dissected from the adventitia of the main body of the aorta.

Figure 14. The nerve mass is held up and a Kelly clamp placed across the main body of the nerve above the bifurcation of the artery. The nerve is then divided.

Figure 15. The surgeon then places a stitch ligature around the Kelly clamp and ligates the main nerve trunk.

Figure 16. This drawing shows what the operative field should look like following the extensive dissection which removes all the ramifications of the nerve. Note that both the common and internal iliac artery and vein are stripped clear of any nerve tissue from the bifurcation of the aorta well down over the promontory and bony surface of the sacrum. Note also that the midsacral vein and its tributaries are intact and that the wound is dry.

Figure 17. To have a satisfactory dissection the operative field should be bloodless. Before the peritoneal incision is closed all bleeding points must be controlled. A running atraumatic catgut suture may be used for closure.

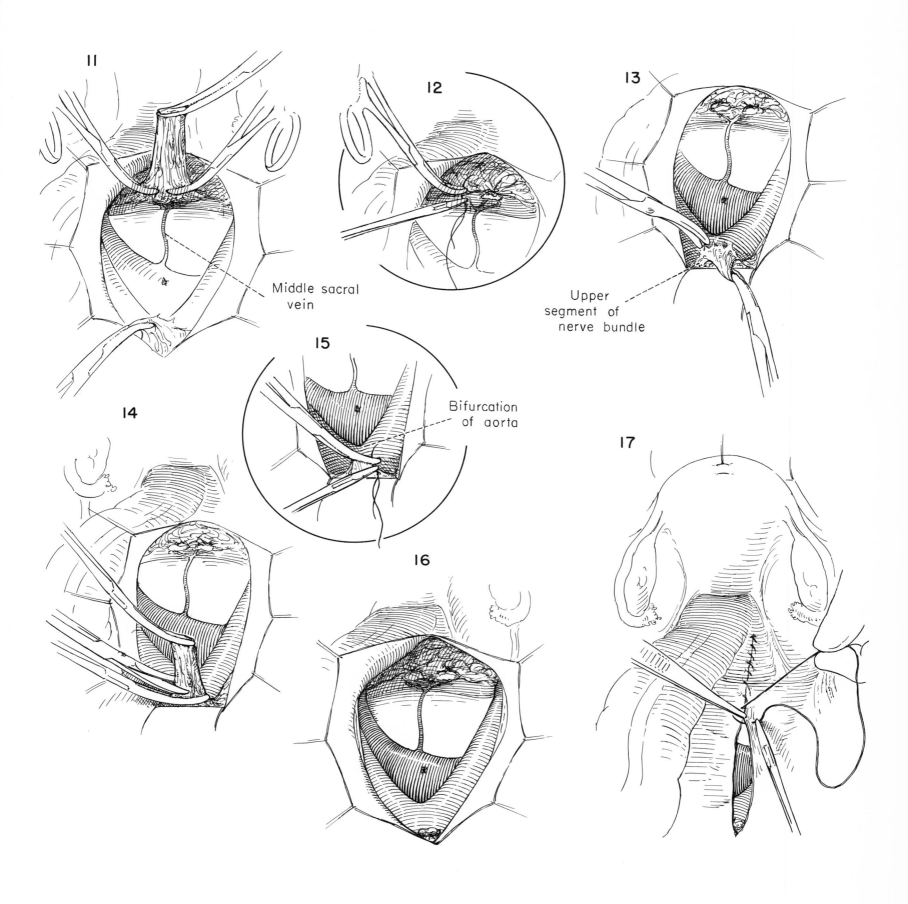

Middle sacral vein

Upper segment of nerve bundle

Bifurcation of aorta

Operations on Tube and Ovary

SALPINGO-OOPHORECTOMY

The majority of operations performed on the tube and ovary are done because of unilateral disease in one or the other. At times, however, the pathological condition demands that both adnexa be removed. In this case the operation of choice is a total hysterectomy and bilateral salpingectomy performed as an en bloc removal.

The operation described here is a salpingo-oophorectomy, which is indicated when the disease process involves a tube and ovary on one side only.

As in all operations on the uterus and adnexa the tube and ovary should be completely mobilized before any attempt is made to remove them. It is also important to remember that when indications call for removal of the tube the isthmial portion must be excised where it transverses the musculature of the uterine horn.

Figure 1. The uterus is held to the left and the tube and ovary elevated by a Kelly clamp in the left hand of the operator in order to expose the infundibulopelvic ligament containing the ovarian artery and vein. The position of the ureter is noted in relation to the vessels and a stitch ligature placed around them under direct vision with complete safety.

Figure 2. The suture is tied by the assistant and held long as the surgeon places a Kelly clamp on the vessels toward the adnexa in order to prevent back bleeding. As the surgeon cuts the vessels, the assistant stands ready to apply another clamp to the cuff beyond the tie.

Figure 3. The first suture is then divided and a second stitch ligature applied. The ovarian vessels are thus doubly ligated. The tube and ovary are pulled toward the midline, and the anterior sheath of the broad ligament below the tube is divided obliquely with scissors up to the point of insertion of the round ligament.

Figure 4. The posterior leaf of the broad ligament below the ovary is incised in similar fashion.

Figure 5. The ovarian branch of the uterine artery lies within the ovarian ligament close to the uterus. This vessel is secured by Kelly clamps, divided and tied with a stitch ligature on the uterine side.

Figure 6. A deep mattress suture is placed in the uterine muscle at the cornu where the tube inserts in the uterus to control a troublesome bleeding vessel which is invariably present at this point.

Figure 7. The tube is removed by a wedge-shaped resection of the uterine wall. The mattress suture is then tied.

Figure 8. The peritoneum is closed by a running suture beginning laterally in order to bury the stump of the infundibulopelvic ligament below the level of the peritoneum.

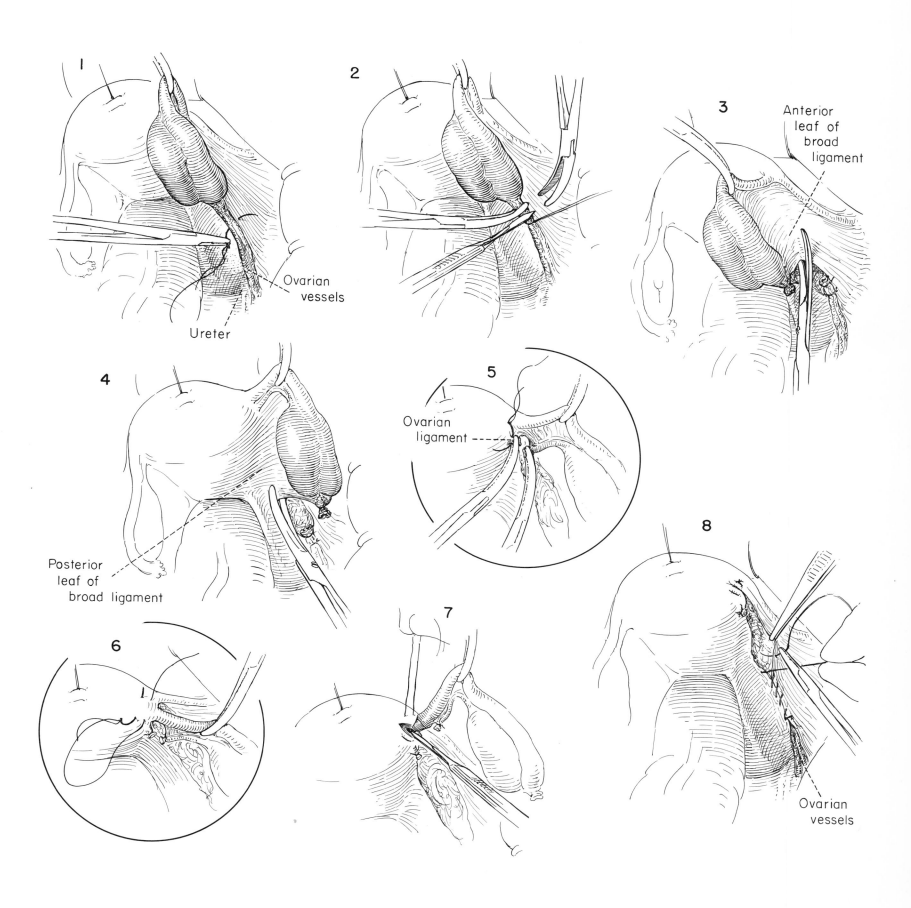

1

Ovarian
vessels

Ureter

2

3

Anterior
leaf of
broad
ligament

4

Posterior
leaf of
broad ligament

5

Ovarian
ligament

6

7

8

Ovarian
vessels

SALPINGECTOMY

For all practical purposes there are few indications for salpingectomy. The chief reason for removing a single tube is, of course, the presence of an ectopic pregnancy. Unilateral pelvic inflammation is a rarity and a one-sided hydrosalpinx should arouse suspicion that the patient might have carcinoma of the tube.

When the underlying pathological state is extensive and is secondary to post-abortal or gonorrheal pelvic inflammation, tuberculosis or endometriosis, the primary disease generally involves the uterus and both adnexa. Under these conditions one might elect to remove the uterus with the tubes but choose to take a calculated risk and leave one or both ovaries.

Figure 1. The uterus is retracted to the left. The tube is elevated between the thumb and forefinger. This exposes the vessels lying in the mesentery of the tube. Two Kelly clamps are placed on the free end of the mesentery close to the tube to avoid injuring the blood supply of the ovary.

Figure 2. The surgeon divides the mesentery between these two clamps. The clamp on the side of the tube simply prevents back bleeding. A stitch ligature is placed around the clamp on the ovarian side and tied.

Figure 3. The first clamp is left in place to provide elevation of the tube. The surgeon then progresses along the mesentery of the tube, repeating the maneuver of clamping, dividing and ligating the vessels. The clamps are placed on the tubal rather than the ovarian side of the mesentery in order to disturb the blood supply to the ovary as little as possible.

Figure 4. The operator elevates the tube to expose the point of insertion in the cornu of the fundus. A deep mattress suture is laid into the uterine muscle beneath the tube. The suture is left long and untied.

Figure 5. The nurse pulls the uterus to the left while the assistant controls the mattress suture in the uterine cornu. The tube is elevated and dissected out of the wall of the uterus in a wedge in the area enclosed by the mattress suture. Tension on this suture controls the bleeding.

Figure 6. The assistant ties the mattress suture. The exposed ends of the ligated vessels may be covered by a running suture in the peritoneum. It is a nice refinement in technique to use interrupted sutures rather than a running stitch, which would tend to pucker the area.

Figure 7. The round ligament is brought over the cornu and sutured to the posterior uterine wall to add additional coverage to the raw area where the tube was excised.

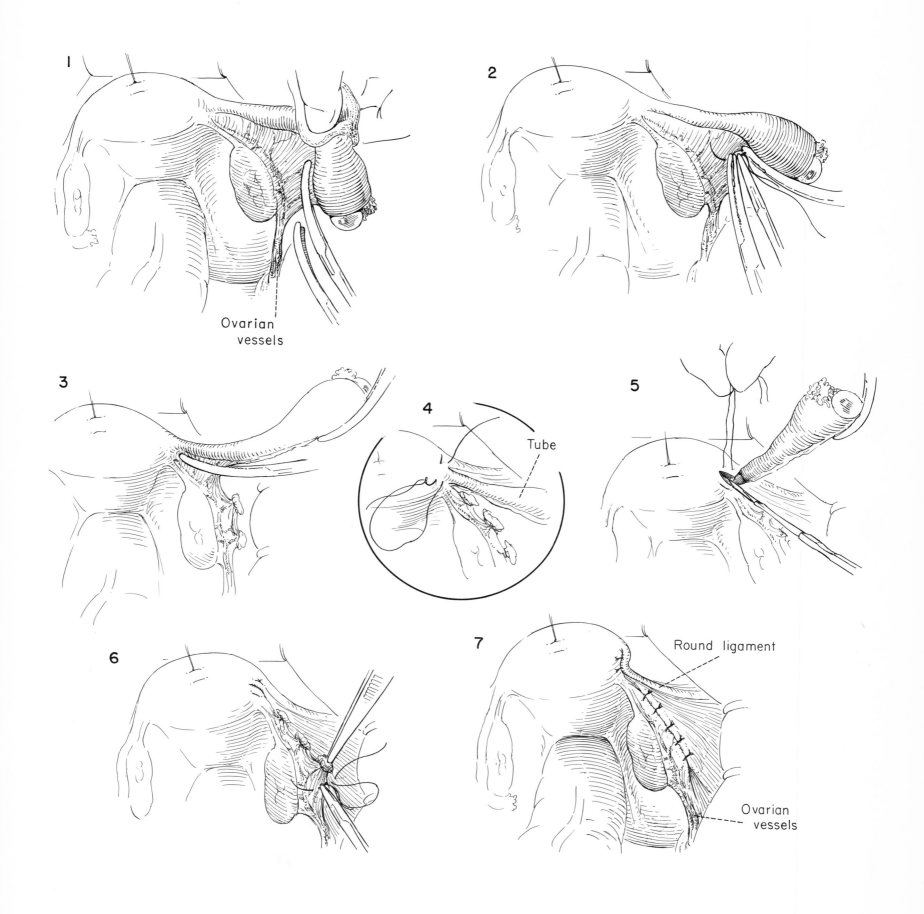

1

Ovarian
vessels

2

3

4

Tube

5

6

7

Round ligament

Ovarian
vessels

REMOVAL OF SMALL OVARIAN CYST

The ovary is a badly abused organ. Because ovarian cancer is on the increase and the majority of ovarian tumors have spread beyond the confines of the ovary when they are first seen, the surgeon tends to sacrifice the ovary too frequently on the sometimes mistaken impression that disease is present.

It is important to be on the alert for the presence of an ovarian tumor, but it is equally important to realize that the ovary is by nature a cystic organ which undergoes physiological enlargement and regression throughout the menstrual cycle. The surgeon, then, must learn to distinguish between a physiological enlargement and a neoplasm before he decides to explore the patient. If the adnexal enlargement persists through three or four menstrual cycles, the patient should be explored for the very good reason that one cannot be entirely sure what the growth is; if it does not regress, it is a space-occupying tumor which is interfering with normal ovarian function.

When the patient is explored and an ovarian cyst of physiological nature or an endometrial type cyst is encountered, the entire ovary need not be removed. These tumors can be shelled out of the ovary. Even a small amount of ovarian tissue may be sufficient to maintain normal menstruation as well as fertility.

Figure 1. The uterus is held on traction to the left while the assistant retracts the tube with Babcock forceps to provide exposure.

Figure 2. The cyst is steadied by the operator's left hand while an incision is made through the capsule close to the base of the cyst. Moist gauze beneath the fingers offers additional traction to permit ease in handling.

Figure 3. A plane of cleavage is readily established which allows the unruptured cyst to be separated from its bed in the main body of the ovary with the knife handle. The assistant applies counterpressure through the Allis forceps placed on the cut edge of the ovary while the surgeon steadies the cyst.

Figure 4. The surgeon grasps the cyst with the thumb and forefinger of the left hand and turns it upward to expose the posterior wall. He then incises the posterior capsule at the base of the cyst.

Figure 5. Continue to pull the cyst upward to expose the cleavage plane. Traction on the incised edge through the medium of a gently applied Allis forceps will help. The separation is readily made with the knife handle.

Figure 6. A Babcock clamp steadies the ovarian ligament while the defect in the ovary is closed with a running atraumatic catgut suture. The stitch passes through the cortex of the ovary to include the depths of the cavity. Exposure is improved by keeping the suture under tension and the edges retracted with Allis forceps.

Figure 7. This suture returns to the point of origin and is tied. Hemostasis is complete, and no raw edge is left uncovered.

OPERATIONS ON TUBE AND OVARY
REMOVAL OF SMALL OVARIAN CYST

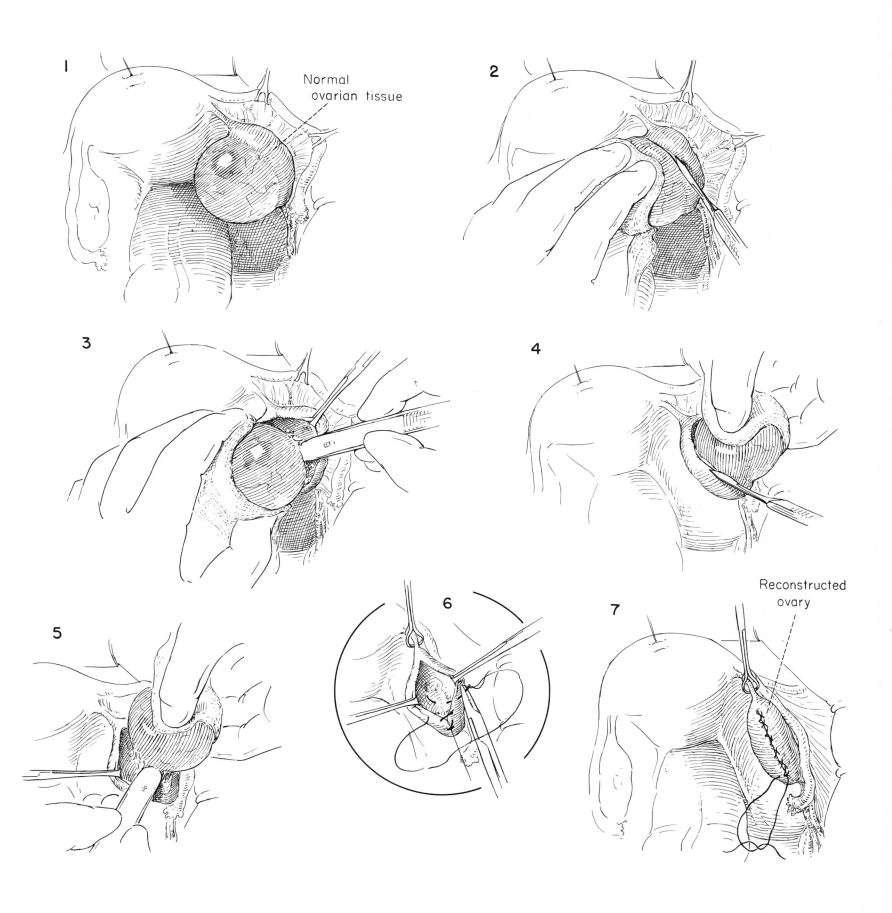

Normal ovarian tissue

1

2

3

4

5

6

7

Reconstructed ovary

INTERLIGAMENTOUS CYSTS

An ovarian cyst in its growth pattern may retain or lose its normal blood supply but continue to expand within the leaves of the broad ligament. The anatomical landmarks, therefore, are obscure because the cleavage planes are not the same as those encountered when the ovarian cyst lies free in the abdominal cavity. In addition to the problems of orientation there are technical difficulties. These focus on the position of the ureter, which frequently lies on the surface of the cyst either on the lateral side or directly beneath it. It is therefore necessary to develop a large operative field so that anatomical landmarks are clearly identifiable before any attempt is made to remove the tumor. To avoid damage to the ureter its course should be traced from the point where it crosses the common iliac artery on downward into the pelvis.

Figure 1. The uterus is placed on traction away from the side of the tumor. The ureter must then be identified and can often be seen and palpated beneath the peritoneum at the point where it crosses the common iliac artery. The peritoneum is incised lateral to the course of the ureter. The ovarian vessels are seen in close proximity to and above the ureter. The operative field must be kept dry. Care should be exercised in handling the vessels.

Figure 2. Exposure is maintained by stay sutures placed on the edges of the incised peritoneum. The ureter is separated from the ovarian vessels as they cross the iliac artery. Unless separated, the ureter may inadvertently be included in the ligation and division of the vessels. The vessels having been identified, they can easily be freed over a short distance. A clamp is placed beneath them and a strand of catgut drawn back through for the first tie.

Figure 3. This maneuver is repeated and the vessels cut and doubly ligated.

Figure 4. In the interest of securing a wider operative field the round ligament is secured with a stitch ligature at a point close to the uterus. The ends of the sutures are left long and the round ligament is divided.

Since the area below the level of the tumor is largely an empty one filled with areolar tissue it is now possible to insert a retractor and have a clear view of the important anatomical landmarks such as the iliac vessels and their branches. It also provides much more space in which to work.

The assistant applies traction to the lateral suture on the round ligament while the surgeon draws the uterus toward him. The surgeon then incises the peritoneal cover on both the anterior and posterior surfaces of the cyst, extending the incision up to the cornu of the uterus.

Figure 5. After first placing a moist gauze sponge on the tumor so that he can obtain better traction the surgeon rotates the tumor toward him and begins to separate the cyst from the overlying peritoneal sheath. Note that the assistant keeps the peritoneum on stretch by traction on the stay sutures. In this fashion the cyst is freed from its bed under direct vision.

Figure 6. A similar plane is easily established beneath the peritoneum on the medial aspect.

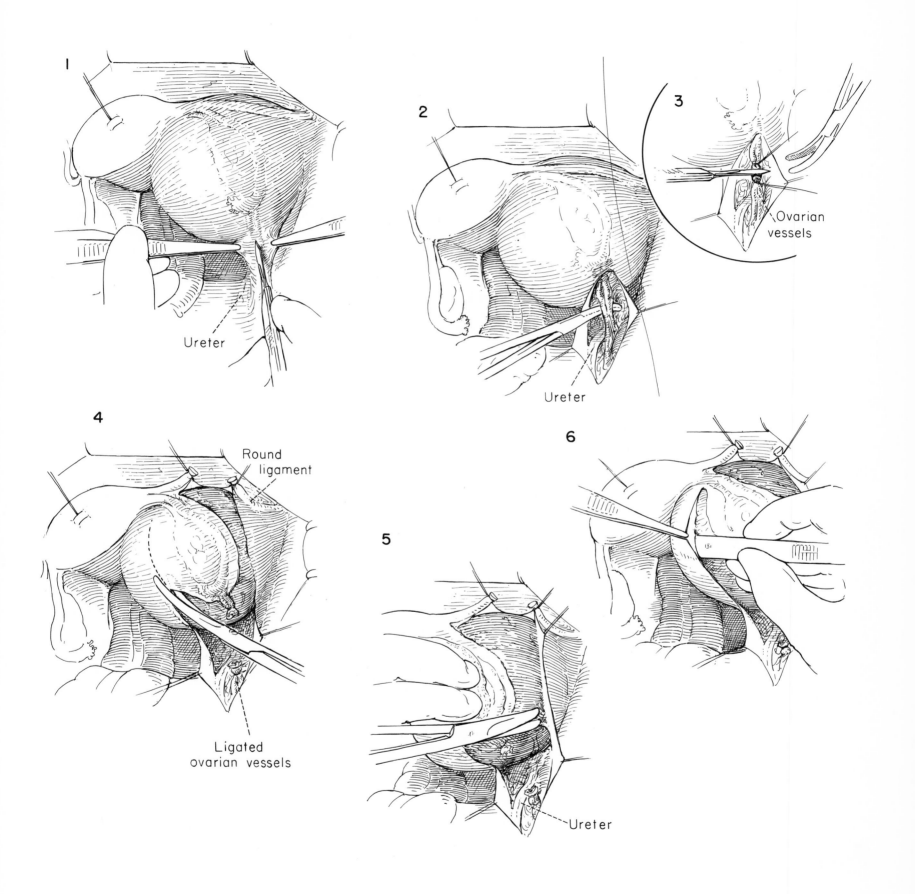

1

Ureter

2

Ureter

3

Ovarian
vessels

4

Round
ligament

Ligated
ovarian vessels

5

6

Ureter

Figure 7. The undersurface of the cyst is exposed and its areolar attachments are freed as the assistant draws the uterus to the opposite side and the surgeon rolls the cyst upward toward the symphysis. Gauze applied to the surface of the cyst permits greater ease in maintaining traction on the tumor. It is of the utmost importance that the operative field be widely exposed so that the blood vessels and the ureter can be kept under direct vision and thereby avoided. Traction on the stay sutures will greatly facilitate the maintenance of an unobstructed operative field.

Figure 8. With the cyst partially free of its bed the surgeon now turns his attention to the ovarian ligament. Within it lies the ovarian branch of the uterine artery. Since the round ligament has been divided it can readily be traced within the broad ligament as it courses along the side of the uterine fundus. A Kelly clamp is applied and the artery divided and secured with a stitch ligature.

Figure 9. A mattress suture is laid in the uterine musculature at the cornu and left untied. The tumor, ovary and tube are drawn away from the uterus, and a wedge is excised at the point of insertion of the tube. The incision is placed within the area enclosed in the mattress suture. The assistant controls the suture while the elliptical incision is carried down to the point of junction of the tube with the endometrial cavity. The suture is then tied to control bleeding from a vessel which is always present at this point.

Figure 10. There are now no major vessels connected with the tumor; it can be safely dislodged from its bed. Any areolar attachments at the base can easily be seen in the wide open field and secured with clamps if need be. The surgeon should be constantly aware of the proximity of the ureter and major vessels.

INSET A. Immediate pathologic appraisal of the removed specimen is mandatory. It must be opened and note taken of the character of the fluid and the gross appearance of the contents. Only when he is certain that no malignant disease is present can the surgeon leave the uterus and the other adnexa intact.

Figure 11. The tumor mass has now been removed in toto. The anatomy of the region is clearly seen. Although the surgeon has taken great care to avoid damaging the ureter, its course should be rechecked and the ureter inspected before the broad ligament is reperitonealized.

Figure 12. The divided ends of the round ligament are re-approximated with interrupted catgut stitch ligatures. A running catgut suture then closes the defect in the peritoneum, extending up to cover the raw area at the uterine cornu where the tube was resected.

Figure 13. If complete peritonealization is not readily accomplished at the uterine cornu the surgeon may elect to bring down the round ligament and suture it to the posterior surface of the uterus with a few interrupted sutures.

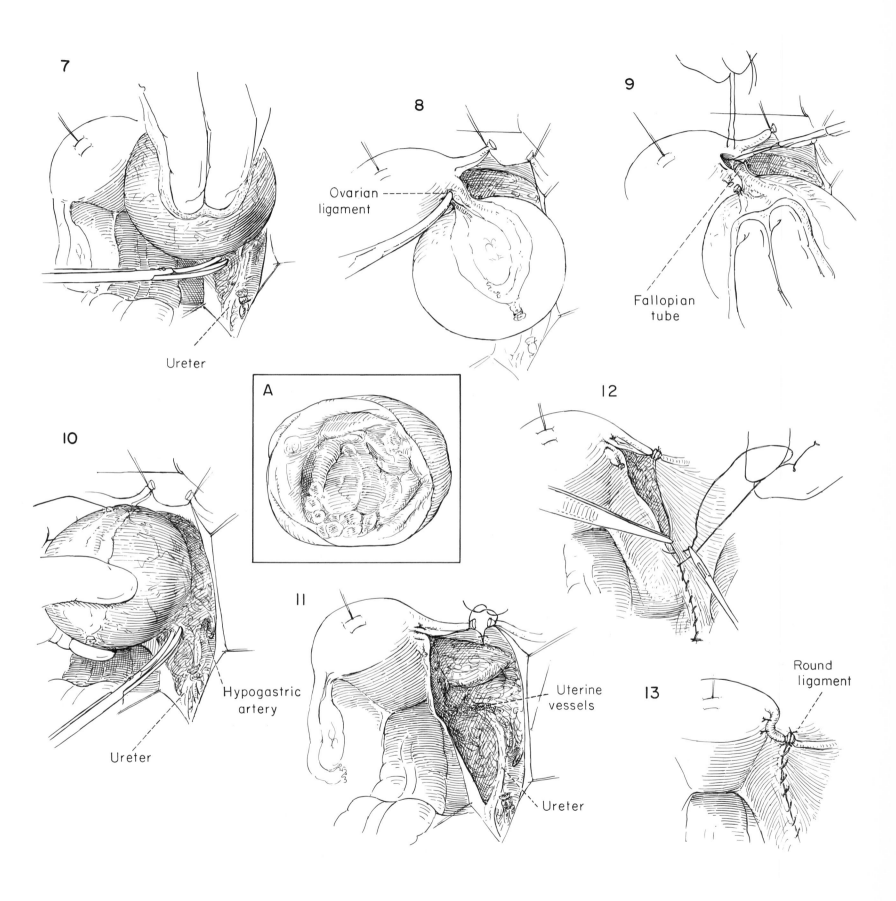

7

8

Ovarian
ligament

9

Fallopian
tube

Ureter

A

10

12

11

Hypogastric
artery

Uterine
vessels

Ureter

Round
ligament

13

Ureter

WEDGE RESECTION OF THE OVARY

In certain physiological disturbances of hormonal nature, such as the Stein-Leventhal syndrome, with prolonged amenorrhea or irregularly profuse bleeding, the ovary has the characteristic appearance of multiple small follicular cysts within its substance and a heavy thick cortical covering. There is no evidence of corpora lutea, either recent or old. Reduction of the bulk of the ovarian substance may correct this condition. This is the so-called wedge resection of the ovary.

Figure 1. The assistant steadies the uterus while the operator grasps the ovarian pedicle and ovary between the index finger and midfinger of the left hand. A generous segment of ovarian substance is outlined, and the thick, heavy fibrous tunica of the ovary is incised.

Figure 2. Allis forceps retract the cut edges, and the dissection is carried well into the substance and the wedge excised.

Figure 3. A Babcock clamp steadies the ovarian ligament medially, and the edges of the cavity are held apart with Allis forceps while the raw edges of the ovary are approximated by a suture which includes the base of the cavity.

Figure 4. The running suture in the ovary is completed by returning to its point of origin. There it is tied. Note that the bulk of the ovarian tissue has diminished.

Since the disease is always bilateral, the same procedure must be carried out on the opposite side.

EXPLORATORY INCISION OF THE OVARY

There are two good reasons for incising the capsule of the ovary and exploring its interior when one or both ovaries are to be left in place, regardless of whether the uterus is removed.

So much of the disease one finds in the ovary tends to occur bilaterally that the surgeon should know what the interior of the ovary looks like when he is removing one adnexa and leaving the other. It is amazing how often disease can be found in the interior of an ovary that appears, on gross examination of the exterior, to be normal.

The second reason concerns itself with ovaries that are to be left in situ following the removal of the uterus for benign disease. There is a tendency to remove both ovaries at the time of hysterectomy regardless of the age of the patient because of the possibility that benign or malignant tumors may later develop in them. The authors are not in sympathy with this point of view. We are in favor of preserving ovarian function unless there is a valid reason for removing both ovaries. If the retained ovaries are sectioned and no gross lesion seen, they are unlikely to develop disease within them at a later date.

Figure 5. The ovary is steadied between the index and middle fingers of the operator's left hand, and a linear incision is made in the long axis and carried directly into the substance of the ovary almost to the hilum.

Figure 6. The two cross sections are thus exposed. The interior of the ovary is inspected, and any suspicious area or cyst is excised for pathological examination.

Figure 7. The ovary is reconstructed with a running atraumatic suture up and back.

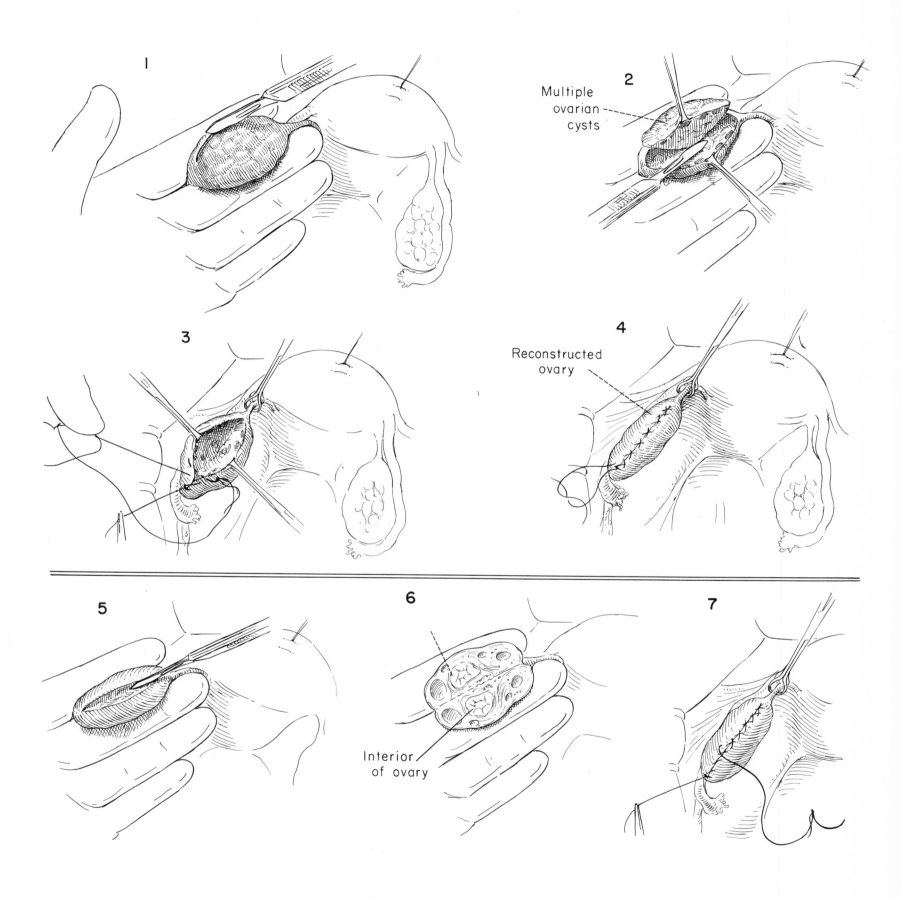

1

2

Multiple
ovarian
cysts

3

4

Reconstructed
ovary

5

6

Interior
of ovary

7

STERILIZATION

For adequate medical reason in the interest of the mother's health, the surgeon may elect to perform a sterilization procedure either at the time of cesarian section or during the postpartum convalescence.

Simple interruption of tubal continuity has not been completely successful as a means of permanent sterilization.

Two methods are in general use: (1) The Irving method avoids any possibility of re-establishment of the continuity of the tubal lumen because the tubes are sectioned and the severed ends are separated. The proximal end is buried in the uterine musculature and the lateral segment in the leaves of the broad ligament. (2) The Pomeroy method is accomplished rapidly with minimal trauma because the tubes are simply tied. The procedure does carry with it the risk of recanalization.

Irving Procedure

Figure 1. The uterus is drawn to the left by a stay suture in the fundus. The surgeon places a stitch ligature around the tube 1 inch from the insertion in the uterus. This suture is held on traction as a similar stitch is passed around the tube ½ inch lateral to it. The tube is divided between ligatures.

Figure 2. The medial segment of the tube is freed from its mesentery and bleeding points are ligated. The posterior uterine wall is incised about ¾ inch from insertion of the tube.

Figure 3. The incision is enlarged by inserting and spreading the jaws of a small straight hemostat.

Figure 4. A needle is threaded on each end of the long suture left on the medial end of the divided tube, carried into the incision and brought out through the peritoneum. Tying draws the cut end below the peritoneal surface.

Figure 5. The lateral end of the tube is depressed beneath the peritoneum of the broad ligament and the peritoneal rent closed.

Figure 6. The procedure is repeated on the opposite side.

Pomeroy Procedure

If the surgeon elects to operate a few days after delivery and before involution of the uterus, Pomeroy sterilization is both simple and effective.

Figure 7. The abdomen is opened through a small midline incision about 2 inches below the umbilicus, exposing the fundus of the enlarged uterus. The edges of the wound are retracted to gain exposure. The surgeon grasps the tube at its midportion and delivers it into the incision with an Allis forceps.

Figure 8. A loop is made in the tube by approximating the distal and proximal arms together. The surgeon holds them together while the assistant applies an Allis clamp to the apex of the loop. The surgeon then ligates a knuckle of tube.

In the past it was customary to apply a crushing clamp to the two limbs before applying the suture. This step has been abandoned because recanalization seemingly occurred with greater frequency when this was done.

Figure 9. The tube is then excised just beyond the ligature.

Figure 10. The long ends of the ligature are cut and the tube replaced in the abdomen.

A similar procedure is carried out on the opposite side.

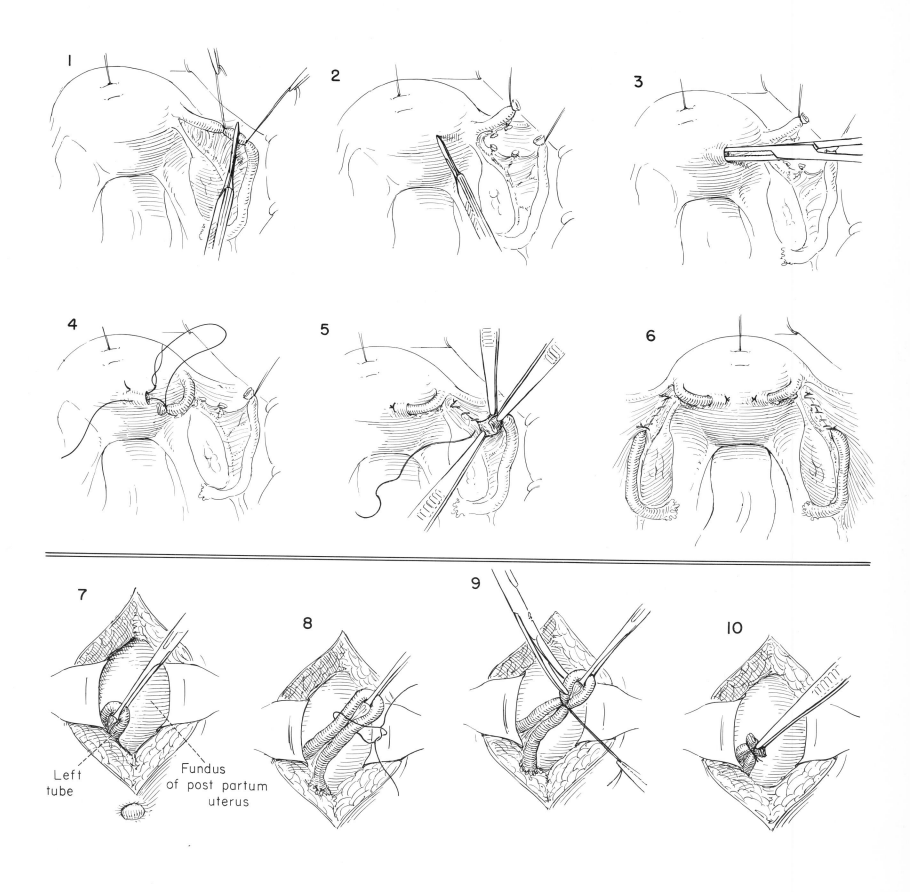

Left tube

Fundus of post partum uterus

Operations to Restore Tubal Patency

There are a variety of pathological entities which affect the tube and influence fertility. Some of them lend themselves to surgical correction. The chances are better when the primary infection has been caused by streptococci rather than by gonococci or the tubercle bacillus. The latter tend to damage the epithelial lining of the tube; streptococci create a perisalpingitis and adhesions which interfere with the motility of the tube, which is essential to physiological transport of the ova into the uterine cavity. Other intra-abdominal infections resulting in pelvic peritonitis would create similar problems. Perisalpingitis is quite common following acute appendicitis or an appendiceal abscess.

When the hysterosalpingogram indicates that there is normal patency of the tubes and lesions are seen on culdoscopy, it is reasonable to assume that they are interfering with tubal motility. It is possible to correct this condition by freeing the adhesions.

THE DISSECTION PLASTIC

Figure 1. A traction suture is placed in the fundus of the uterus, which is held on tension and drawn toward the operator's side of the table. The open fimbriated ends of the tube lie on the surface of the ovary, but it is apparent that the mesosalpinx is foreshortened because of adhesions binding the tube to the surface of the ovary.

Figure 2. Continuing the traction on the uterus the surgeon and assistant gently hold the tube on tension with blunt-end, smooth forceps as the surgeon gently divides the adhesions with fine dissecting scissors of the Metzenbaum type.

Figure 3. After the adhesions have been separated the mesosalpinx comes into view and the open end of the tube lies free. The motility of the tube is restored.

DISSECTION OF THE CLOSED TUBAL FIMBRIA

When preliminary investigative studies of the tube with gas insufflation indicate a block somewhere in its course, the hysterosalpingogram will demonstrate the area of obstruction. In this instance the point of obstruction is obvious and occurs at the fimbriated end of the tube, with patency up to this point. The chances of future pregnancy will improve materially if a simple plastic procedure is done on the closed ends.

Figure 4. Again a stay suture of the figure-of-eight type is placed in the fundus of the uterus and held on traction. The assistant draws the uterus toward the surgeon while the latter incises any peritubal adhesions and demonstrates the closure of the fimbriated ends of the tube.

Figure 5. With the uterus still held on traction the surgeon picks up the tube between thumb and forefinger to steady it as he incises the peritoneum and the adhesions covering the fimbriated end.

Figure 6. With the tube still held firmly in the fingers of the surgeon and the incision made, the undamaged tubal epithelium comes into view. The surgeon then gently inserts the blunt ends of a Kelly clamp into the lumen and exerts gentle lateral pressure by opening the blades of the clamp, thereby enlarging the ostia. A minor degree of trimming recreates the fimbria.

Figure 7. The operation is now complete. The tube is free of any peritubal adhesions which might interfere with its motility and the patency of the tube is restored by the plastic operation which opened the fimbriated end.

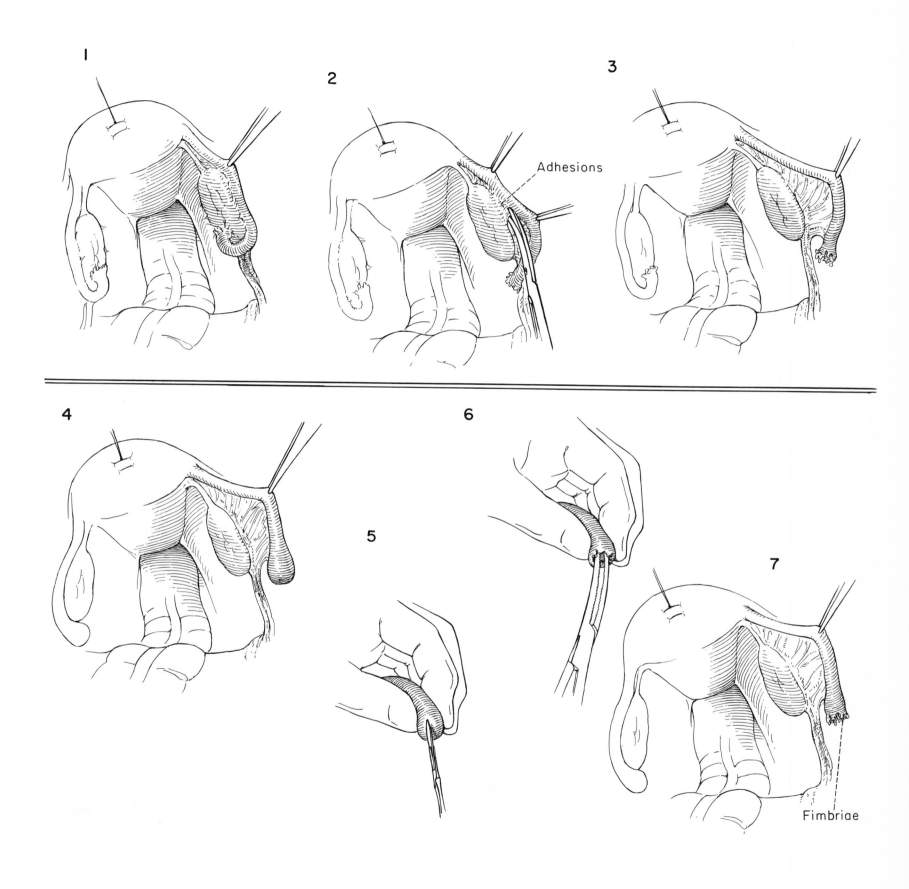

1

2

Adhesions

3

4

6

5

7

Fimbriae

FIMBRIAL RECONSTRUCTION

Although the hysterosalpingogram may indicate that the block in the tubal lumen takes place at the fimbriated end, it is still difficult with the tube in hand to evaluate the extent of the normal tube. It is important to know this before any attempt is made to perform a plastic operation. The necessary knowledge can be obtained by employing an insufflation apparatus fixed in place and controlled from outside the operative field. This maneuver, however, is cumbersome. It is possible to get the same information, rather simply, by closing the cervix with a large clamp and injecting air or fluid into the endometrial cavity.

Figure 1. The assistant holds the uterus on tension as the surgeon evaluates the extent of the disease. While the mesosalpinx is free the fimbriated ends of the tube are closed.

Figure 2. A large clamp with a broad right-angle base encompasses the entire uterus. When the clamp is closed it will seal off the lower end of the endometrial cavity. The surgeon then injects a solution of indigo carmine or methylene blue into the endometrial cavity. Direct inspection of the tube indicates the point of obstruction.

Figure 3. The surgeon grasps the fimbriated end of the tube, steadying it by the index finger and thumb as he incises the adhesions over the closed ends.

Figure 4. Still steadying the tube with thumb and forefinger the surgeon identifies the lumen. He then introduces the blades of the Kelly clamp into the open end.

Figure 5. If the damage is so extensive that simple opening of the tube will be insufficient to keep the ostia open permanently, it is necessary to perform a plastic operation on the fimbria. The assistant holds the tube on tension with a noncrushing clamp. The surgeon steadies the open end while he introduces a nerve hook into the lumen to grasp the interior wall of the tube.

Figure 6. As the hook is withdrawn it is turned to allow firm traction on the endosalpinx.

Figure 7. Continued traction will now cuff back the fibrous end of the fallopian tube.

Figure 8. To facilitate the placing of fine interrupted sutures on the everted tubal cuff it is essential to keep all structures on tension. The operating nurse holds the uterus on tension while the assistant grasps the tube with forceps and applies traction. The surgeon then places the first of the fine interrupted sutures in the leading edge of the everted tubal epithelium and sutures it to the anterior peritoneal surface of the tube at the lateral angle.

Figure 9. A similar suture is placed on the medial angle.

Figure 10. This figure shows the completed operation with the tubal cuff everted and the sutures placed circumferentially.

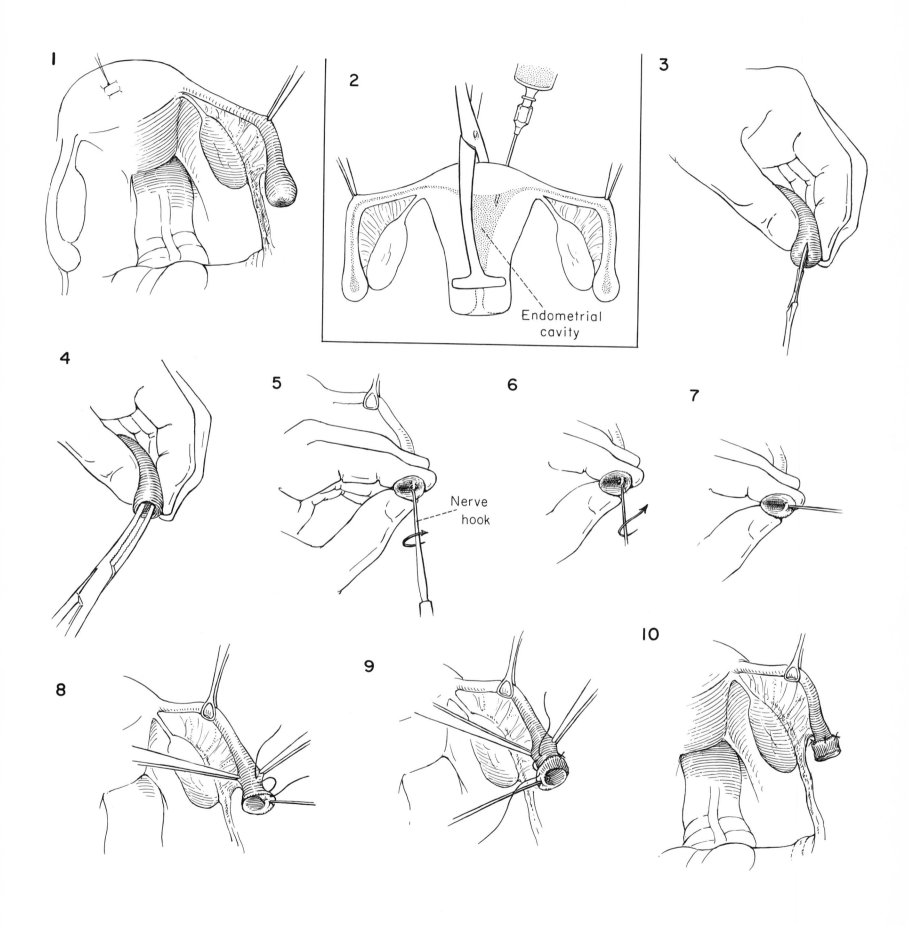

FIMBRIAL PLASTIC WITH HOOD

INSET A. Although a plastic reconstruction has been performed on the open end of the tube the surgeon may wish to ensure patency of the tube during the reparative phase by preventing adhesions from forming around the newly fashioned ostium. This can be accomplished by inserting a long polyethylene tube through the tubal lumen into the canal. Attached to the tubing is a plastic hood which will fit over the reconstructed fimbriated end of the tube. When sutured into position it will serve as a protective barrier to prevent adhesions from the operative area until it has time to heal. The silastic material is prone to pick up lint; the hood should be kept in its container until it is used.

Figure 1. The nurse applies traction on the stay suture on the uterine fundus while the assistant stretches out the tube by holding it with smooth forceps. The surgeon then inserts the polyethylene tubing into the tubal lumen and advances it with a smooth forceps. It need be only long enough to lie comfortably in the distal half of the tube.

Figure 2. The nurse steadies the uterus and the assistant the tube. The surgeon holds the flanged plastic hood between his fingers as he places the first of the sutures which will hold it in place. The suture passes through the outer end of the hood from without inward. It is then led through the interior of the hood and in turn sutured to the cuplike end of the tube. It returns through the hood at a point very close to its site of entry.

Figure 3. After placing three sutures in similar fashion the surgeon prepares to advance the hood into its final position. The nurse steadies the uterus with traction on the stay suture. The assistant grasps the tube near the cornual end with forceps while he steadies the outer portion of the tube between thumb and finger just below the newly constructed ostium. The surgeon applies traction to the sutures he has just applied and gently advances the plastic hood in the direction of the tubal opening. When this is impossible, a wire frame that will stretch the bell of the hood can be used.

Figure 4. With the hood in position all the sutures are tied.

Removal of the Hood

When the surgeon feels that complete healing has taken place and that the danger of adhesions forming around the ostium is over, the plastic hood and polyethylene tubing must be removed. In most instances two or three months are allowed to elapse before the second operation is done.

Figure 5. A stay suture is again placed in the fundus and held on traction to steady it. The assistant holds the tube on tension with a Babcock clamp and thumb forceps while the surgeon gently separates, with fine scissors, any filmy attachments the surface end of the hood may have acquired from the adjacent peritoneum.

Figure 6. The sutures which originally held the hood in position are divided.

Figure 7. The plastic hood and the polyethylene tubing are then gently removed. The tubal ostium is now patent and lies free without adhesions or attachments to other structures.

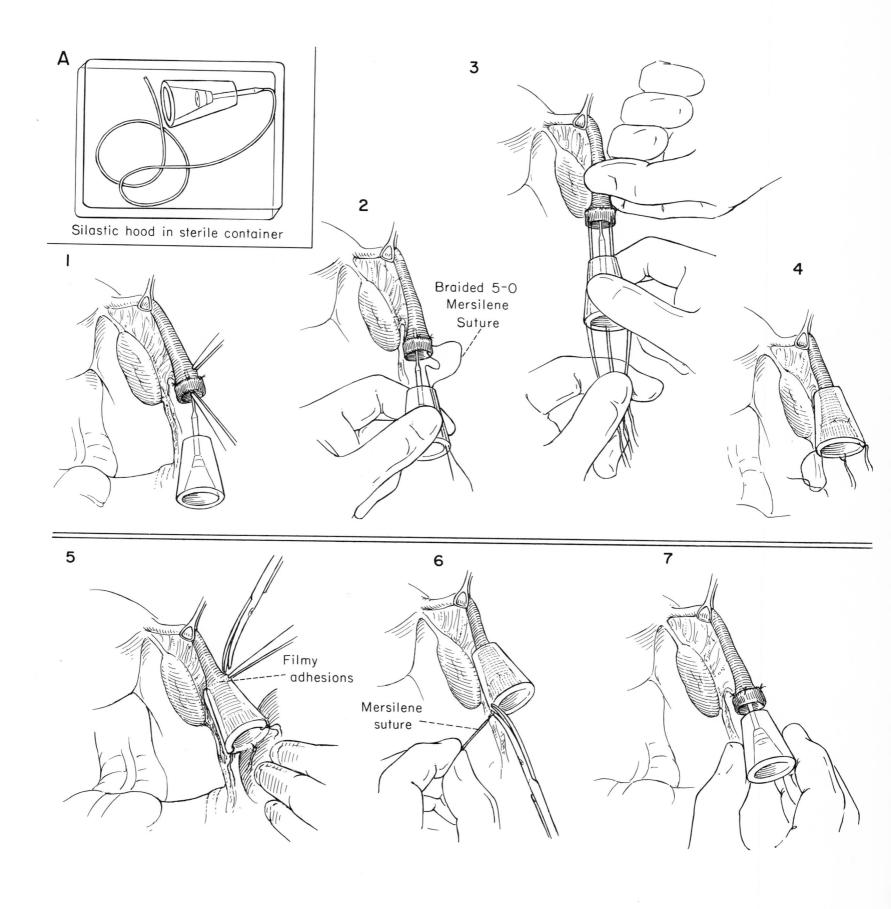

A

Silastic hood in sterile container

1

2

Braided 5-0 Mersilene Suture

3

4

5

Filmy adhesions

6

Mersilene suture

7

CORNUAL RESECTION

The preoperative investigations may indicate that block is present at the cornual end of the tube. Although there is no way of knowing it prior to operation, the remaining portion of the tubes may be normal. Resection of the cornual end of the tube with establishment of a new lumen into the endometrial cavity is a reasonable method of reconstituting tubal patency.

Figure 1. Although the surgeon observed that gas did not seem to pass through the tube at the time of insufflation or the hysterosalpingogram failed to show any dye in the tubal lumen, the surgeon will be well advised to test the patency of the tube at the time of operation. The block could have been due to spasm of the tube at the isthmial portion where it goes into the endometrial cavity.

The clamp is applied to the cervix, closing off the endocervical canal. The surgeon then injects into the endometrial cavity under pressure. The assistant holds the tube and inspects the fimbriated end to see whether any dye comes through.

Figure 2. The tube is then divided at a point lateral to the obvious areas of obstruction. Two stay sutures are placed on the proximal end of the tube. They are clamped and left long. The suture on the distal end of the tube is left long and is held on tension as the surgeon applies a clamp on the mesentery below the tube and close to the uterus. The tissues included in it are divided and secured with a stitch ligature.

Figure 3. The uterus and distal end of the divided end of the tube are held on tension as the surgeon dissects the cornual portion of the tube out of the uterine muscle. This is literally coned out.

Figure 4. The nurse holds the uterus on traction while the assistant applies tension on the stay sutures left long on the divided end of the tube. The surgeon then introduces a small metal probe into the tubal opening, advancing it in the direction of the uterus. A segment of fine tubing is then pushed firmly over the tip of the probe and drawn back through the tube. This is generally easier and less damaging than trying to thread tubing proximally.

Figure 5. Allis clamps are applied on the divided muscle edges of the opening into the uterine cavity. The polyethylene tubing is inserted after preparing a loop at the end and firmly tying it.

Figure 6. An end-to-end anastomosis between the cut end of the tube and the endometrial opening is performed with fine, interrupted, atraumatic, chromic catgut sutures.

Figure 7. The muscle is gently closed on either side of the tube and the peritoneum reconstructed.

Figure 8. This reperitonealization includes any defect left in the broad ligament.

Figure 9. Subsequent removal of the plastic tubing is easily done in the office with a crochet hook inserted through the cervix. In bilateral reconstruction one segment of tubing with the loop in the center will do the job.

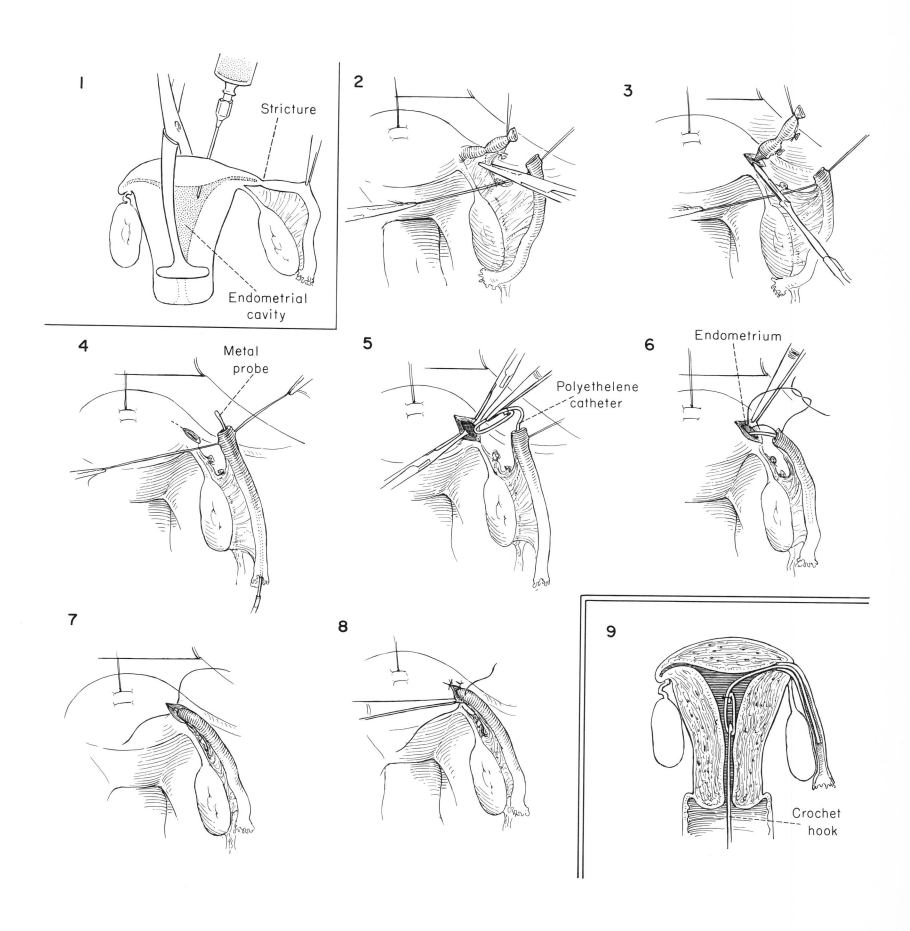

Operations Involving the Intestine

Pathological processes primary in the uterus or adnexa may involve the small intestine either by direct extension of the disease or as a result of inflammation which causes the intestine to become adherent to the other abdominal organs. If the disease is of invasive nature the surgeon may elect to resect the intestine. When the intestine is simply adherent he may choose to separate one from the other. In such instances there is very real danger that the bowel wall may be damaged and will require immediate repair.

REPAIR OF INJURED SMALL INTESTINE

It is always wise to repair the damage to the bowel wall as soon as the surgeon recognizes that it has occurred. As a general rule, the bowel heals readily. Serosal agglutination occurs in a few hours. Shallow breaks in the serosa are usually harmless, but when doubt exists it is always best to close the defect.

When the tear or perforation is small it can be closed successfully with a simple purse-string suture without narrowing the intestinal lumen. If such a closure produces obvious restriction of the caliber of the bowel cavity, it should be abandoned and the technique for repair of the larger vent employed.

Figure 1. The purse-string type of suture closure is made with fine silk or atraumatic catgut. The surgeon picks up the serosa and the muscle wall of the bowel in a series of bites surrounding the defect, taking care not to enter the bowel cavity.

Figure 2. The suture is then drawn tight and tied. A second stitch encircling the first is laid in place and when tied can be depended upon to keep the closure intact until the bowel wall heals.

REPAIR OF A LARGER RENT

Figure 3. To avoid narrowing of the lumen in closing a larger tear, the suture line should cross the bowel at right angles to the long axis. A longitudinal laceration is converted into a transverse one by traction on Allis clamps placed on the edges of the opening.

Figure 4. An atraumatic, fine, chromic catgut suture is started at one end, includes all layers, and is placed and tied just beyond the opening to be closed.

Figure 5. A straight snap grasps the short end of the stitch.

Figure 6. The suture is continued in simple over-and-over fashion.

Figure 7. At the lower end, one final stitch is placed to lie entirely on one side of the rent and just beyond the opening.

Figure 8. The loop and free end of the suture are tied together and the Allis clamp removed as this is done.

Figure 9. A straight snap on one end of this suture is kept on tension to steady the bowel, and a series of vertical silk or cotton mattress stitches is started. The first is carefully placed to lie just beyond the end of the inner suture line.

Figure 10. The first silk tie is kept long and the end of catgut cut off at the knot. Each subsequent mattress stitch is carefully placed and tied to approximate two narrow serosal surfaces without cutting through.

Figure 11. This shows the completed closure.

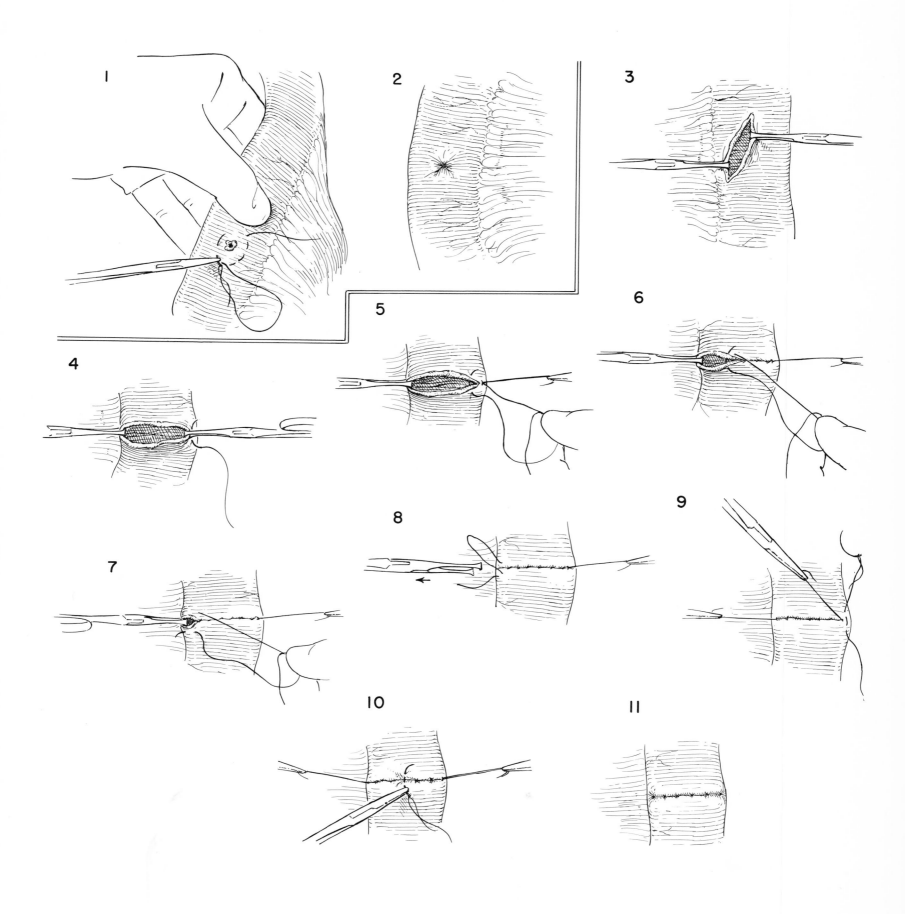

EXCISION OF A MECKEL'S DIVERTICULUM

Excision of an asymptomatic diverticulum, discovered as an incidental finding at the time a laparotomy is being performed for other disease, comes very close to being meddlesome surgery.

At times, however, it may justly be considered as a possible source of the pelvic symptoms or give indication that it may create trouble in the future. When either of these two conditions exists, excision is warranted.

The surgeon should remember that occasionally these pouches are lined with gastric epithelium. It is possible then for perforation to occur as the acid secretions irritate and ulcerate the adjacent epithelium of the bowel. The basic problem is to be sure that the excision is extensive enough to include all the mucosa and that the closure does not produce any constriction of the bowel lumen.

Figure 1. The diverticulum arises in the ileum within 2 feet of the ileocecal valve on the side directly opposite the mesenteric attachment. Vessels in the mesentery of the diverticulum should be freed from the bowel near the base by blunt dissection with the tip of a hemostat and doubly clamped.

Figure 2. The vessels are cut and secured with fine ties.

Figure 3. The diverticulum is held on tension by traction on an Allis clamp applied to the blind end and two light Kocher clamps are placed across the base, with care that the lower one is flush with the bowel.

Figure 4. Moist gauze is laid across the field beneath the clamps, and the bowel is cut across with the cautery.

Figure 5. The Kocher clamp is removed, and Allis clamps are applied to the full thickness of the cut edge of bowel on either side.

Figure 6. By traction, this longitudinal opening is converted into a transverse one, and closure is effected by the method illustrated in detail on page 101.

Figure 7. An inner row of running catgut is secured at one end and carried to the other, completely closing the opening in the gut.

Figure 8. The snap on the end of this suture is held toward himself by the surgeon, and the first mattress stitch of silk is carefully placed a little beyond it. The catgut is cut and a snap placed on the ends of the silk tie to maintain traction.

Figure 9. The outer row of interrupted fine silk stitches is continued to ensure approximation of an adequate serosal surface and to bury the first suture line.

Figure 10. This shows the completed closure, watertight and with no tendency to narrow the bowel.

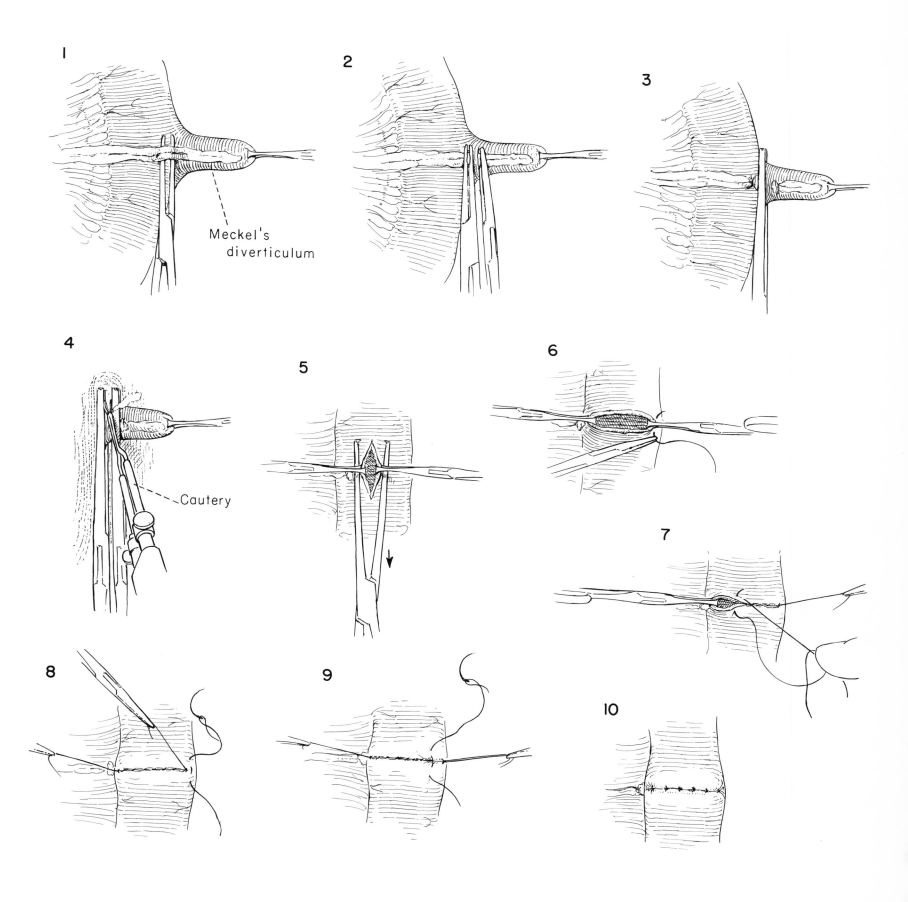

ENTEROENTEROSTOMY (Side-to-side Anastomosis)

When the patient presents evidence of obstruction to the flow of intestinal contents within the small bowel it is usually wise to resect the bowel and restore continuity with an end-to-end closure.

On occasion, however, the surgeon may elect to short-circuit the intestinal flow. The simplest way to accomplish this is to perform a side-to-side anastomosis. It is a particularly useful procedure when the disease is such that resection will not contribute to cure and only palliation is indicated.

As in all bowel surgery the surgeon must adhere to the basic principles: (1) that the blood supply to the healing area is not compromised, (2) that the serosal surfaces are apposed without tension, and (3) that the integrity of the bowel lumen is maintained and the free passage of intestinal content is assured.

In this operation the two-layer type of closure, employing an inner row of chromic catgut and an outer layer of interrupted silk, is illustrated.

Figure 1. The loops selected for anastomosis are brought out of the incision. A rubber-shod clamp is applied, the gas and liquid contents are expressed from the segment selected for operation, and the clamp is closed just tightly enough to prevent reflux.

Figure 2. The two selected loops are brought to lie comfortably side by side and the entire field is protected with moist gauze, including a strip beneath the loops of bowel.

Figure 3. The rubber-covered clamps afford an easy means of holding the bowel in any position desired. Here the first assistant approximates them carefully as the surgeon prepares to join them with the first posterior row of sutures.

Figure 4. This is composed of a series of interrupted mattress stitches of fine silk or cotton. Each is tied and cut at once except for the first, which is held long in a hemostat. This suture line is to lie parallel to the long axis of the bowel, but with a calculated drift at either end which will result in a long ellipse, with the stoma in the center of it and just opposite the point of mesenteric attachment. The last stitch is tied and left long like the first.

Figure 5. The bowel is opened in two steps: first, an incision is made with the scalpel parallel to the suture line and about 1 cm. from it. The serosa and muscularis cut easily and retract, allowing the mucosa to bulge slightly.

Figure 6. As soon as the mucosa is opened, it collapses, and further incision is best made with scissors. An opening 2 inches or more in length is made in each loop.

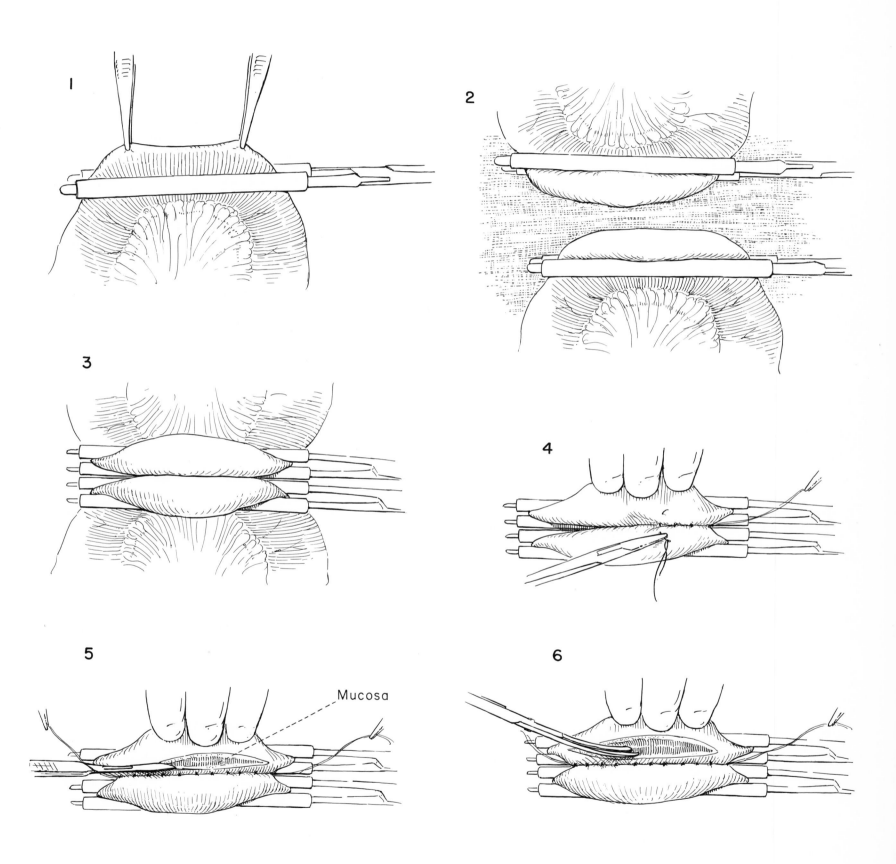

1

2

3

4

5

Mucosa

6

Figure 7. The full thickness of bowel wall around these openings is now approximated with a running suture of fine catgut on an atraumatic needle. Turning the corners presents the only technical problem; therefore, the suture is started at the center point posteriorly.

Figure 8. As the corner is reached, the stitch is carried out on the serosal surface at a point just beyond the angle and definitely on the anterior surface.

Figure 9. The Connell method is used to continue closure along the anterior aspect of the stoma. Each bite of the stitch is taken from the serosal side and includes the full thickness of bowel close to the edge of the opening.

Figure 10. By moving alternately from one side to the other, one brings the serosal surfaces of bowel neatly together.

Figure 11. This suture is discontinued as the center point is reached and held on tension to maintain approximation of the bowel. A second stitch is begun at the posterior midline and carried around the opposite corner and back along the anterior edge of the stoma exactly as was its predecessor.

Figure 12. This row is calculated to end just opposite the other. The two free ends are tied, completing the inside suture.

Figure 13. The rubber-shod clamps can be released now without fear of spillage. Since they inevitably interfere with the circulation, they should be loosened and removed at the earliest possible moment.

The outside row of interrupted silk sutures is completed with fine mattress stitches approximately 0.5 cm. apart. The bowel is easily held steady by the assistant if he makes traction on the two end silks which were left long from the first posterior row.

Figure 14. This shows the completed anastomosis just before the corner stitches are cut.

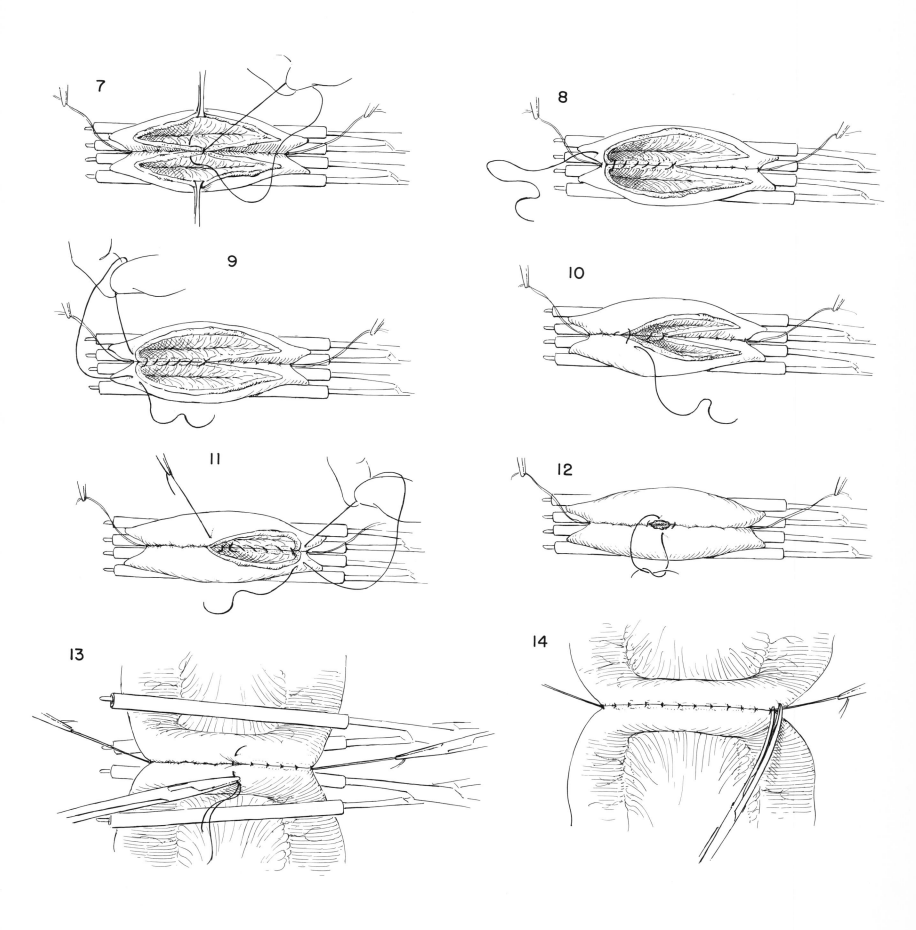

RESECTION OF SMALL INTESTINE AND SIDE-TO-SIDE ANASTOMOSIS

The surgeon operating in the pelvis for disease in the uterus, tube or ovary may be confronted with the necessity of removing a section of small intestine. The situation may arise for a variety of reasons; the most common cause is extensive damage to or devascularization of the bowel occurring in the course of an operation performed on the uterus or adnexa. At times small intestine is found adherent to a previous operative site or secondary to a pre-existing pelvic inflammatory process. If an element of strangulation is present or seems probable in the future it may be prudent or essential that the bowel be resected. Finally, the surgeon may discover a benign tumor within the small intestine or a malignant process in the uterus or adnexa that has invaded the small intestine. Resection is then mandatory.

The illustrations on this page show in detail the technique of isolating and resecting a loop of bowel. It is first delivered into the wound. All other structures are isolated and protected with gauze. The segment of bowel to be removed is then outlined.

Figure 1. The surgeon supports bowel and mesentery with the fingers of the left hand and opens the peritoneum with scissors close to the bowel and at a point where no vessels can be seen.

Figure 2. This opening is carried to the bowel wall, and mesenteric vessels are clamped and cut as they are encountered.

Figure 3. These bites are secured with stitch ligatures.

Figure 4. The wedge of mesentery to be removed is completely freed between clamps, which are replaced by ligatures before the next maneuver is begun.

Figure 5. Kocher clamps are now applied to the bowel in pairs, exactly at the sites where the mesentery has been opened. An effort should be made to distribute bowel evenly across the jaw of the clamp with the teeth at the end well beyond the intestinal wall and exactly in line with the plane of the mesentery.

Figure 6. The normal bowel is carefully covered with moist gauze and a cautery is used to transect the intestine flush with the edge of the clamp. A similar procedure at the other site completes the removal of the segment of bowel.

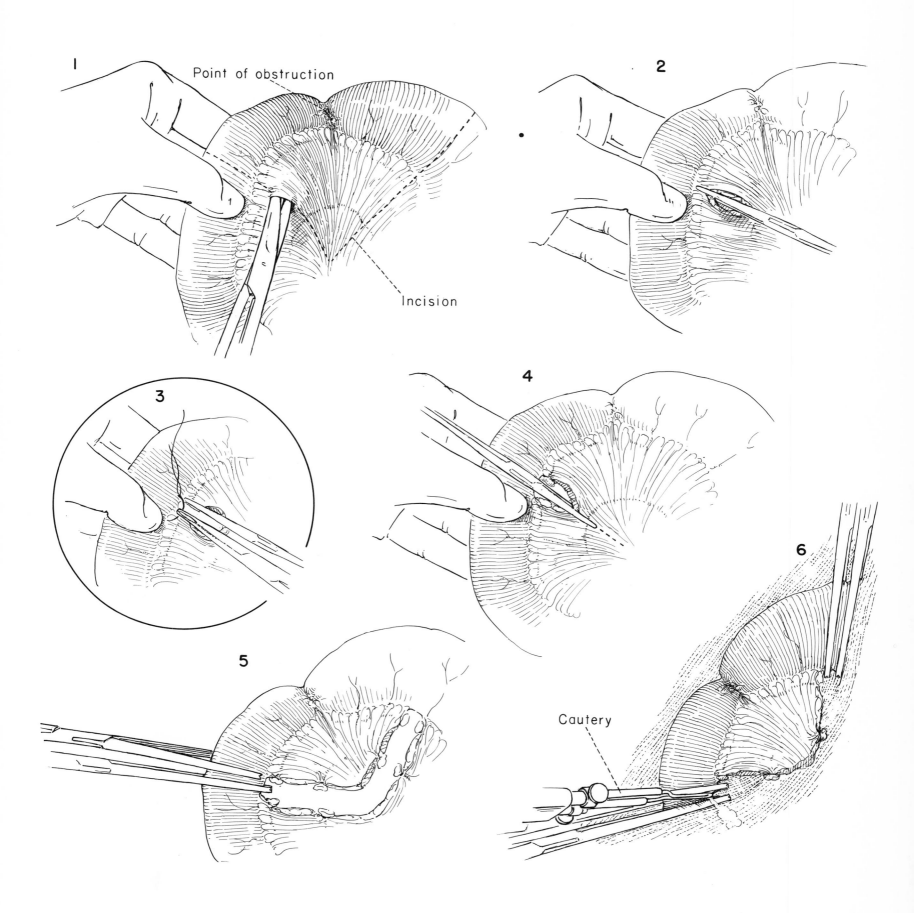

1

Point of obstruction

Incision

2

3

4

5

6

Cautery

If there is much distention or disproportion in size between the two resected loops of small intestine the surgeon will be well advised to close the ends of the two sections of bowel and perform an enteroenterostomy. The resulting stoma is large and there is much less risk of having it constrict and create a potential point for subsequent obstruction. The actual opening in the two loops of bowel should be made proximal to the closed ends to avoid leaving a blind pocket.

Although resection takes longer to perform because of the added number of suture lines it is probably the safest method of reconstructing the intestinal canal after removal of a full segment of bowel. It is the first choice when there is a doubt about the success of an end-to-end suture.

Figure 7. Before the anastomosis is begun, the two ends of the bowel are closed. A running catgut suture on an atraumatic needle starts at one end, and bites are placed alternately in the bowel wall on either side of the Kocher clamp.

Figure 8. When this row is complete, a gentle pull is applied to the two ends in the same axis as the clamp, and the clamp is opened and withdrawn. The tension on the suture should bring the opposing bowel serosal surfaces together.

Figure 9. The stitch is carried back as a second running row just outside the first and tied to the free end when it reaches it.

Figure 10. An outside row of interrupted silk or cotton mattress sutures is used to reinforce the closure. Both limbs of intestine are handled in identical fashion.

Figure 11. The side-to-side anastomosis proceeds as shown on pages 105 and 107. Rubber-covered clamps prevent spillage of intestinal content while the bowel is open. The stoma is carefully placed close to the turned-in ends of bowel to leave no blind pouches. The two loops are brought together in such fashion that the closed ends are not adjacent and the cut edges of mesentery overlap slightly.

Figure 12. The first posterior row of interrupted silk mattress stitches has been completed, and the bowel is being opened.

Figure 13. An inner layer of closure is accomplished with a running over-and-over suture which starts at the posterior midpoint, turns the corner, and continues along the anterior edge of the stoma as a Connell stitch.

Figure 14. A similar stitch closes the right half. The rubber-shod clamps are loosened and the final anterior row completed with interrupted silk. The assistant holds the bowel steady by supporting the end sutures.

Figure 15. Additional silk sutures approximate the leaves of the mesentery and close the hiatus where the bowel lies against bowel.

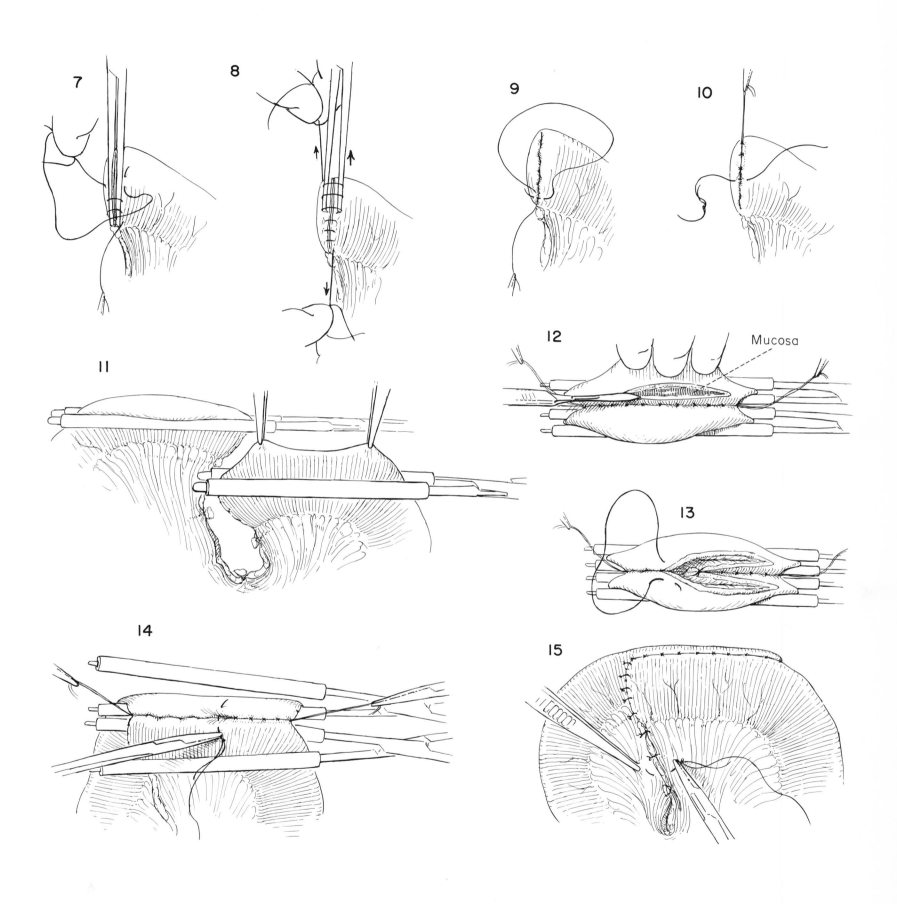

RESECTION OF SMALL INTESTINE AND
END-TO-END ANASTOMOSIS

In the absence of any disproportion in size between two involved loops of bowel, resection followed by end-to-end suture is the procedure of choice. It carries less danger in the convalescent period since only one suture line is needed. When properly done it restores the normal architecture so successfully that it may be impossible in later years to determine the actual site of the anastomosis.

The secret of successful closure depends on the amount of attention paid to the basic principles of any intestinal anastomosis: (1) the blood supply to the cut ends of the bowel must be adequate; (2) the two ends of the bowel must approximate without tension; and (3) there must be no diminution in the size of the bowel lumen.

On completion of the anastomosis the size and patency of the stoma should be checked before the intestine is replaced within the abdomen.

The technical steps involved in the resection of the intestine are performed in the identical manner described in the plates concerned with resection and side-to-side anastomosis. As illustrated here the individual steps appear in condensed fashion.

Figure 1. The bowel is delivered into the wound and steadied with the left hand, and an avascular spot in the mesentery is selected to begin the dissection.

Figure 2. With the mesentery completely freed and the vessels ligated, Kocher clamps are placed on the bowel.

Figure 3. All normal tissues are protected by wet gauze and the bowel transected with the cautery.

Figure 4. The two segments to be joined are held in close approximation by the assistant. The clamps are rotated slightly to expose the posterior bowel wall.

Figure 5. The first posterior row of sutures is in progress. The stitches should be placed as close to the clamp as possible and still permit their being tied without cutting through. Silk or cotton is usually used, and the first and last stitches are tied but not cut.

Figure 6. The bowel is steadied by holding up on these two sutures, and the Kocher clamps are removed. Usually the crushing has been forceful enough to glue the two sides together, and it will be necessary, as in the illustration, to establish the lumen by applying and pulling on an Allis clamp.

INSET A. If there is dilatation of the intestine with danger of spill when the end is opened, it is advisable to exclude the area temporarily by means of rubber-covered clamps placed lightly across the bowel before the Kocher clamps are removed.

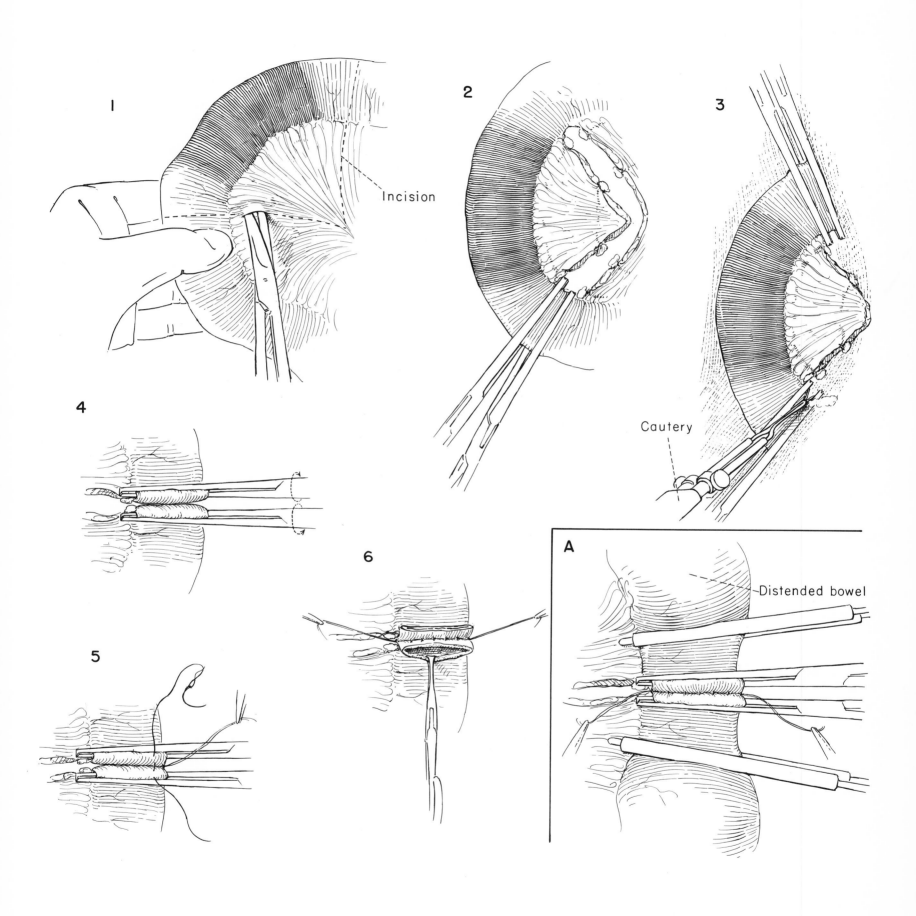

1

Incision

2

3

Cautery

4

6

5

A

Distended bowel

Figure 7. Note that the two divided ends of the bowel come together without tension. Traction is exerted on the two stay sutures which were left at each end of the transverse line of closure of the serosal surfaces of the bowel posteriorly. The anterior edge of the bowel is held open by Allis clamps to provide exposure of the posterior edge composed of muscle and mucosa which must be sutured.

The closure begins in the midline. In any end-to-end type suture there is always the danger that narrowing of the caliber of the bowel may occur. Interrupted sutures then are preferable to a running lock stitch. The mucosa and muscle wall are included in each interrupted double zero atraumatic catgut suture.

Figure 8. A series of interrupted sutures are placed on the posterior edge, moving from the center toward one corner. This type of suture permits easy identification of the tissues to be sutured at the corners.

Figure 9. The interrupted sutures are placed serially, continuing up on the anterior wall of the bowel until they reach the point which corresponds to the initial suture on the posterior wall.

Figure 10. The surgeon now turns his attention to the posterior wall again and continues to place a series of interrupted sutures, beginning in the midline and continuing toward the open corner. Each suture is held on tension after being tied as the next one is being placed. It is then divided while the next suture is being tied.

Figure 11. The interrupted sutures continue serially around the corner and up on the anterior wall until they meet, in the midline, the sutures previously placed on the opposite side. The continuity of the bowel has been restored. If rubber clamps have been placed on the bowel to prevent spillage they should be removed at this time.

Figure 12. The primary closure is reinforced by a series of interrupted silk mattress sutures placed in the seromuscular coats of the bowel; they are similar to those placed initially in the posterior wall.

Figure 13. Although there is far less danger of narrowing the lumen when interrupted sutures are used, the size and patency of the stoma must be checked. This is accomplished by grasping the two limbs of the bowel between the thumb and forefinger and introducing a finger through the stoma.

Figure 14. Finally, the defect in the bowel mesentery must be closed. This is best done with a series of interrupted silk sutures. Care should be exercised in placing the sutures to avoid injury to the vessels within the mesentery.

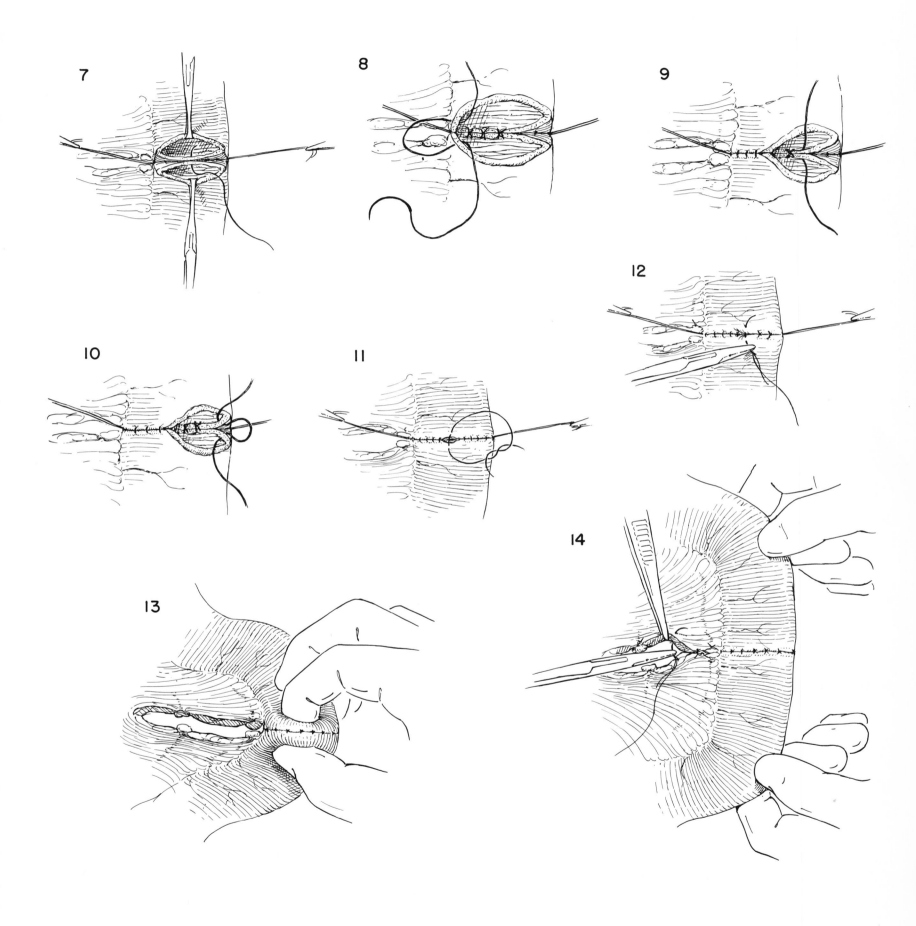

ILEOTRANSVERSE COLOSTOMY

Despite the adequacy of the preliminary investigative studies for what was believed to be disease primary in the uterus or adnexa, the surgeon may find himself confronted with disease in the cecum, terminal ileum or ascending colon.

Although one prefers to resect the ascending colon and perform an ileocolostomy at one stage, the two stage procedure has much to recommend it. This is particularly true when it is essential that an extensive operation be performed in the pelvis. The surgeon would be wise to complete the pelvic portion of the operation, perform a short-circuiting ileotransverse colostomy and leave the final resection of the ascending colon to a later date.

It is also well to remember that anastomoses from the terminal ileum to the ascending colon frequently fail because of inadequate blood supply in the cecum. If it is necessary to resect the terminal ileum and impossible to do an end-to-end suture, it is wiser to do an ileotransverse colostomy.

Although an ileocolostomy can be accomplished by a simple lateral anastomosis between two segments of bowel, the subsequent management of the case is usually made much easier if the bowel is divided and an end-to-side anastomosis performed. Complete defunctioning of the bowel is assured if this is done.

Figure 1. The mesentery of the terminal ileum is opened at a selected point, in an area free of vessels.

Figure 2. This opening is enlarged by clamping and cutting the mesenteric vessels.

Figure 3. It is also further extended toward the root of the mesentery.

Figure 4. Kocher clamps are placed across the bowel, the area protected with moist packs, and the intestine cut across with the cautery.

Figure 5. The blind stump of ileum adjacent to the cecum is closed. First a continuous catgut suture is laid in place over the clamp.

Figure 6. This is drawn together as the clamp is removed and is then brought back as a continuous mattress suture and tied at the point at which it started.

Figure 7. An outside row of interrupted silk completes the closure.

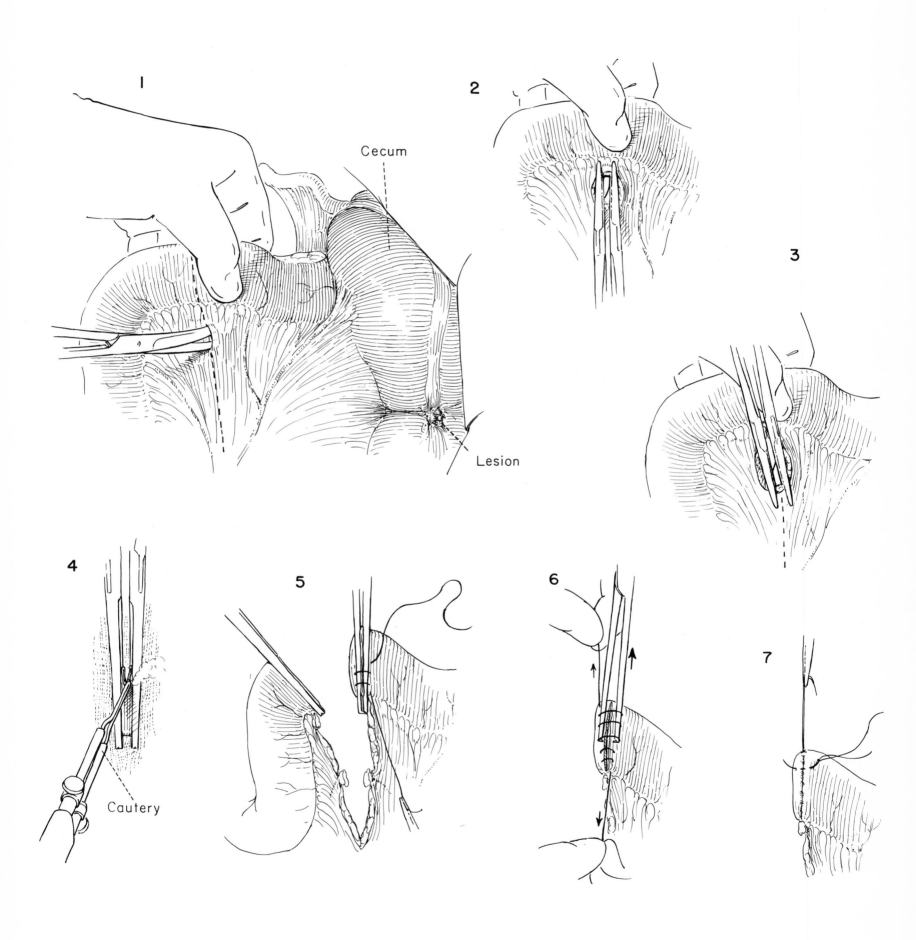

1

Cecum

Lesion

2

3

4

Cautery

5

6

7

Figure 8. Note that the divided end of the terminal ileum is being brought to the transverse colon for an anastomosis. The following illustrations will demonstrate the end-to-side ileocolostomy.

A point is selected on the transverse colon comfortably distal to the hepatic flexure yet lateral to the midcolic vessels which provide the major blood supply to the transverse colon. This is important if a right colectomy is to be done later.

The anastomosis should be made through the tenia of the colon. After the proper site for the anastomosis has been selected the full thickness of the bowel at the tenia on the superior surface of the bowel is picked up with Allis forceps. A Kocher clamp is applied across this fold of colon. It is extremely important that the amount of colon included in this clamp should match the size of the cut end of the small intestine.

Figure 9. The surrounding bowel is packed off with gauze and the operative site isolated. The surgeon applies traction on the Allis clamp, elevating it so that he can remove the knuckle of the bowel above the clamp with a cautery. These precautions are particularly desirable when the surgeon had not anticipated the necessity for performing any such procedure and consequently had not prepared the bowel for resection prior to operation.

Figure 10. The anastomosis then proceeds in standard fashion. The two Kocher clamps are rolled outward, exposing the serosa of both loops of bowel. A series of interrupted silk or cotton sutures are then placed in the seromuscular coats until a posterior suture line is completed.

Figure 11. Before removing the Kocher clamps and opening up the edge of the small bowel which must be sutured to the opening in the colon, a rubber-covered clamp is applied to prevent spillage of the bowel content.

Figure 12. Similarly, a rubber-covered clamp is placed across the colon in the long axis below the point of the anastomosis to prevent an escape of fecal matter from the colon. The two ends of bowel are then opened up and Allis clamps are applied to the leading edges of the respective loops of bowel.

Again to minimize the chance of compromising the caliber of the bowel, interrupted atraumatic catgut sutures are employed rather than a running lock stitch type of suture.

The first interrupted suture is placed in the midline. A series of such sutures are placed, tied and cut, proceeding from the midline toward both corners.

Figure 13. The interrupted sutures continue around the corners and up on the anterior surface of the bowel until they meet in the midline. The first line of the anastomosis is now complete.

Figure 14. Since the continuity of the bowel lumen has now been restored there is no longer need for the rubber-covered clamps.

A second layer of interrupted silk or cotton sutures is placed in the seromuscular coats of the anterior portion of the bowel wall. The new lumen should now be tested to ensure patency.

Figure 15. This illustrates the finished anastomosis. A real effort should be made to close the opening under the proximal loop where the mesentery was divided. This is best done with interrupted silk or cotton sutures approximating the edge of the mesentery to the posterior peritoneum.

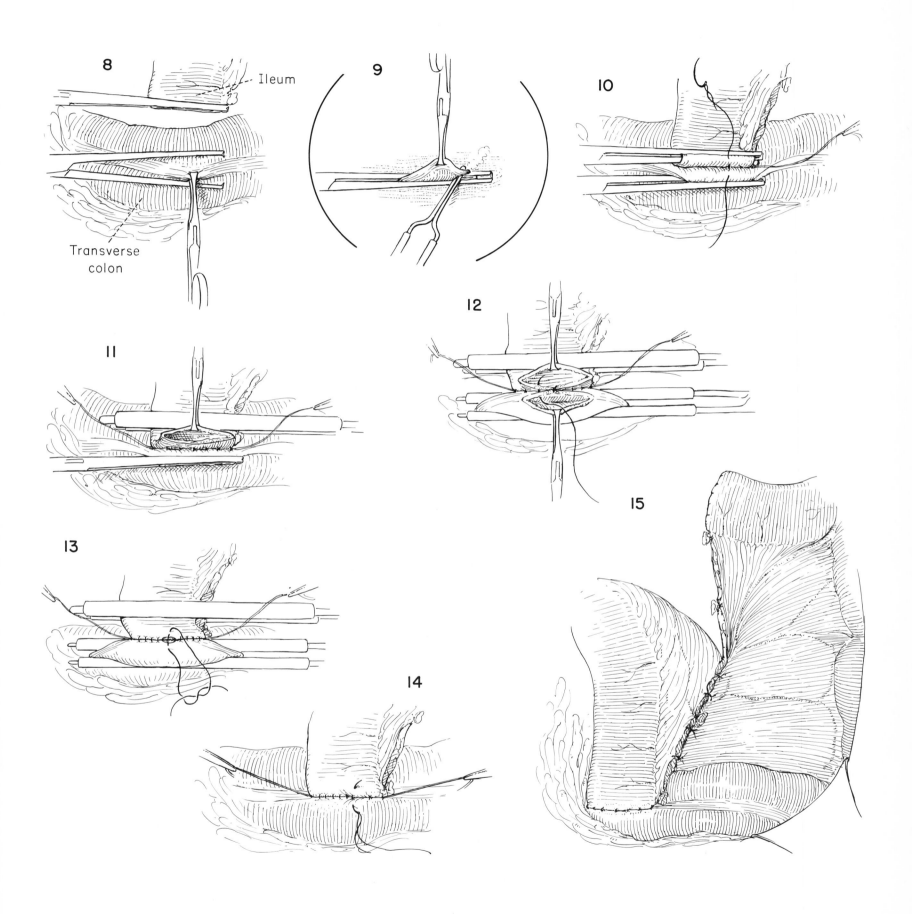

LARGE BOWEL RESECTION AND ANASTOMOSIS

Damage to or involvement of the intestine at the time of pelvic surgery or invasion of the bowel from a primary genital source is not confined to the small intestine alone. The sigmoid colon is often adherent to either uterus or ovary. This is particularly true when there has been previous surgery in the lower pelvis or when the pathological condition is due to either pelvic inflammation or endometriosis.

If the sigmoid has been extensively damaged or implicated in a disease process, the involved segment may have to be isolated and resected between clamps. There is no place for side-to-side suture; it must be made end to end. Should there be a disproportion in size of the two segments of bowel as a result of either obstruction within the bowel lumen or infection around the bowel it would be much safer to perform a defunctioning colostomy proximal to the involved area, preferably in the region of the transverse colon, and to leave the final reconstruction of the sigmoid to the time of a second operation.

The same general principles of preservation of the blood supply, approximation of the two loops without tension and the maintenance of an adequate lumen, which were applicable in surgery on the small intestine, are even more important when resections are made on the rectum or sigmoid. The suture line in the sigmoid resection must withstand greater pressures than is true in the small intestine. If leakage at the suture line occurs and the contents extravasate, the convalescent period is prolonged by the resulting septic complications. The open anastomosis performed on the sigmoid is less subject to stricture or obstruction. Nevertheless, it is often wise to perform a defunctioning loop type of colostomy proximal to the anastomosis. This maneuver will provide maximum protection to the patient until the reparative process is complete.

Figure 1. The sigmoid loop has been selected to illustrate this operation. The lateral peritoneal attachments in the left iliac fossa are first cut to permit full mobilization of the bowel. This preliminary dissection to the point of complete mobility is essential whenever the bowel is to be resected, for the two cut ends must come together easily in all cases.

Figure 2. The sigmoid has been retracted to the left and the mesentery opened with scissors against the pressure of the supporting fingers.

Figure 3. This opening is extended to the bowel by clamping, cutting and tying the vascular arches.

Figure 4. A wedge of mesentery has been isolated and thin Kocher clamps placed across the bowel. The field is protected with wet gauze and the intestine cut across with the cautery.

Figure 5. The cut ends are held in approximation by the assistant, and a posterior layer of interrupted silk mattress sutures is placed.

Figure 6. Rubber-covered clamps are applied to prevent escape of gas and feces before each Kocher clamp is removed.

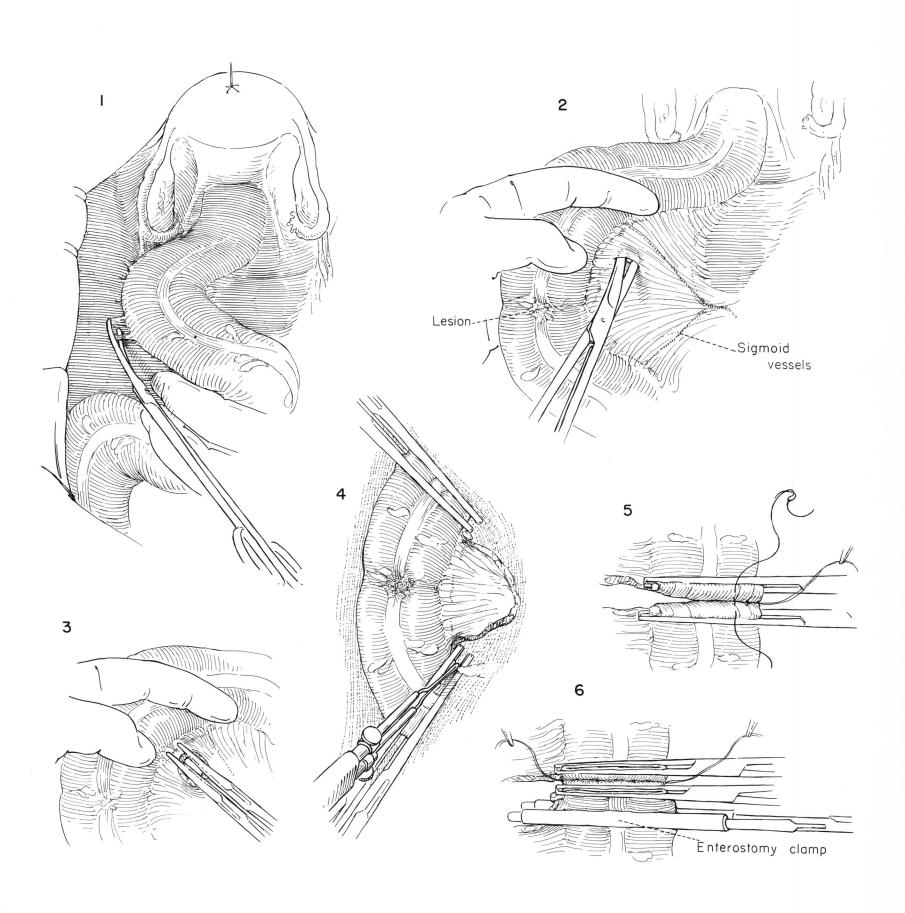

1

2

Lesion

Sigmoid
vessels

4

5

3

6

Enterostomy clamp

Figure 7. Spillage from the sigmoid is much more likely to be followed by low grade sepsis than is true of similar episodes in surgery on the small intestine. It is therefore wise to wall off the operative area with gauze and to apply rubber-covered clamps on either side of the area of anastomosis.

With the ends rolled outward to expose the seromuscular coats of the two loops, a series of interrupted silk or cotton sutures are placed and tied. The two most lateral sutures are left long to provide traction. The adherent ends of the bowel, left when the Allis or Kocher clamps are applied, are opened up and held apart by Allis clamps placed on the cut edges. This is done on both loops. The posterior or anterior edge of the bowel which must be sutured then comes into direct unobstructed view.

Figure 8. The first step in the open type of anastomosis is to suture the mucosa and muscle in the midline with an interrupted type of atraumatic chromic catgut suture. This is tied and held on tension as the next suture is applied and then cut. A series of interrupted sutures begins in the middle and proceeds to the corners of the apposed loops of bowel.

Figure 9. The interrupted chromic catgut sutures continue around the corners onto the anterior wall of the intestine. It is advisable to begin in the midline and to complete one half of the bowel suture before starting on the other side. This is done in the interest of better exposure.

Figure 10. When the two series of interrupted sutures meet in the midline, the initial suture line is complete.

Figure 11. The rubber-shod clamps may now be removed. The assistant and the surgeon maintain traction on the two end sutures as the operator places a series of interrupted silk or cotton sutures in the seromuscular coats of the bowel. When the initial suture line has been tied it is reinforced and buried. A double layer closure results.

Figure 12. Although the open type of anastomosis rarely restricts the caliber of the bowel lumen, it is always wise to test the patency of the stoma by holding up the anastomotic area between thumb and forefinger and passing a finger through the stoma.

Figure 13. The opening in the mesentery is closed with more interrupted sutures of silk or cotton.

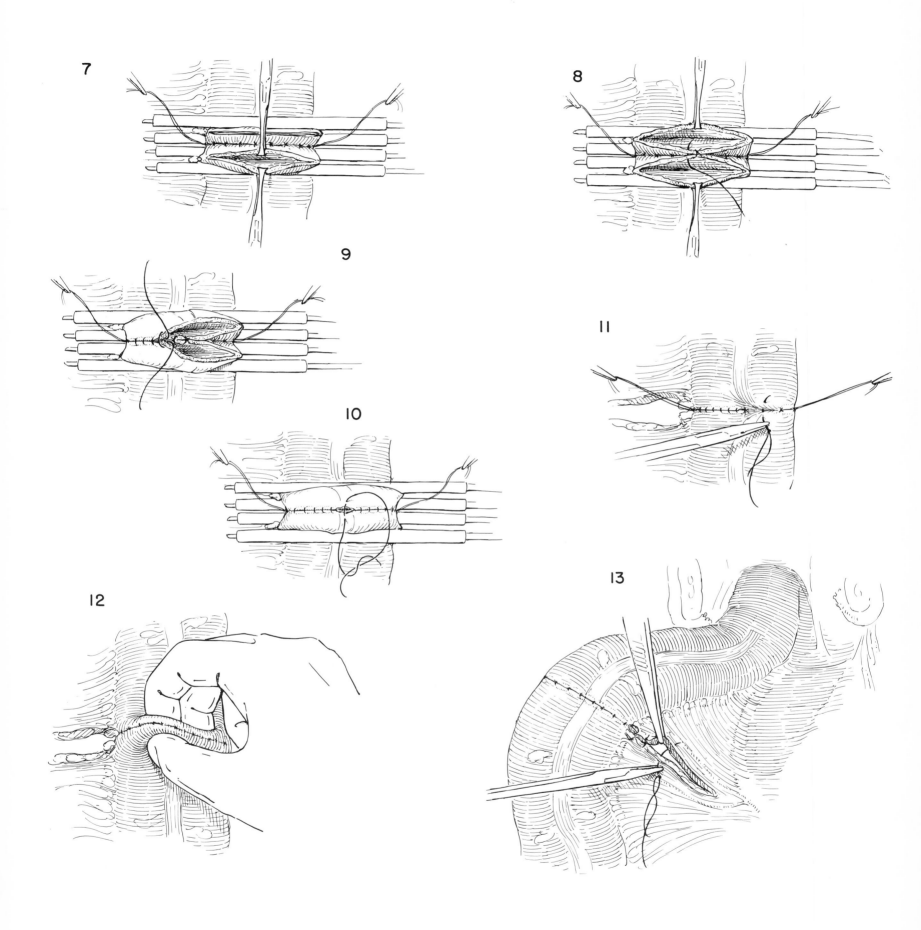

COLOSTOMY

It is often desirable to decompress the large bowel by means of a colostomy proximal to a point of obstruction in the large bowel or a recently constructed suture line following resection of the obstructed or damaged area. Taking the fecal stream away from such areas allows the distention to subside in the presence of obstruction or the inflammation to quiet down. It also avoids strain on the new area of anastomosis and minimizes the chance of leakage from the suture line. The operation can be performed rapidly and with little risk to the patient.

The operation described here is a temporary or loop colostomy. When the obstruction below is relieved or the suture line solidly healed, it can be closed and the continuity of the bowel restored. Only the anterior surface of the bowel need be opened to ensure adequate function.

The loop colostomy may be performed on the sigmoid colon if no further surgery is contemplated in the pelvis. If an inflammatory process is present in the pelvis or tumor blocks the lumen to such an extent that there is disproportion in size between the two loops, it is wiser to perform a temporary colostomy and leave the resection to a later date.

When this condition is present it is better to place the colostomy in the transverse colon. The placement of the colostomy in the upper abdomen creates a cleaner, more unencumbered field for the subsequent resection in the pelvic area.

In the illustration shown here a segment of transverse colon is exteriorized.

Figure 1. A separate, short, transverse skin incision should be made about 2 inches above the umbilicus and just to the right of the midline. The transverse colon and its omentum are delivered, and the omentum is turned upward and dissected free of the colon by cutting filmy, avascular attachments in the line of the tenia.

Figure 2. A full 3 inches of bowel and its mesocolon are completely separated from the overlying omentum.

Figure 3. The omentum is drawn down over the bowel again and opened vertically where it will expose the area of previous dissection, then replaced within the abdomen.

Figure 4. The bowel and its mesentery are elevated with the left index finger, and the mesentery is opened in a bloodless area adjacent to the intestine.

Figure 5. A glass rod is passed through under the loop by letting it follow the finger as it is withdrawn.

Figure 6. The loop is held up by an assistant, and the wound is closed in layers around it, sufficiently snugly to prevent herniation of other bowel loops, yet loose enough to avoid any tendency to obstruct the colostomy itself. One should be able to introduce one finger beside the colon. A length of rubber tubing is now forced over the two ends of the glass rod to prevent accidental dislodgment. The bowel is opened with a cautery in 24 hours by a transverse incision on the anterior two-thirds of its circumference at a point slightly nearer the active limb.

INSET A. If a prolonged period of intestinal defunctioning is anticipated, the two stomas produced when the bowel is cut across will separate slightly and lie comfortably if a tongue of skin is fashioned on one side under the loop.

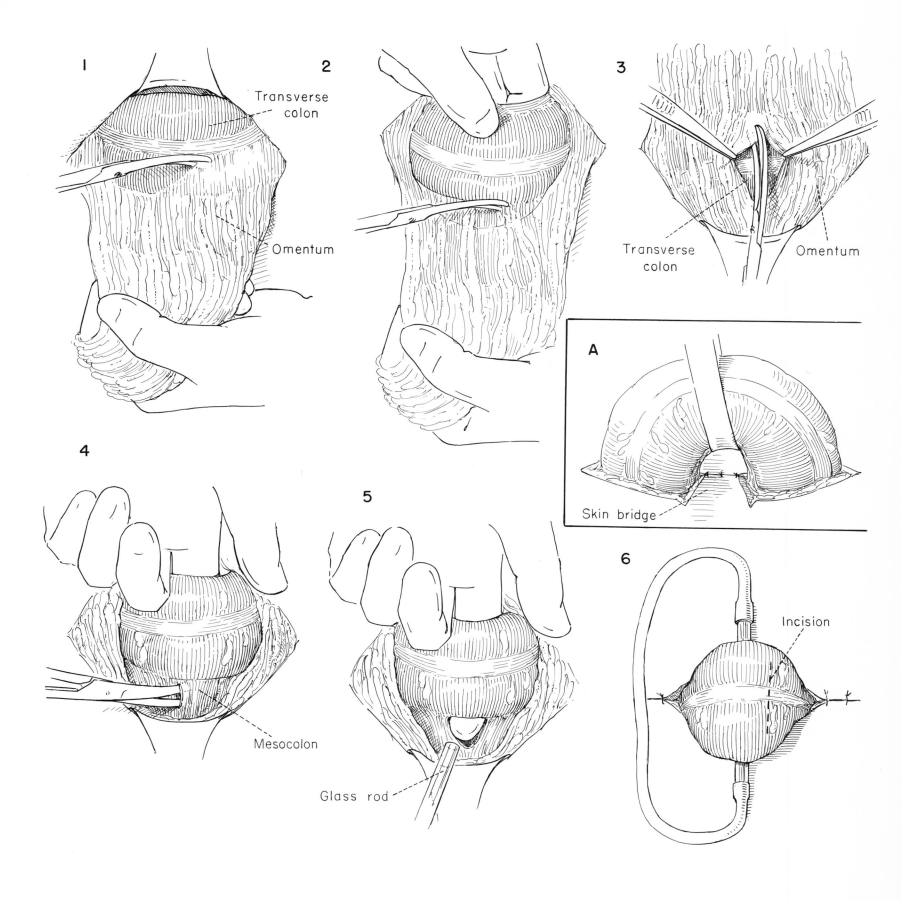

1

Transverse colon

Omentum

2

3

Transverse colon

Omentum

A

Skin bridge

4

Mesocolon

5

Glass rod

6

Incision

CLOSURE OF COLOSTOMY

The closure of a temporary colostomy must be done according to the general principles applicable to other intestinal operations. Inasmuch as tension at the suture line is of basic importance, the colostomy opening must be dissected free and be fully mobilized before any attempt is made to close the defect in the bowel wall. Failure to do this is a common mistake.

Closure of the colostomy should not be attempted until the surgeon is assured that there is no obstruction in the bowel lumen distal to the colostomy. The barium enema should demonstrate a free passage of material through a previous anastomosis prior to the closure of the colostomy.

Great care must be taken that the blood supply is in no way compromised and that no narrowing results from the repair. Any obstruction at the point of closure during the period of healing increases the risk of leakage and the formation of a fecal fistula.

The technique shown here is that of closure of a simple loop colostomy opened on its anterior aspect.

Figure 1. A 2-mm. collar of skin is left all around the bowel.

Figure 2. Scissor dissection is carried down to the surface of the bowel until the rectus fascia is reached.

Figure 3. The fascia is exposed for a centimeter or more on all sides of the bowel. The Allis clamps placed on the skin collar offer an easy means of holding the bowel on tension.

Figure 4. The fascia is opened at a point adjacent to the bowel and completely freed from it. This incision is extended at either end in the line of the original wound.

Figure 5. The peritoneum is opened and separated in similar fashion. The loop of bowel can now usually be delivered farther out of the abdomen.

Figure 6. The collar of skin at the stoma and any scar present at the line of juncture between mucosa and serosa are trimmed away.

Figure 7. Allis clamps on the edges of the stoma keep the bowel up while a closure in two layers and transverse to the axis of the bowel is carried out. First we use an inner layer of running catgut.

Figure 8. A second row of interrupted silk is also used, and care is taken that it extends well beyond the original opening at either end.

Figure 9. The bowel has been returned to the free peritoneal cavity and the peritoneum closed.

Figure 10. Because the wound is potentially contaminated, interrupted catgut sutures rather than silk or cotton are used to close the fascia.

The superficial fascia and skin are loosely approximated and a dressing is applied.

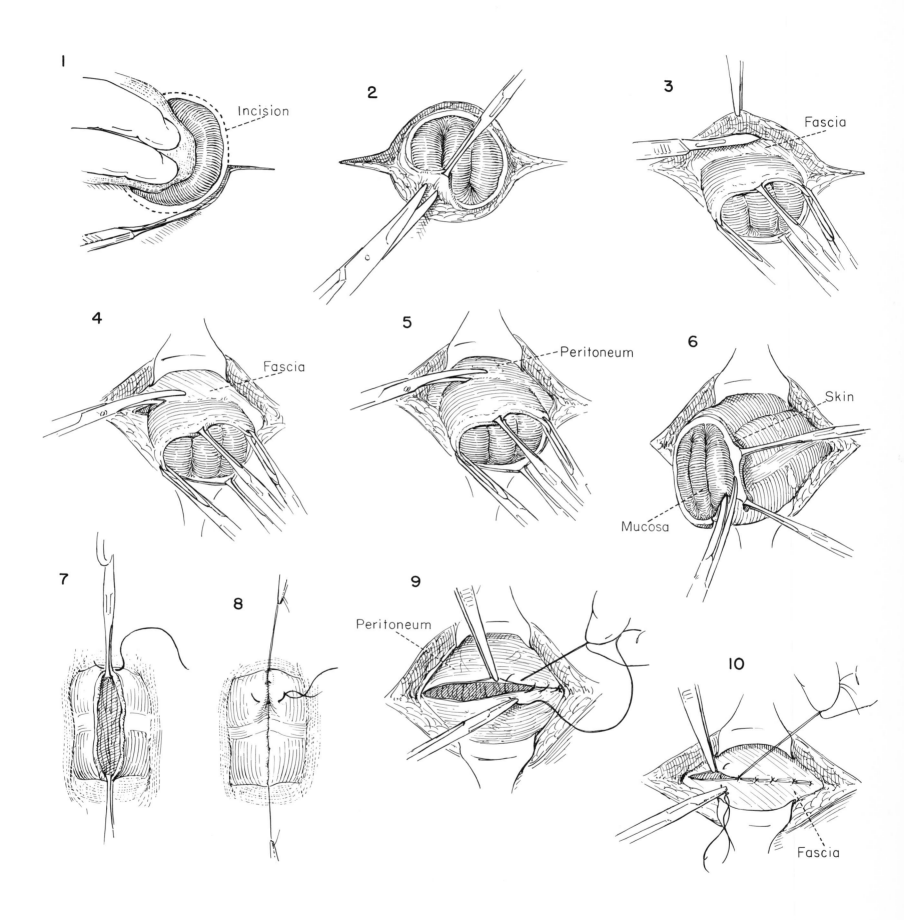

APPENDECTOMY

It is customary when performing definitive operations in the pelvis, particularly those on the uterus or adnexa, to remove the appendix as an adjunctive procedure.

The operation described in this plate has the advantage of simplicity in performance. It has proved itself from repeated usage. Other methods are undoubtedly equally rapid and effective.

Figure 1. The appendix is easily controlled by a curved hemostat applied to the mesentery near the tip of the organ.

Figure 2. A series of bites is taken across the mesappendix, aiming for the point of juncture with the cecum.

Figure 3. The tissue is cut as it is clamped. It is usually advantageous to tie these bites before proceeding.

Figure 4. The appendix base is crushed with a straight snap.

Figure 5. A plain catgut tie is secured at the level of the crush, and the snap is removed as the tie is made.

Figure 6. The ends of this tie are held close to the knot with a snap. A second crushing clamp is placed about 5 mm. distal, and the appendix is cut across with a knife blade moistened in carbolic acid. A deliberate effort is made to cauterize the cut end of the appendix with this solution; the cecum beneath is carefully protected with dry gauze while this is done.

Figure 7. Excess carbolic is neutralized by wiping the stump with a cotton swab dipped in alcohol.

Figure 8. Various methods of burying the stump are used. This figure illustrates the placing of a Z stitch of chromic catgut. It is essentially a figure of eight which picks up the bowel at the four corners as a shallow mattress.

Figure 9. The stitch is tightened, puckering the appendix site. The stump is simultaneously buried by poking it down in the center of the pucker with the snap which is still on the base tie.

Figure 10. The stitch is tied as the snap is released and removed.

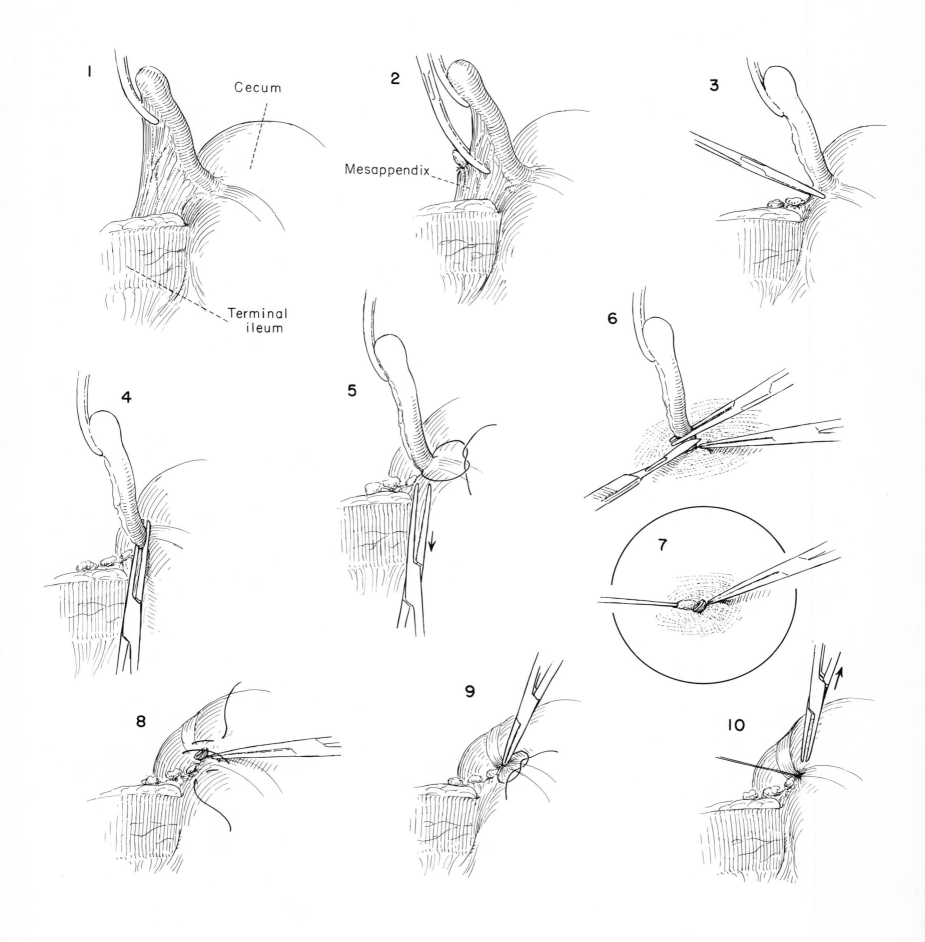

1

Cecum

Terminal ileum

2

Mesappendix

3

4

5

6

7

8

9

10

Operations Involving the Urinary Tract

BLADDER DAMAGE

The bladder may be damaged in the course of many gynecological operations. On rare occasions the bladder may be entered in separating the peritoneum from the anterior wall. The most likely area of injury, however, is the base of the bladder. This can occur in a number of different ways. The commonest time of injury is during the dissection of the posterior surface from the underlying cervix or vagina. The chances of damage compound if any previous operations have been performed in this area either abdominally or through the vagina. It is particularly prone to happen when the Wertheim type of radical hysterectomy is done for carcinoma of the cervix or endometrium. If preoperative radiation has been given, the likelihood increases.

The misadventure of entering the bladder is not a serious matter provided the surgeon recognizes that a perforation has occurred and takes immediate steps to repair it or to reinforce any weak spots.

When the rent is small, simple layer closure will suffice. Interrupted catgut sutures avoid the problem of including too much bladder wall and creating distortion. Most perforations or weakness of the bladder wall at the base can be satisfactorily repaired without danger of including the ureters, provided the surgeon recognizes they are in close proximity.

If the defect is at all extensive the surgeon will be well advised to do a concomitant suprapubic cystotomy.

Figure 1. The defect is shown on the bladder dome.

Figure 2. Catgut rather than linen or silk should be used in the repair to avoid a nidus for subsequent stone formation. The reparative sutures should not enter the mucosa, but include only the serosal and muscle layers. The surgeon and assistant prepare to place the first suture.

Figures 3, 4, 5, 6. The first layer is reinforced by a second layer of interrupted catgut sutures. The suture enters the outer surface and muscle and emerges at the edge of the defect on either side. Tying of the sutures inverts the tissue, thereby strengthening the closure.

SUPRAPUBIC CYSTOTOMY

Suprapubic cystotomy provides an excellent means of diverting the urinary stream when it is desirable to prevent bladder distention and undue strain on a suture line after repair of extensive damage. It is an essential part of many urological procedures.

Figure 7. In most instances the bladder will have been exposed previously. Here the operation begins with a centrally placed lower abdominal skin incision.

Figure 8. The skin, muscle and fascia are divided in the midline halfway to the umbilicus.

Figure 9. The peritoneum is cleaned from the undersurface of the rectus muscle with the knife handle.

Figure 10. A retractor is placed in the lower angle of the wound at the symphysis.

Figure 11. The surgeon lays the right hand flat on the peritoneofascial surface. By gentle upward pressure and flexing of the fingers the peritoneal fold is retracted and the prevesical space exposed.

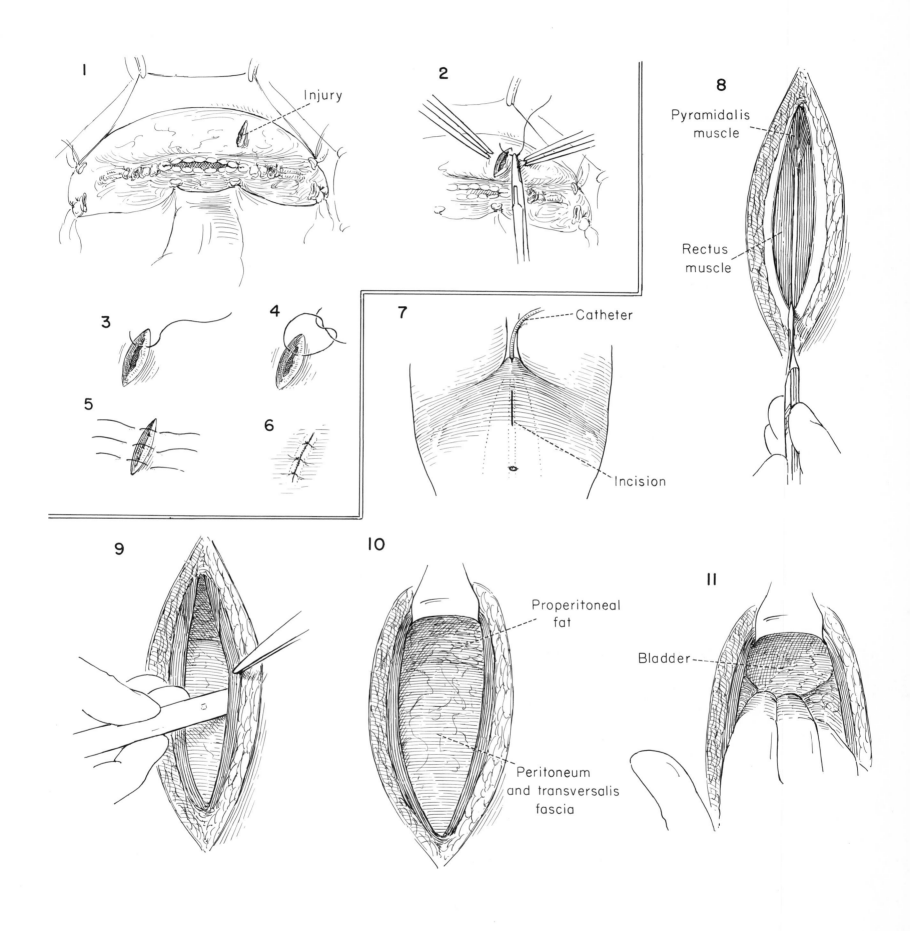

1

Injury

2

3

4

5

6

7

Catheter

Incision

8

Pyramidalis
muscle

Rectus
muscle

9

10

Properitoneal
fat

Peritoneum
and transversalis
fascia

11

Bladder

Figure 12. The anterior surface of the bladder forms the floor of the prevesical space. Retractors are placed in both ends of the wound to aid in exposure. Allis clamps are placed on the bladder wall at either side of the midline just below the peritoneal reflexion. The surgeon and assistant elevate the clamps as the incision into the bladder is made. If the bladder is empty, the mucosa may have a tendency to recede.

Figure 13. To avoid unnecessary spillage of urine the assistant inserts a suction tip into the bladder through the incision. The bladder is sucked dry.

Figure 14. The Allis clamps are shifted to include the full thickness of the bladder wall on either side of the incision. Traction is applied to the clamps as the surgeon inserts a Pezzer or large Foley catheter into the bladder interior.

Figure 15. The defect in the bladder wall is closed around the catheter with interrupted catgut sutures which pass through the full thickness of the wall of the bladder but avoid penetrating the mucosa.

Figure 16. The sutures are tied. This illustration shows an empty Penrose drain being placed in the lower end of the wound to minimize the danger of sepsis caused by any urinary leakage.

Figure 17. Proper placing of the drainage tube in the bladder is important. To avoid a possible osteomyelitis or permanent fistula the tube should be brought out well above the symphysis and out of contact with it. The rectus muscles are brought together in the midline with interrupted catgut sutures. The drain in the prevesical space is led out through the lower end of the abdominal wound. The prevesical space should always be drained.

Figure 18. Interrupted catgut sutures then complete the closure of the fascia around the catheter and drain.

Figure 19. The drain and the catheter are fixed to the sutured skin edges. Firm upward traction is applied to the catheter as it is being fixed to the skin. This keeps the Foley balloon firmly against the roof of the bladder. In this position it cannot impinge on the bladder base and produce any obstruction to the ureters.

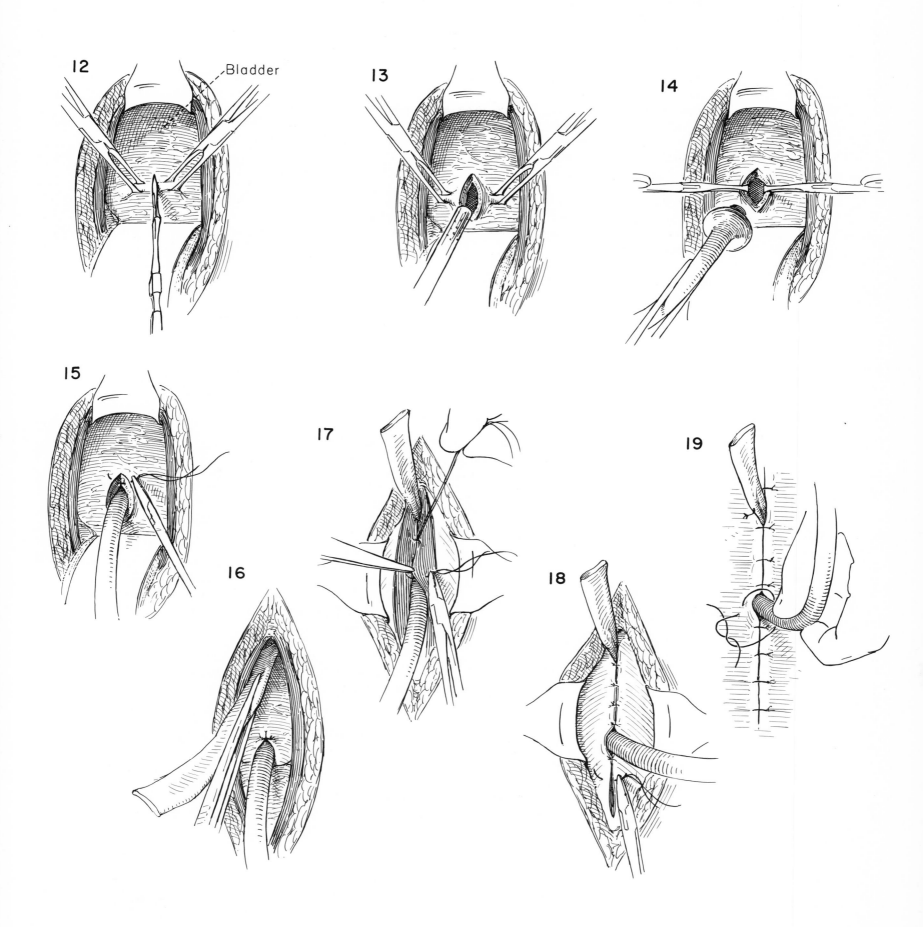

Bladder

12

13

14

15

16

17

18

19

END-TO-END REPAIR OF DAMAGED URETER

However careful the surgeon may be in performing surgery in the pelvis there is always the potential risk of damaging a ureter either by severing it, nicking it or by including it in a stitch ligature.

The anatomical areas in which damage to the ureter is most likely to occur are (1) at the level of the uterosacral ligaments in close proximity to the uterine vessels, and (2) at the point where the ureter and ovarian vessels cross the common iliac artery. The surgeon should exercise great care in applying clamps to control bleeding in these areas.

The damage to the ureter may be recognized at the time it is done or may become evident during the convalescent period. The optimum time to correct any damage arises when the surgeon realizes that the ureter has been injured. Although the steps employed to repair the injury are basically the same, the surgeon will experience greater difficulty in mobilizing the ureter from the surrounding scar when the repair is undertaken at a later date.

The end-to-end type of repair is most useful when the ureter has been divided but there is no loss of tissue length and the divided ends can be brought together without tension. The ureteral anastomosis is usually made around an inlying catheter, which acts as an internal splint.

Immediate repair of damage to the ureter above the level of the ligated uterine vessel is illustrated.

Figure 1. An incision in the posterior peritoneum lateral to the ureter exposes the entire length of pelvic ureter lying on the medial flap.

Figure 2. Stay sutures are placed on the peritoneal edges to widen the operative field. The periureteral tissue is gently elevated and the ureter dissected free from the underlying attachments.

Figure 3. To avoid handling the ureter with instruments, stay sutures are placed in the tissue adjacent to the ureter on either side.

Figure 4. If the ureter is deliberately sectioned on the oblique, the largest possible opening will be available for anastomosis. The dotted line indicates the proposed excision. The barest minimum of tissue should be removed.

Figure 5. The stay sutures are held on tension and the lower segment cut with a single decisive incision.

Figure 6. The edge of the divided upper ureteral segment is similarly treated.

Figure 7. Stay sutures steady the ureter as the surgeon grasps a ureteral catheter in smooth forceps and introduces the tip into the lumen of the upper ureter as far as the kidney pelvis.

Figure 8. The assistant steadies the ureter by traction on the stay sutures while the surgeon introduces the catheter into the bladder where the excess curls up in the interior.

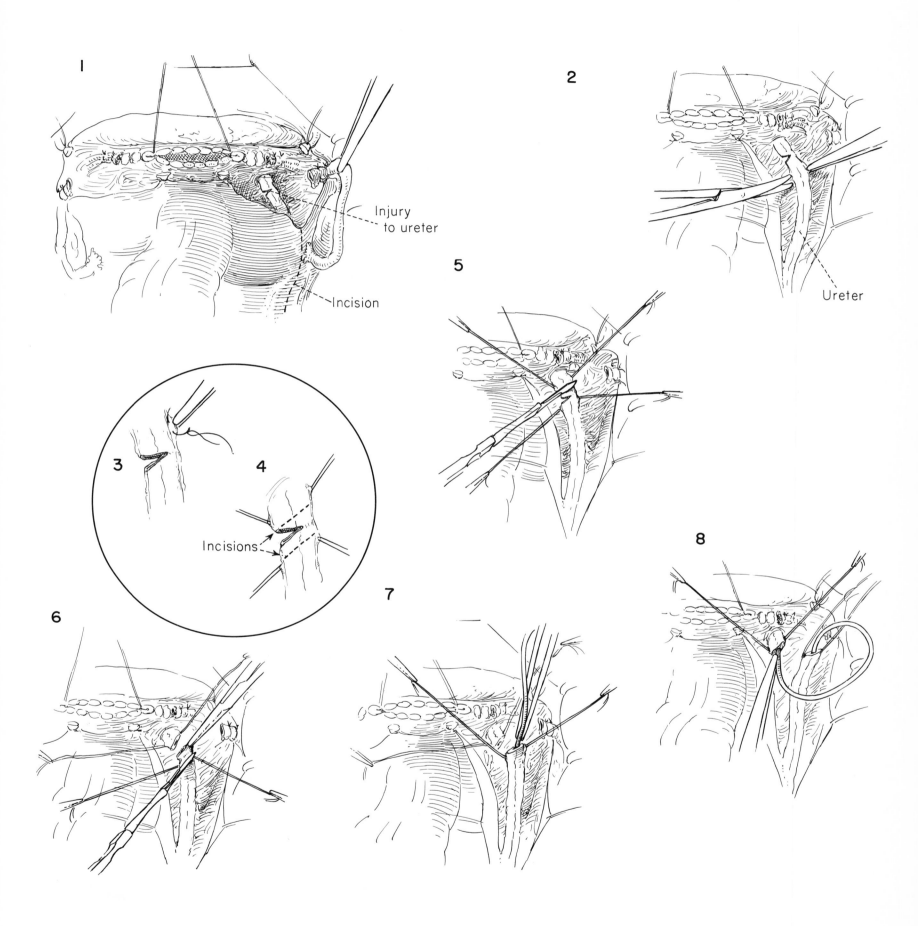

1

Injury
to ureter

Incision

2

Ureter

3

4

Incisions

5

6

7

8

Figure 9. Stay sutures placed in the periureteral tissue but not in the wall of the ureter itself will reduce the use of instruments to a minimum when the sutures are held on traction. If the anastomosis is to be successful the ureter must be handled very gently to avoid trauma to both the intrinsic and extrinsic blood supply. The anastomosis is usually made around an inlying catheter which serves as a splint.

Figure 10. The success of the entire end-to-end suture procedure depends on the accuracy with which the severed ends are approximated.

Fine atraumatic No. 00000 chromic catgut sutures are placed in the anterior wall of the ureter at both angles. Nonabsorbable suture material should not be used because of the likelihood of producing a fistula.

When the angle sutures are tied they are left long and held on tension to facilitate the placing of the remainder of the interrupted sutures. The periureteral stay sutures may now be removed to avoid further trauma to the blood vessels in the periureteral tissue.

Figure 11. With the assistant steadying one angle suture and the surgeon the other, a series of interrupted atraumatic chromic catgut sutures are placed in the ureteral wall of both segments. They are individually tied and cut.

Figure 12. The surgeon now turns his attention to the placement of the sutures in the posterior wall of the divided ureter. This is accomplished by rotating the sutures placed on the angles so that the posterior edge comes in view. A row of interrupted sutures similar to those on the anterior wall are now placed in the posterior wall. When they are tied and divided the ureteral edges are approximated and lie without tension on the suture line.

Figure 13. To further reduce the tension on the suture line the surgeon now places two lateral sutures in the periureteral tissue above and below the suture line on both sides of the ureter. When these are tied they serve to steady the ureter in much the same way they do when a tendon is repaired. Any tension will come on these lateral sutures and not on the suture line.

Figure 14. Since these illustrations indicate the immediate repair of a damaged ureter at the time of hysterectomy the surgeon now reconstructs the pelvic floor and closes the peritoneum.

Figure 15. The inlying catheter has been placed in the ureteral lumen and passed down into the bladder cavity. It must now be recovered. This is done by introducing an operating cystoscope. The free end of the catheter coiled in the bladder is grasped, pulled through the urethra and sutured to the skin.

Alternate Method of Splinting the Ureter

INSET A. Stay sutures have been placed on the divided ends of the ureter. A grooved director is inserted into the lumen of the ureter and the anterior ureteral wall incised about ½ inch from the cut end, avoiding the intrinsic blood vessel.

INSET B. The distal arm of a small T tube is inserted into the stab wound in the ureter and advanced toward the bladder with forceps. The maneuver is repeated on the upper arm. If a V-shaped section is removed opposite the long arm of the tube, the arms will collapse when it is subsequently removed, thus avoiding trauma to the ureteral wall.

INSET C. The distal arm extends through the completed anastomosis as a splint. The main portion of the catheter leads out retroperitoneally through a stab wound in the lower abdominal wall.

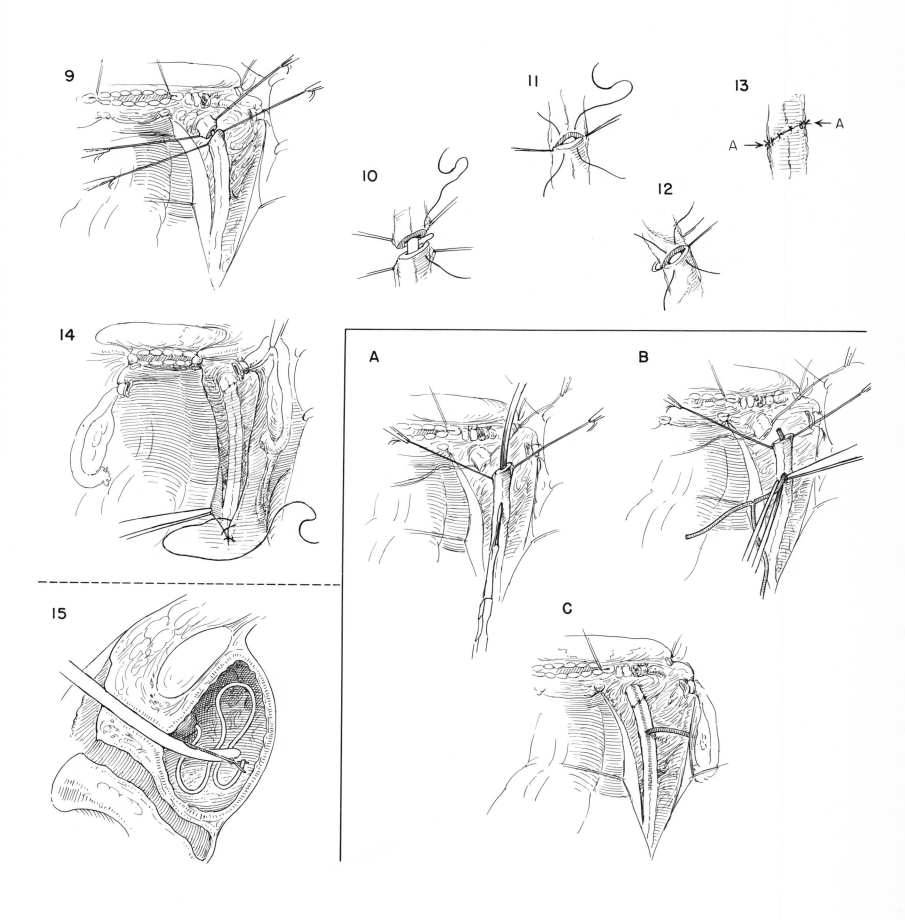

TRANSPLANTATION OF THE URETER INTO THE BLADDER

The end-to-end type of suture of the severed ends of the ureter can be employed only when there is no loss of tissue length. Frequently the loss of tissue substance is so great that the ends of the ureter cannot be sufficiently mobilized to permit them to be approximated without tension.

If the injury in the ureter has been in its pelvic portion and the upper segment of the ureter has adequate length it may be transplanted into the dome of the bladder. If the extent of the injury is recognized at the time of the initial surgical procedure the transplantation can be done at that time.

In most instances the damage is not known until complications appear during the convalescent phase. At the second operation the point of the division of the ureter must be identified and the degree of lost continuity determined. If the ureter can then be mobilized and enough proximal length remains, the upper end can be transplanted into the bladder dome. When the above conditions do not prevail the surgeon must decide whether he wants to (1) perform a skin ureterostomy, (2) transplant the ureter into the bowel, or (3) tie off the ureter and hope that the kidney will stop functioning.

This series of drawings shows the technical steps to be used when the damage to the ureter has been discovered during the postoperative period. These reconstructive steps are the same as those that would be used had the loss of ureteral length been noted at the time of the primary surgical procedure.

When the injury has occurred late the actual extent of damage to the ureter is not known and can only be revealed when the traumatized ureter is dissected free. The continuity of operative steps in this series of drawings will proceed as though the damage were discovered during convalescence.

Figure 1. The normal course of the ureter is determined by following it down into the pelvis from the point of identification at the level of the common iliac artery.

The surgeon then divides the posterior parietal peritoneum overlying the ureter as the assistant aids in elevating the peritoneum with forceps.

Figure 2. Stay sutures are placed on the severed peritoneal edges to widen the operative field. The assistant picks up the peritoneum overlying the reconstructed bladder flap as the surgeon incises it.

Figure 3. The surgeon and assistant elevate the cut peritoneal edge with stay sutures so that the bladder can be mobilized from beneath.

Figure 4. The round ligament previously sutured to the stump of the vaginal canal is isolated and the index finger passed beneath it.

Figure 5. Suture ligatures are placed in the round ligament close to the vaginal attachment. These are held on tension while the surgeon divides the ligament between them. The lateral suture on the round ligament is left long and allowed to hang outside the abdominal incision. In this fashion, supplemented by the stay sutures on the lateral edge of the peritoneum, a wide open operative field is created.

Figure 6. The surgeon then begins to dissect the damaged ureter from the surrounding fibrosis. Particular care must be taken not to jeopardize the blood supply to the ureter. As far as possible, the dissection should be carried out in the periureteral tissue, with the use of instruments reduced to a minimum.

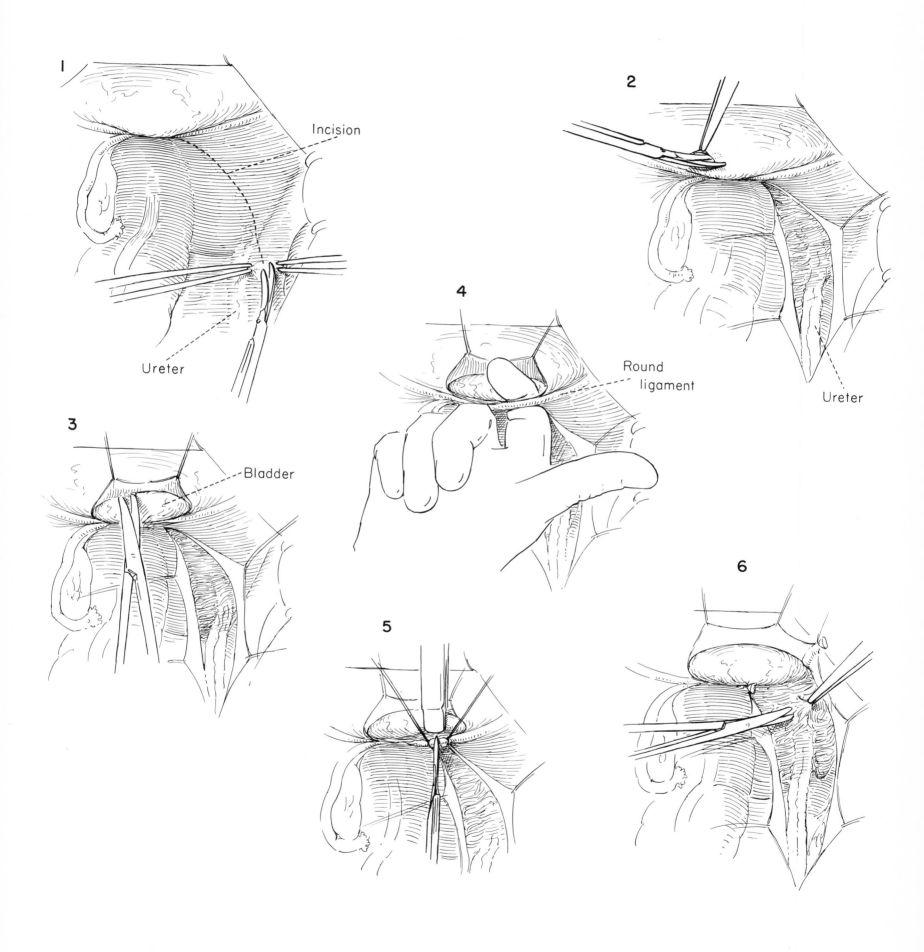

Figure 7. The dissection continues in the scar tissue around the damaged ureter. The field must be kept absolutely bloodless. Continuous saline irrigation and suction may ensure this more effectively than routine sponging.

Figure 8. The extent of the damage to the ureter is now evident. The lower segment of the ureter is represented by a fibrous cord. The surgeon must now make the decision whether end-to-end suture is possible or whether transplant into the bladder is feasible. In this instance, the decision has been made to transplant the ureter into the bladder. Stay sutures are passed into the periureteral tissue, the ureter elevated, and a ligature of silk drawn underneath it with a clamp.

Figure 9. The ureter is singly tied and transected at the most distal normal portion.

Figure 10. As the assistant applies traction to the Kelly clamps placed on the lower peritoneum, the surgeon uses the palmar surface of the fingers to gently separate the bladder from the symphysis in a bloodless areolar area. A Deaver retractor placed in the lower angle of the wound exposes this prevesical space, with the bladder presenting on the posterior surface.

Figure 11. Allis clamps support the dome of the anterior bladder wall in the midline as the surgeon incises the wall between the forceps.

Figure 12. Small curved retractors keep the incision widely open to reveal the trigone with the ureteral orifices as well as the posterior wall of the bladder.

Figure 13. Traction on the Kelly clamps is maintained upward. The surgeon then places the left index finger beneath the bladder from the abdominal side. Elevation of the bladder base gives a firm foundation on which to incise the posterior bladder wall at a point where the ureter can be brought to it without tension.

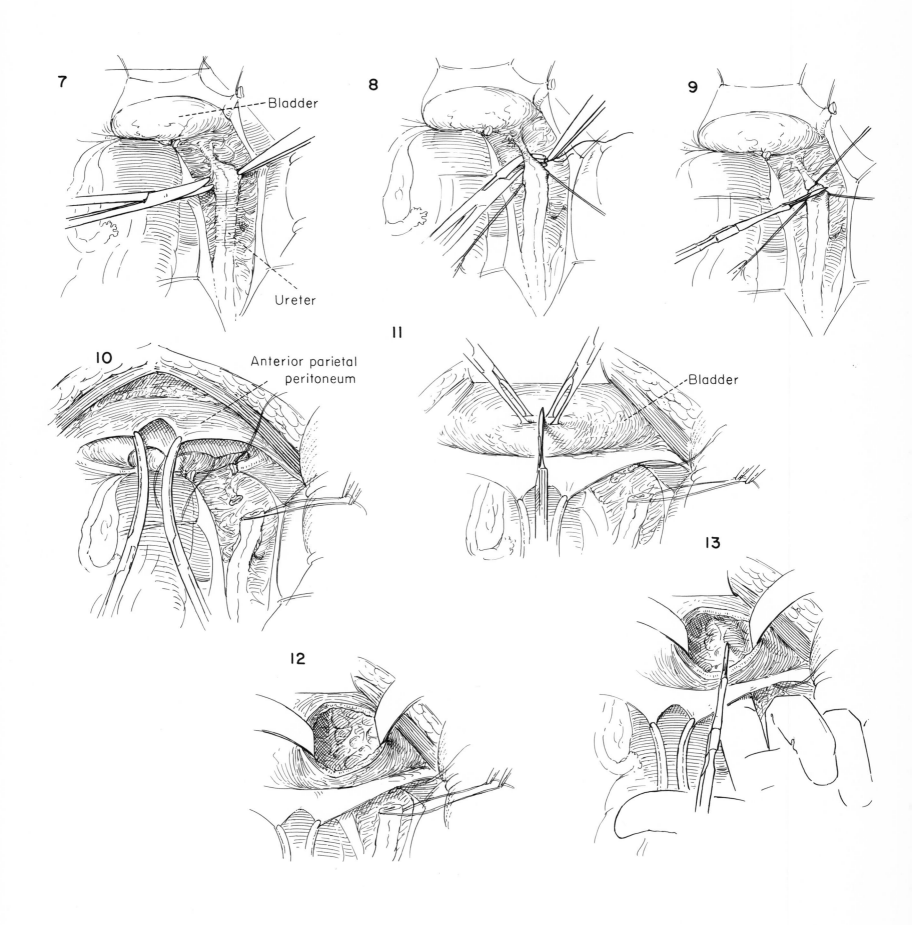

7

Bladder

Ureter

8

9

10

Anterior parietal peritoneum

11

Bladder

12

13

Figure 14. The incision in the posterior lateral bladder wall is exposed by applying traction to the stay sutures on the lower peritoneum. The surgeon introduces a Kelly clamp into the interior of the bladder and out through the opening to grasp the stay sutures on the ureter.

Figure 15. By traction on the stay sutures the ureter is now led through the opening in the bladder wall. The curved retractors in either angle of the bladder aid in the exposure.

Figure 16. Stay sutures held on countertraction steady the ureter while the surgeon incises the ureteral wall in the longitudinal axis in an area free of blood vessels. This enlarges the ostium. When the ureter lies comfortably without tension or rotation in the long axis, the anastomosis is begun.

Figures 17 and 18. The surgeon steadies the stay sutures on the ureter and places the first of a series of interrupted catgut sutures which fix the cut end of the ureter to the opening in the bladder wall. The suture includes the bladder muscle and mucosa and the full thickness of the ureter.

Figure 19. The complete anastomosis results in an elliptical ostium.

Figure 20. The assistant elevates the stay sutures on the peritoneal bladder flap to expose the incision on the posterior bladder wall on the abdominal side. The defect is closed with interrupted catgut sutures, the last of which includes the periureteral tissue to help fix the ureter. The closure should be snug without compressing the ureter.

Figure 21. The assistant applies traction on the peritoneal clamps to expose the incision in the anterior bladder wall. The incision is then closed with interrupted sutures except for the upper portion. Through this opening a Pezzer or Foley catheter is inserted into the bladder to provide drainage while the anastomosis heals. The catheter is fixed in place in the manner used following suprapubic cystotomy.

Figure 22. The operation is completed by reconstruction of the pelvic floor and peritonealization of the raw areas.

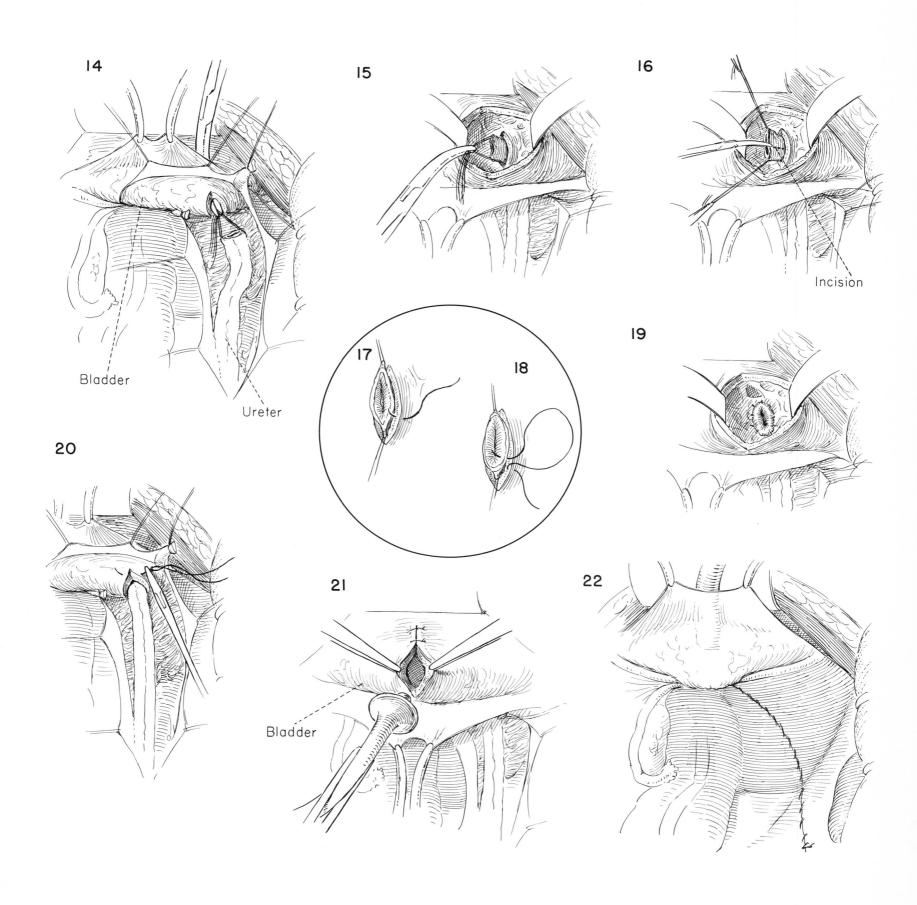

14

15

16

Incision

17

18

19

Bladder

Ureter

20

21

22

Bladder

URETERO-INTESTINAL ANASTOMOSIS

When there has been too much loss of ureteral length through operative trauma, either end-to-end suture or transplantation into the bladder may be impossible. In the interest of trying to save the kidney the surgeon may elect to divert the urinary stream into the sigmoid colon by creating a uretero-intestinal anastomosis. Although the operation may be employed when extensive damage is produced at the original operation, it is best adapted to the situation in which signs of ureteral obstruction or ureterovaginal fistula have appeared, and the presence of which has been confirmed by cystoscopy and intravenous pyelogram. Preliminary preparation of the colon by mechanical cleansing or antibiotic agents is desirable.

To obtain the optimum result with the fewest complications the surgeon must adhere to the cardinal principles for any type of uretero-intestinal anastomosis. The sigmoid must be brought to the ureter and not the ureter to the sigmoid. Any tension on the suture line may cause the ureter to pull out of the bowel and any malalignment can produce obstruction to the urinary flow.

This operation may be done for extensive damage to the ureter, irreparable vesico- or ureterovaginal fistula or as part of extensive surgical procedures for pelvic malignant lesions.

Figure 1. The surgeon identifies the ureter as it crosses the common iliac vessels and divides the peritoneum lateral to it with scissors.

Figure 2. The operative field is kept open by placing stay sutures on the incised peritoneal edges. The ureter lies on the medial peritoneal flap. The ureter is carefully dissected out of the dense area of fibrosis. The common and internal iliac arteries lie beneath and are often firmly adherent to the ureter as it courses down toward the bladder. This can be a difficult dissection. To avoid damage to the artery and maintain the blood supply to the ureter, a dry field is a "must."

Figure 3. The ureter has now been successfully dissected free of the encasing fibrosis. The extent of damage to the ureter is evaluated.

Figure 4. The surgeon then gingerly dissects the proximal ureter free from underlying attachments. This area may be treacherous, for at this point the ureter crosses the common iliac artery, shown beneath the ureter.

Figure 5. A stay suture is placed in the periureteral tissue on either side of the ureter. With the separation accomplished, a Moynihan clamp is passed beneath the ureter and a silk tie inserted in the open ends of the clamp as the assistant elevates the stay sutures.

Figure 6. The silk is then tied about the distal ureter. The suture is left long for the moment. The assistant elevates this tie while the surgeon applies similar traction to the stay sutures on the proximal ureter and divides it.

URINARY TRACT OPERATIONS
URETERO-INTESTINAL ANASTOMOSIS

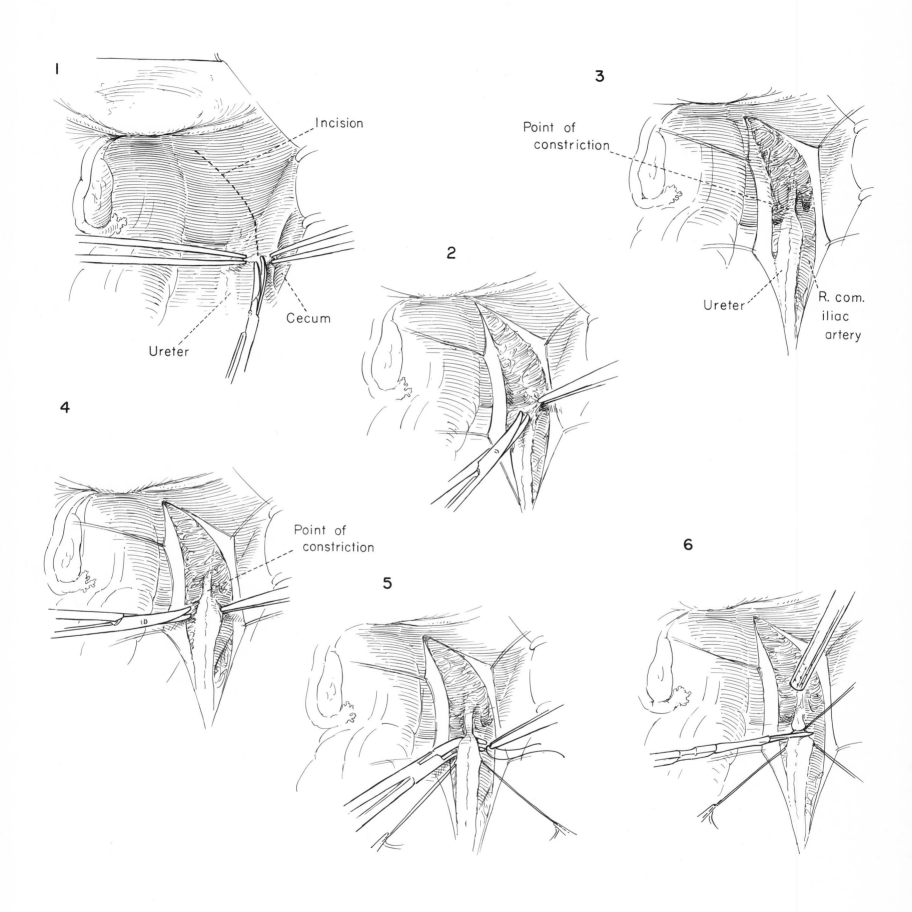

1

Incision

Cecum

Ureter

2

3

Point of constriction

Ureter

R. com. iliac artery

4

Point of constriction

5

6

Figure 7. The surgeon elevates the stay sutures as he gently dissects the ureter away from the underlying artery under direct vision. The object is to free the ureter on the underside while preserving its attachment to the anterior peritoneum.

Figure 8. The ureter has been mobilized posteriorly and freed from the anterior peritoneum for a distance of about 1 inch. The medial leaf of the peritoneal flap is placed on tension as the surgeon sections the peritoneum transversely about 3/4 inch below the most distal excursion of the ureter.

Figure 9. The assistant now pulls the stay sutures toward the symphysis, and the surgeon incises the peritoneum medial to the ureter in an upward direction. The result is a peritoneal flap with ureter adherent to its undersurface.

Figure 10. The peritoneal flap with attached ureter is evident. The sigmoid is then brought over to meet the severed end of the mobilized ureter. A longitudinal incision is made in the anterolateral surface of the sigmoid in the long axis at a point where the sigmoid lies in proximity to the ureter without tension.

Figure 11. The sigmoid is elevated with the left hand and steadied as the surgeon incises the serosal and muscle coats down to but not through the mucosa. The incision extends for a distance of about 1 inch.

Figure 12. Fine-tooth forceps and eye scissors are needed for the meticulous dissection necessary to separate the sigmoid mucosa from the overlying muscle. The assistant keeps the seromuscular coat on tension while the surgeon divides the fine tissue bands holding the mucosa to the muscle. A flap approximately 1/2 inch wide should be developed on each side. Great care must be taken not to perforate the mucosa. A seromuscular trough has been created in the bowel wall.

Figure 13. With a grooved director as a guide and the ureter on tension the open end of the ureter is enlarged by incising the posterior wall upward in the long axis for a distance of about 1/4 inch.

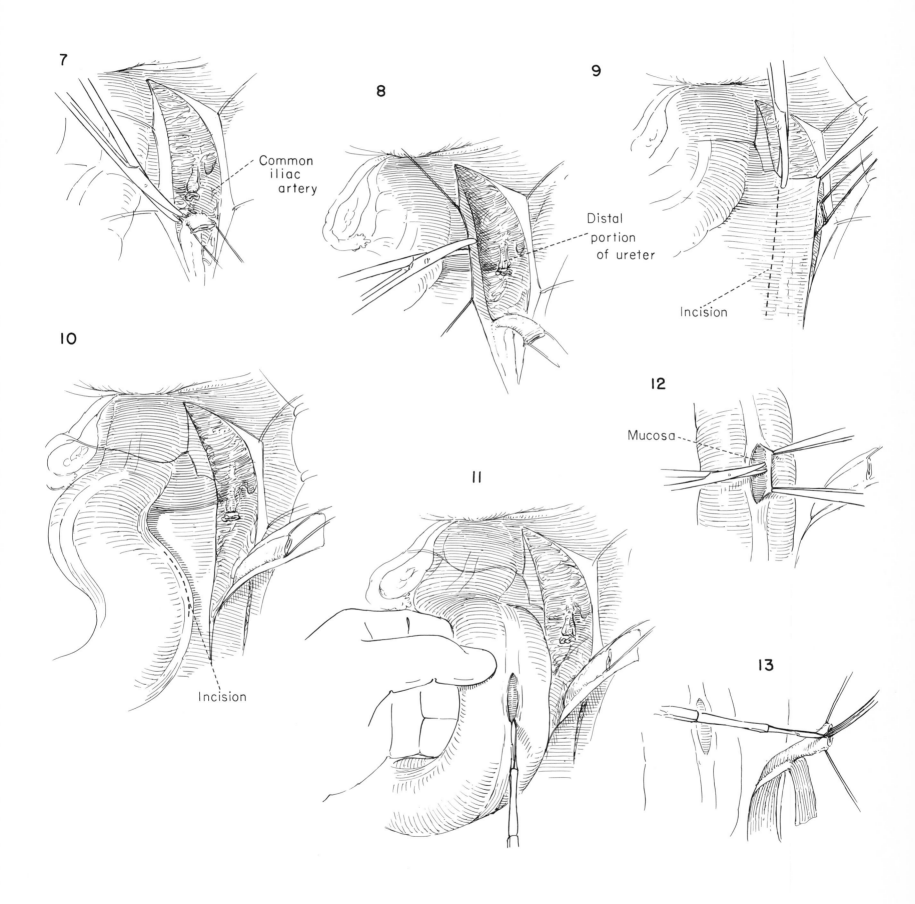

7

8

Common
iliac
artery

9

Distal
portion
of ureter

Incision

10

Incision

11

12

Mucosa

13

Figure 14. The surgeon places a fine atraumatic suture at the upper end of the incision in the ureter, through the entire thickness of the wall, as the assistant holds the ureter on stretch.

Figure 15. The bowel lumen is entered by incising the mucosa for about ¼ inch at the lower end of the trough previously fashioned in the sigmoid.

Figure 16. The fine atraumatic suture which passed from the outside of the ureteral wall into the lumen of the ureter now enters the inside of the bowel to emerge on the outer side of the mucosa. This suture is tied.

Figures 17 and 18. These show the series of interrupted sutures in such a manner that full thickness of ureter is sutured to sigmoid mucosa. This is slow, painstaking work.

Figure 19. The uretero-intestinal anastomosis is now complete. The seromuscular edges of the trough are now loosely closed over the ureter with interrupted sutures. The ureter must lie in the bed without tension or compression and without suggestion of constriction at the point where it enters the serosal tunnel. The peritoneal flap hangs free.

Figure 20. The cut edge of the peritoneal flap covering the ureter is then sutured to the sigmoid wall with interrupted silk sutures. The flap must lie easily as a patch over the ureter without kinking. For this reason the distal end of the peritoneal flap is placed first.

Figure 21. Interrupted silk sutures are placed at spaced intervals to complete the peritonealization of the ureter. The peritoneal flap not only covers the ureter and seals the anastomosis, but also serves to fill the cardinal principle of all uretero-intestinal anastomoses that the sigmoid must be brought to the ureter and fixed.

Figure 22. The fixation of the sigmoid may be further enhanced by interrupted sutures of catgut to the right lateral pelvic peritoneum both below and above the flap.

The operation is completed by closing the defect in the peritoneum with a running atraumatic catgut suture.

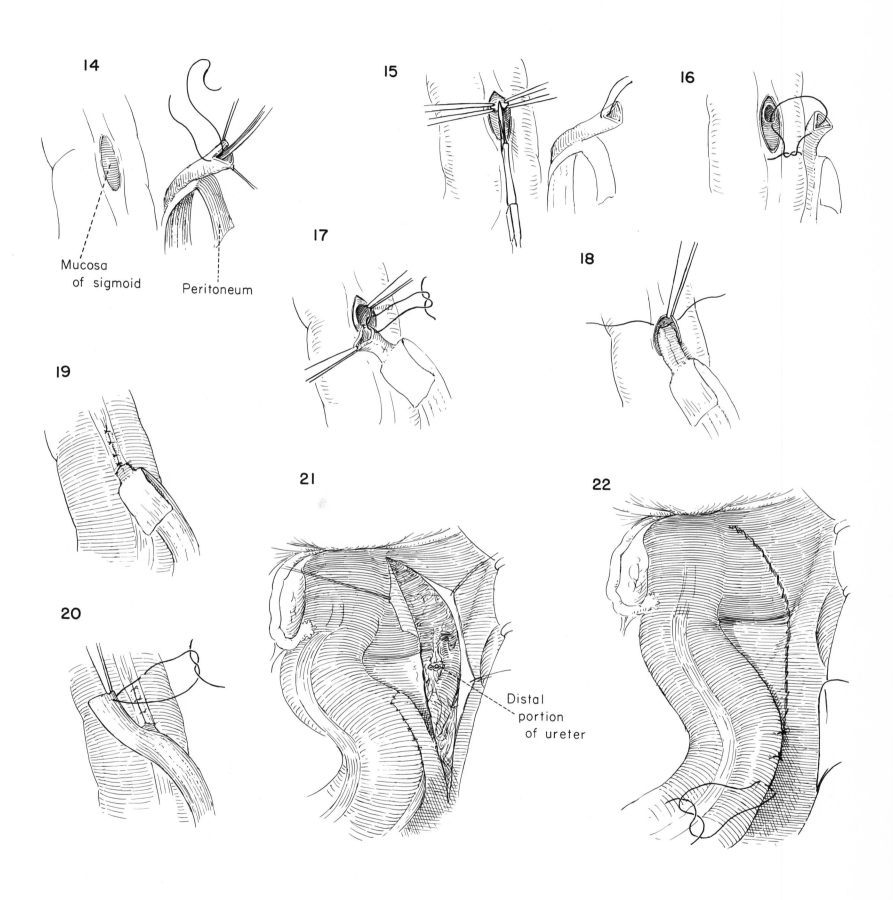

14

Mucosa
of sigmoid

Peritoneum

15

16

17

18

19

20

21

Distal
portion
of ureter

22

SKIN URETEROSTOMY

The surgeon is confronted with a severe problem when the ureter is badly damaged at a level which makes either an end-to-end suture or a transplant into the bladder impossible. There are several alternatives left to the operator: (1) He may take a calculated risk and transplant the damaged ureter into the sigmoid, despite the fact that the bowel has not been adequately prepared with antibiotic drugs. (2) He may deliberately ligate the divided ureter provided he has reasonable evidence that the kidney pelvis is not infected. If the kidney does flare up, a nephrectomy will be required later; if it does not, the kidney will atrophy silently. (3) He may elect to do a nephrectomy rather than divert the urinary stream to the bowel. (4) He may attempt a skin ureterostomy.

Adequate length of ureter is essential in deciding for or against creating a skin ureterostomy. An excess length is an asset for there is a marked tendency of the ureter to retract. Obstruction, usually at the fascial level, is not uncommon. This is less often seen with a dilated ureter than with a normal one. The surgeon will be well advised to leave a ureteral catheter in place and to change it at regular intervals in the convalescent period. This may cut down on the complications arising from the obstruction.

The same technique for fashioning a skin ureterostomy may be used for diverting the urinary stream in the radical extirpation operations for pelvic cancer.

Figure 1. The technical problems are more troublesome on the left side because of the presence of the sigmoid. The sigmoid is retracted toward the midline and steadied by an assistant. The common iliac artery is identified. No ureter can be seen at this point. The assistant steadies the sigmoid while the surgeon picks up and divides the posterior parietal peritoneum above the level of the artery in the course of the normal path of the ureter.

Figure 2. Stay sutures are placed on the divided edges of the peritoneum. The dilated proximal end of the ureter is found and traced to the narrow point of obstruction.

Figure 3. The periureteral tissue is dissected as the assistant keeps the ureter under tension, and instruments are used as gently as possible.

Figure 4. A cleavage plane between the ureter and surrounding bed is developed and a heavy silk suture passed beneath the ureter. This is tied and held long, stay sutures are placed, and the ureter is divided with a sharp knife. To reduce the amount of spillage, a suction tip should be available.

Figure 5. The assistant elevates the ureter gently out of its bed by traction on the stay sutures as the surgeon mobilizes the ureter from the underlying tissue. Here, as in other operations on the ureter, the surgeon should try to establish the cleavage plane in the tissues around the ureter, staying away from the actual ureter itself in order to protect its blood supply. It may, however, be necessary to free up the ureter as far as the kidney pelvis.

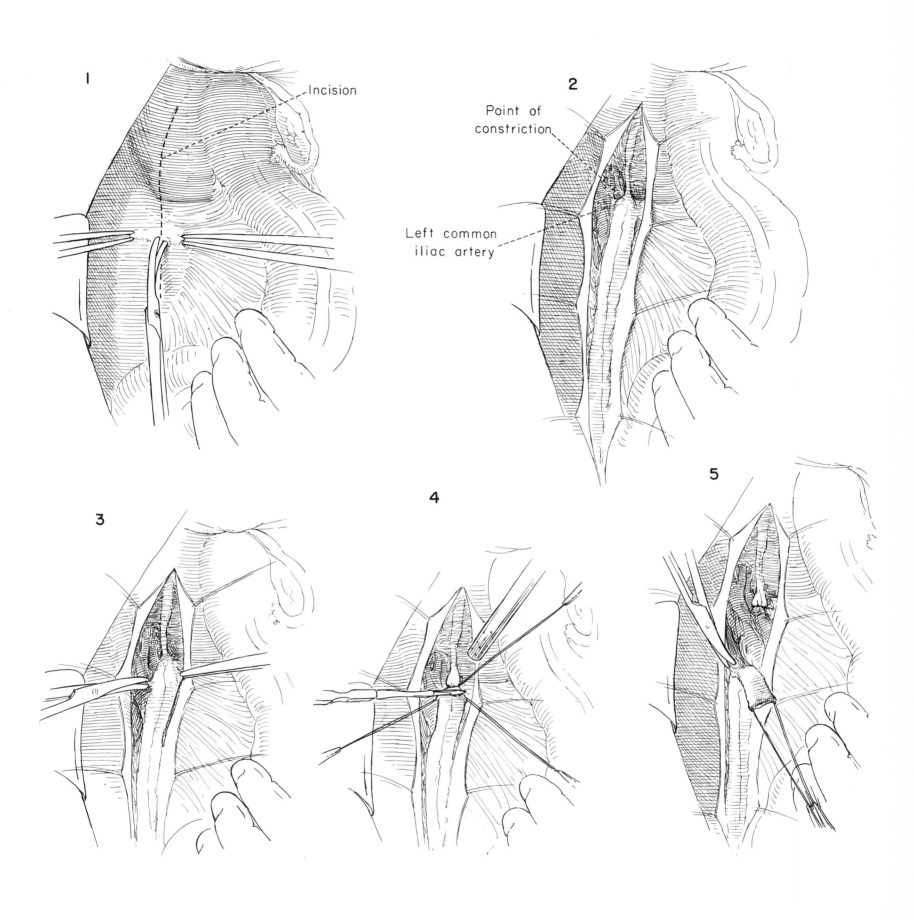

1   Incision

2   Point of constriction   Left common iliac artery

3

4

5

Figure 6. With the ureter thoroughly mobilized the surgeon now directs his attention to the anterior abdominal wall. Kelly clamps are placed at widely separated intervals on the peritoneum. With the handle of the knife the surgeon then peels the peritoneofascial layer away from the abdominal wall musculature.

Figure 7. The peritoneum has been separated from the muscles for a considerable distance. A Kelly clamp is then inserted in the tissue plane created by the separation of the peritoneum. The tip of the clamp emerges from beneath the peritoneum at the site of the ureteral dissection. The surgeon then grasps the stay sutures on the ureter and pulls it into the retroperitoneal tissue plane.

Figure 8. The site of the ostium for the skin ureterostomy will be determined by the thickness of the abdominal wall in relation to the length of available ureter. The optimum position would be on the anterior abdominal wall at about the level of the anterior superior spine in the nipple line. If the ureter is short it may be necessary to place it higher up and more to the lateral side.

With the proper landmark established the surgeon picks up the skin with a clamp and excises a full thickness disc with a knife.

Figure 9. The incision is carried down through the fat of the abdominal wall and enough is removed to expose the underlying rectus fascia.

Figure 10. Small curved retractors in the edges of the skin incision help in obtaining exposure of the fascia. Since skin ureterostomies are prone to constrict at the fascia level it is important that a circular section of the fascia be removed. To facilitate this a cruciate type of incision is made in the fascia.

Figure 11. The surgeon then grasps the full thickness of the abdominal wall with his left hand while he guides a Kelly clamp through the skin incision and into the retroperitoneal space.

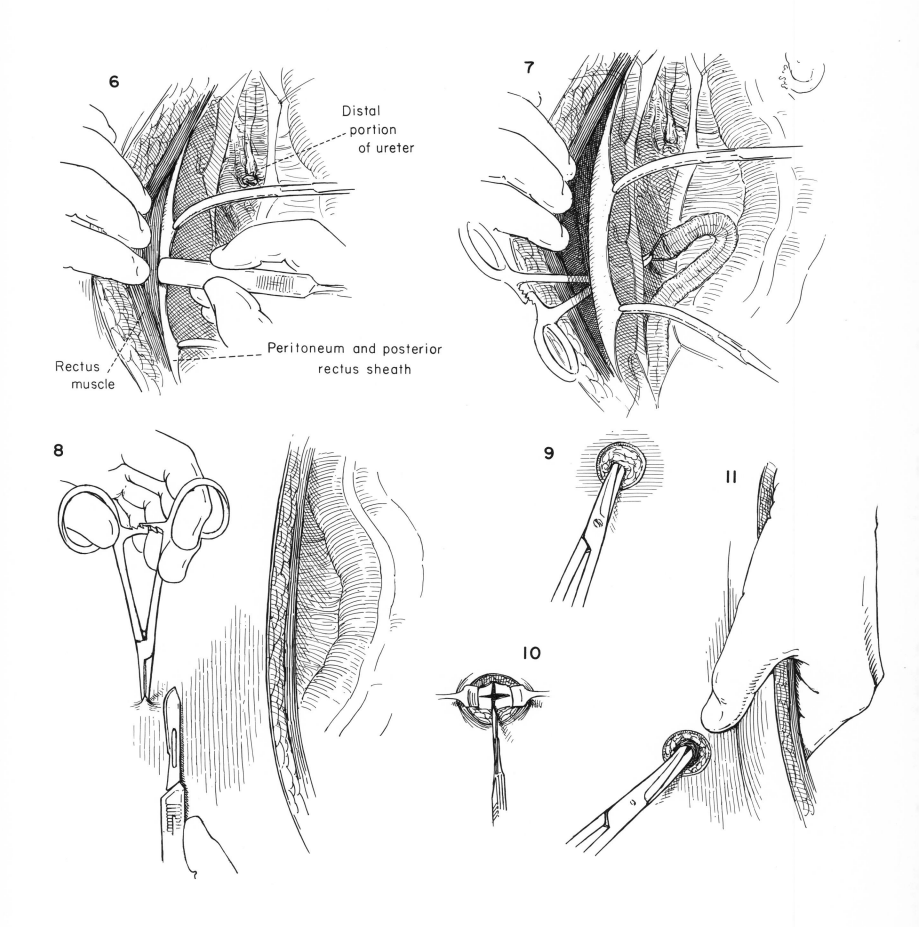

6

Distal
portion
of ureter

Rectus
muscle

Peritoneum and posterior
rectus sheath

7

8

9

10

11

Figure 12.   To provide exposure of the retroperitoneal space the assistant applies traction medially while the surgeon retracts the full thickness of the abdominal wall. The ureter with the stay sutures attached to the end can be seen lying in the depths of the wound. The Kelly clamp enters the retroperitoneal space to grasp the sutures left on the severed proximal end of the ureter. The ligated distal cut end of the ureter can be seen in the upper portion of the illustration lying behind the divided posterior peritoneum. Stay sutures are in place on the edges of the medial leaf.

Figure 13.   The Kelly clamp now pulls the ureter gently through the opening created in the muscle and fascial layers of the abdominal wall.

Figure 14.   The caliber of the normal ureter is too small to permit it to be fixed to the skin. It must be fixed or retraction will occur regardless of the length of the ureter. To widen the ostium a longitudinal incision is made in the wall on the side opposite the one containing the blood supply as the assistant keeps the ureter on tension.

Figure 15.   The ureteral end, after the incision has been made in the long axis, has now a spatula-like appearance. Traction is exerted on the sutures to obtain adequate length. The end of the ureter should come through the opening with ease.

Figure 16.   Fine sutures of chromic catgut are placed in interrupted fashion along the periphery of the ureter, anchoring the full thickness of the ureteral edge to the skin.

Figure 17.   The ureteral ostium is now complete. It is always advisable to insert a fine bore Foley type ureteral catheter in the skin ureterostomy. It is advanced upward as far as the kidney pelvis and is left in place.

Figure 18.   Before inflation of the balloon attachment the position of the catheter within the ureter should be checked. This is done by injecting saline solution into the catheter lumen. If there is any obstruction to the passage of fluid, or blood appears, the catheter is too far into the kidney pelvis and must be withdrawn until a free flow occurs. The balloon is then inflated to hold the catheter in place and to counteract the force of normal peristalsis.

Figure 19.   A silk suture is placed around the catheter, several turns are taken and it is then fastened to the skin.

Figure 20.   The wound edge is held back with a retractor as the posterior peritoneal incision is closed with a running catgut suture. The ligated distal end of the ureter is seen at the upper end of the illustration behind the peritoneum.

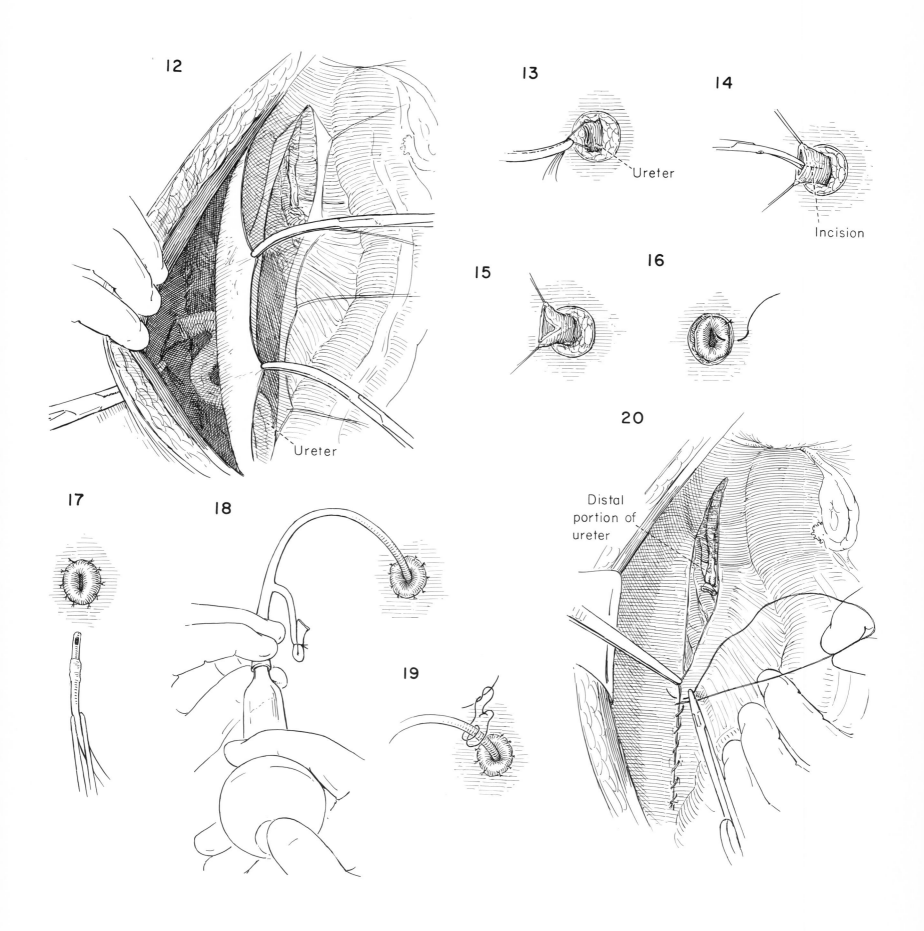

12

13

Ureter

14

Incision

15

16

20

Distal portion of ureter

Ureter

17

18

19

Operations on the Abdominal Wall

PFANNENSTIEL INCISION

The paramedian incision is generally used when it is necessary to enter the abdomen for pelvic pathology. Among other advantages, such as providing opportunity to thoroughly explore the abdomen, it permits wider latitude in carrying out procedures in the pelvis over and above those originally planned.

When the symptoms and physical findings suggest that disease is confined to the uterus and adnexa, the surgeon may elect to perform a transverse lower abdominal incision of the Pfannenstiel type. Procedures such as myomectomy, salpingectomy, oophorectomy, suspension operations and hysterectomy when the uterus is freely movable and there is no question of associated disease can all be satisfactorily managed through a Pfannenstiel incision. Though the skin is incised in a transverse direction, the muscles are separated but not sectioned. The cosmetic effect is excellent and the resulting wound strong. It has the psychological advantage of being hidden from view and is not a constant reminder to the patient that she has had a pelvic operation. It is also a very comfortable incision.

Any exposure beyond the pelvis, however, is difficult and the surgeon will be wise if he restricts its use to patients who are not fat and whose pelvic disease will not require extensive lateral dissection or the removal of large masses.

Figure 1. A curved incision is made just above the hairline, extending beyond the border of the rectus muscles on both sides. If it is placed near the symphysis, the subcutaneous fat interferes with clean wound healing. The lateral extension of the incision provides mobility of the skin flap that must be turned up.

Figure 2. The bleeding vessels are secured and tied and skin towels applied. The assistant holds up on Kelly clamps placed on the superior edge of the incised fascia on either side of the linea alba as the surgeon completes the section of the fascia in the midline.

Figure 3. Another Kelly clamp is placed on the lower fascial edge and elevated to expose the lateral margin of the rectus. The surgeon then extends the fascial incision laterally.

Figure 4. Kelly clamps placed on the lower fascial edge are elevated by the assistant as the surgeon separates the sheath from the underlying lower rectus muscles with the knife handle. The pyramidalis muscle remains attached to the fascia.

Figure 5. The upper segment of anterior rectus sheath is freed from the underlying muscles in a similar manner.

Figure 6. Individual vessels can be seen arising in the muscle and perforating the fascia. These vessels must be clamped, divided and tied as they are encountered.

Figure 7. The separation of fascia from muscle proceeds in the direction of the umbilicus, as the assistant continues to elevate the Kelly clamps. The dissection is carried upward far enough to permit an adequate midline longitudinal incision.

ABDOMINAL WALL PROCEDURES
PFANNENSTIEL INCISION

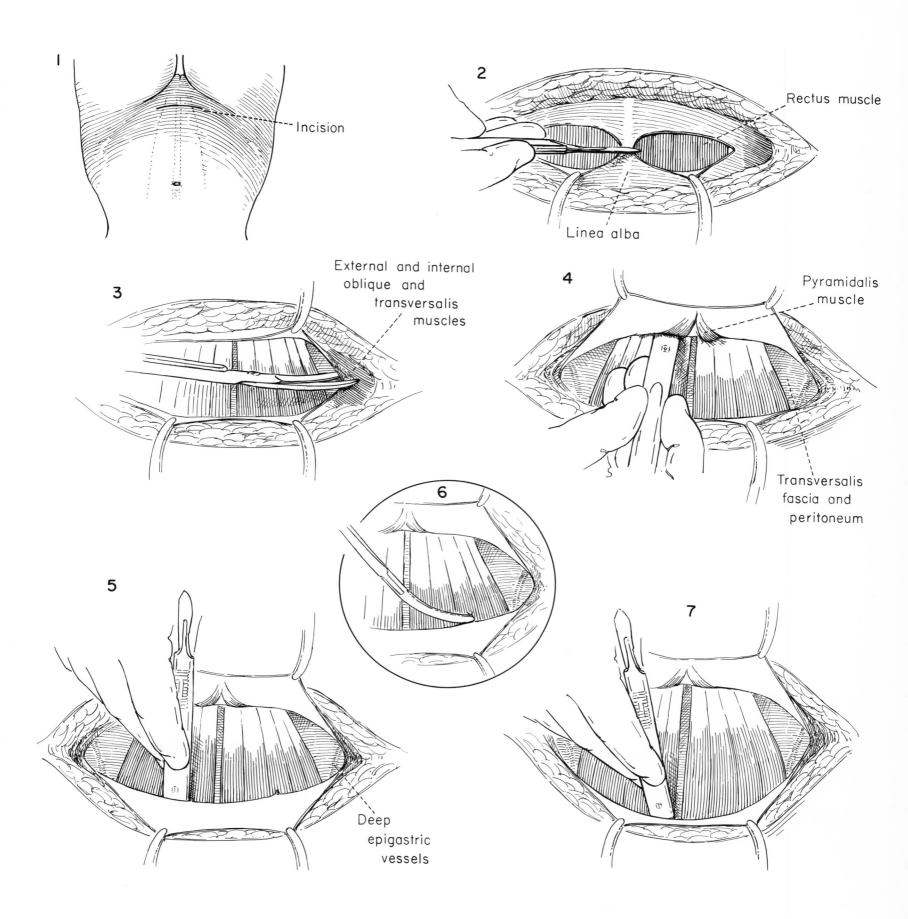

1

— Incision

2

Rectus muscle

Linea alba

External and internal
oblique and
transversalis
muscles

3

4

Pyramidalis
muscle

Transversalis
fascia and
peritoneum

6

5

7

Deep
epigastric
vessels

Figure 8. The rectus muscles are separated from the transversalis fascia and peritoneum in the midline by elevation of the medial borders with forceps and gentle dissection with the knife handle.

Figure 9. The assistant and surgeon pick up the fascia and peritoneum with toothed forceps opposite one another as the surgeon begins the incision into the abdominal cavity. This should be well above the symphysis pubis to avoid the possibility of damage to the bladder.

Figure 10. A Deaver retractor is placed in the upper margin of the wound to expose the extent of the separation of anterior sheath from the muscles. Kelly clamps are placed on the peritoneal edges and the peritoneum divided in upward and downward directions as the surgeon provides protection to the small bowel by inserting the index and middle fingers beneath the peritoneum in the line of incision.

Closure of the Pfannenstiel Incision

Figure 11. Closure of the peritoneum and transversalis fascia begins at the upper end of the wound. A running atraumatic chromic catgut suture approximates serosal surfaces of the peritoneum as the assistant keeps the suture on tension and the surgeon elevates the incised edges of the two layers with toothed forceps.

Figure 12. A stronger closure will result if the rectus muscles are approximated in the midline by interrupted plain catgut sutures.

Figure 13. Any bleeding points beneath the fascial flap must be secured and the wound must be completely dry before the fascial defect is closed. It is closed with interrupted silk sutures. The assistant leaves each suture long until the next is tied, and elevates each one in turn to aid the surgeon in placing the next stitch. Small drains should be placed in the lateral angles of the wound beneath the fascia level, since these wounds carry the potential danger of hematoma formation. The drains should be removed in 48 hours.

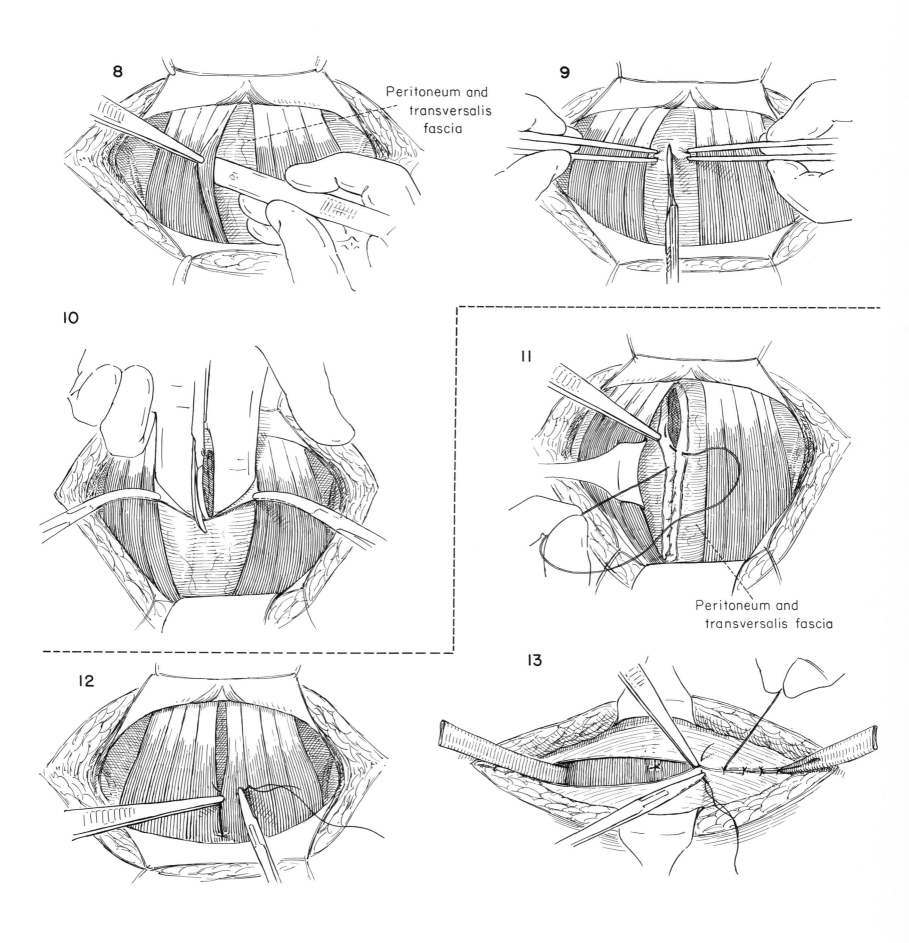

TRANSVERSE INCISION

When there is no question that the disease process is localized in the lower pelvis, the transverse low abdominal incision dividing the rectus muscles has much to recommend it. The chief advantages are that, after division of the muscle, little retraction and packing back of the intestine are necessary. This incision gives a much wider exposure to the deep pelvis than can be obtained by the Pfannenstiel approach.

The advantages over the Pfannenstiel type of incision include the following: (1) Because of the division of the rectus muscles, the incision tends to gape open and a maximum amount of exposure is obtained with a minimum amount of retraction. (2) With the patient in Trendelenburg position the bowel shows little tendency to get in the way and very little gauze is needed to keep the intestine out of the operative field. The sparse use of gauze minimizes the handling of intestine, a cause of postoperative gas pains. (3) The Trendelenburg position makes anesthetization easier.

The transverse incision has definite disadvantages, however. These center around the necessity to divide the rectus muscle. The incision is difficult to close and the chances of hernia are correspondingly greater. There is also a tendency for the muscle to bleed, which increases the likelihood of hematoma formation and wound sepsis despite the use of drains in the angles of the wound.

When used electively, the advantages tend to outweigh the disadvantages.

Figure 1. The transverse incision is made in the abdominal wall approximately 2 inches above the symphysis pubis; it extends to the inguinal ligament on both sides.

Figure 2. The skin and subcutaneous fat are divided down to fascia, bleeding vessels are controlled, and protective towels are applied to the wound edges. The assistant and the surgeon retract the skin edges as the surgeon incises the fascia overlying each rectus muscle.

Figure 3. The surgeon divides the linea alba while the assistant holds the upper border of the fascial edge on tension with Kelly clamps placed to either side of the midline.

Figure 4. To completely expose the lateral border of the rectus muscle, clamps are placed at the angles of the fascial incision, and the incision is carried laterally to the full extent of the fascial envelope which encloses the rectus muscle.

Figure 5. The surgeon then separates the transversalis fascia and peritoneum from the undersurface of the rectus by gently passing the gloved index finger beneath the muscle. Occasionally the thin, adherent transversalis fascia may interfere with complete exposure by the fingertip. In this case the surgeon then lightly incises the fascia with a knife as he pushes the fascia upward to bulge into the wound.

Figure 6. The index finger of the surgeon's left hand is then inserted beneath the right rectus muscle from the lateral side to the midline. The surgeon elevates the muscle as he begins to divide its fibers transversely.

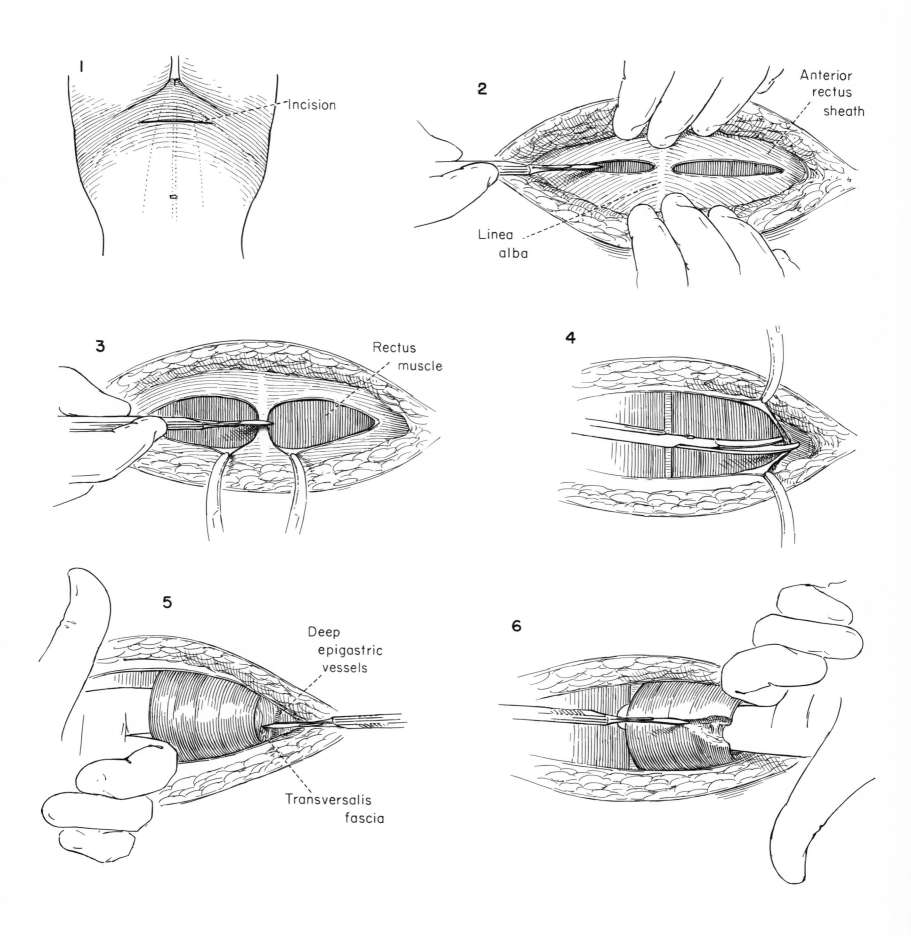

1 — Incision

2 — Anterior rectus sheath — Linea alba

3 — Rectus muscle

4

5 — Deep epigastric vessels — Transversalis fascia

6

Figure 7. The assistant secures any bleeding vessels as they appear in the transection of the muscle and ties them. Because of the absence of any posterior sheath at this level, the upper end of the muscle bundle will retract sharply if it is completely divided at this stage. This will make the reconstructive phase more complicated. The index finger is placed beneath the muscle bundle as the surgeon divides it to the point where only a few muscle fibers remain.

Figure 8. To keep the divided muscle and anterior rectus sheath together as one bundle and avoid the retraction, mattress sutures are placed through the overlying fascia and muscle at the medial and lateral angles. The sutures are left long and clamped with hemostats. Only the upper end need be handled in this way.

Figure 9. The surgeon elevates the remaining muscle fibers and divides them, completing the incision through the entire bundle.

Figure 10. Bleeding points are sought for and controlled. The assistant then elevates the lateral stay sutures while the surgeon places a third mattress suture in the midportion of the divided muscle. The same steps are carried out on the left rectus muscle.

Figure 11. The surgeon and the assistant then pick up the peritoneofascial layer with toothed forceps in the center of the exposure. The forceps and incision should be placed in the middle of the exposed layer in order to avoid the dome of the bladder, which lies just beneath. The obliterated hypogastric vessels can be seen lying on the peritoneum on either side of the midline. The surgeon then prepares to divide the peritoneum between the elevated forceps.

Figure 12. The abdominal cavity has been entered. The surgeon and the assistant now provide further exposure by inserting gloved fingers into the opening of the peritoneum and elevating it. The peritoneal incision is then continued laterally in both directions. Care must be taken not to damage the deep epigastric vessels which lie on the peritoneum at the lateral margins of the wound.

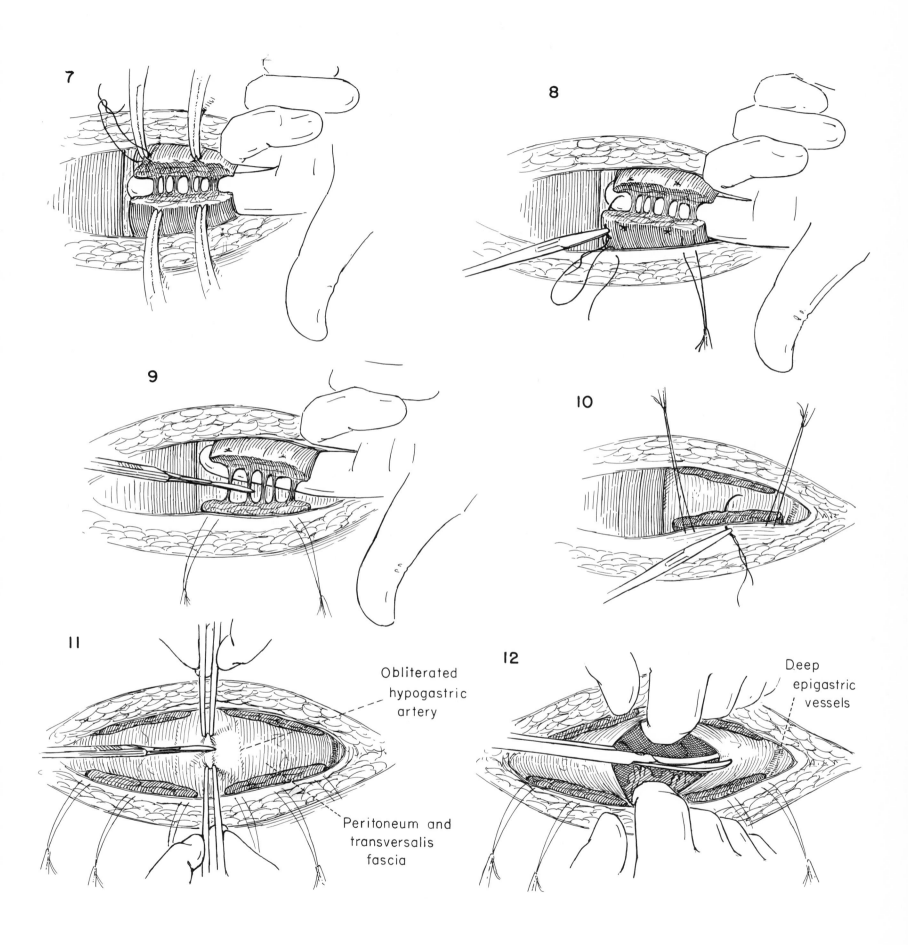

7

8

9

10

11 Obliterated
hypogastric
artery

Peritoneum and
transversalis
fascia

12 Deep
epigastric
vessels

Closure of Transverse Incision

The abdominal operation has been completed and the wound is now ready for closure.

The repair portion of the transverse type of incision is the most difficult stage of the procedure. There is unquestioned disadvantage in dividing rather than separating the muscles as is done in the Pfannenstiel incision. The operator must be most meticulous in the reconstructive phase of the operation to prevent subsequent development of a hernia. For gynecological operations the muscles are usually divided a short distance above their attachment to the symphysis. At this point there is no posterior fascial sheath to keep the deeper portions of the muscle bundle from retracting. The wound must be kept very dry and all bleeding vessels controlled to prevent a hematoma and potential wound sepsis. If the surgeon is aware of these facts and exercises great care, the muscles can be satisfactorily apposed and a successful closure obtained.

Figure 13. The surgeon closes the peritoneum and transversalis fascia with a running chromic catgut suture.

Figure 14. The assistant now elevates the stay sutures previously placed through the muscle and fascia of the upper rectus muscle. The surgeon begins to place the first mattress suture through the fascia and muscle of the upper bundle, beginning at the lateral margin.

Figure 15. The first leg of the mattress suture then continues to the lower muscle bundle, is carried from beneath the muscle to the superior surface of the fascia, and is then returned through the fascia and muscle about ¼ inch away.

Figure 16. The assistant again elevates the upper rectus muscle with the traction sutures as the surgeon begins to return the mattress suture through muscle and fascia from the inferior surface of the muscle. The mattress suture is completed as the needle emerges on the superior surface of the fascia approximately ¼ inch medial to the point of origin and parallel to it.

Figure 17. An entire series of these mattress sutures is placed through the upper and lower muscle bundles on both sides. The initial stay sutures have been removed and the mattress sutures have been tied on the right side.

Figure 18. The fascial edges are then brought together over the approximated rectus muscle bundles with interrupted catgut sutures.

Figure 19. The fat is approximated with interrupted sutures. Small drains are placed in the lateral angles of the wound beyond the rectus muscles, and are removed within 48 hours. The skin is closed in the usual way.

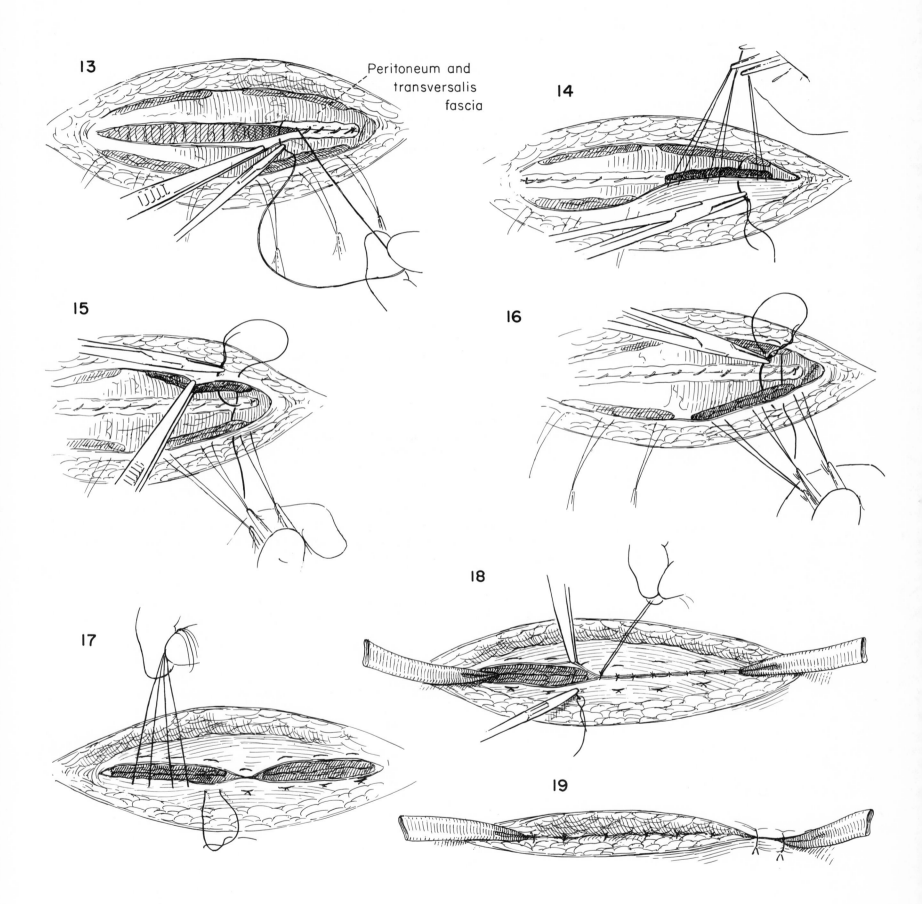

Peritoneum and transversalis fascia

13

14

15

16

17

18

19

INCISIONAL HERNIA

An abdominal operation performed through a longitudinal incision may so weaken both the fascia and the muscle of the lower abdominal wall that the peritoneum and abdominal contents herniate through the defect. The hernia may include the entire incision, but more commonly is located in the lower portion of the wound.

The basic principle in attacking any hernia is to establish normal anatomical landmarks before attempting to dissect out the hernial sac. The best way to do this is to identify normal fascia lateral to the hernial sac. The dissection is then carried out on all sides of the hernia. The surgeon now turns his attention to the sac itself. This is then freed up from the underlying fascia, moving medially toward the central defect. Since an adequate repair depends on reapposition of the muscles in the midline without tension, the extent of lateral excursion of the muscles must be determined and the muscle bundles mobilized so they will fall easily into place.

Figure 1. The old scar is to be excised. The redundancy of the skin will determine the amount to be sacrificed.

Figure 2. Bleeding vessels are clamped and tied. The old skin incision with attached fat is dissected from the normal fascia in the lower portion of the wound. It is important to identify the normal fascia in relation to the central defect.

Figure 3. Inasmuch as the hernia may have lateral extension, the dissection must proceed with care. The assistant draws the hernial defect toward him to permit the surgeon to dissect the lateral prolongation of the hernia from the underlying fascia.

Figure 4. The central defect in the fascia has been identified throughout its circumference. The fat of the abdominal wall is being dissected back laterally.

Figure 5. The surgeon draws the peritoneum overlying the hernia taut as he outlines the lateral extent of the hernia and divides the fascia, exposing the medial edge of the rectus muscle beneath. The extension of the incision will follow the dotted lines.

Figure 6. The surgeon elevates the divided fascial edge and mobilizes the rectus muscle from the fascia above as well as the peritoneum below. The muscle is then freed around its entire circumference.

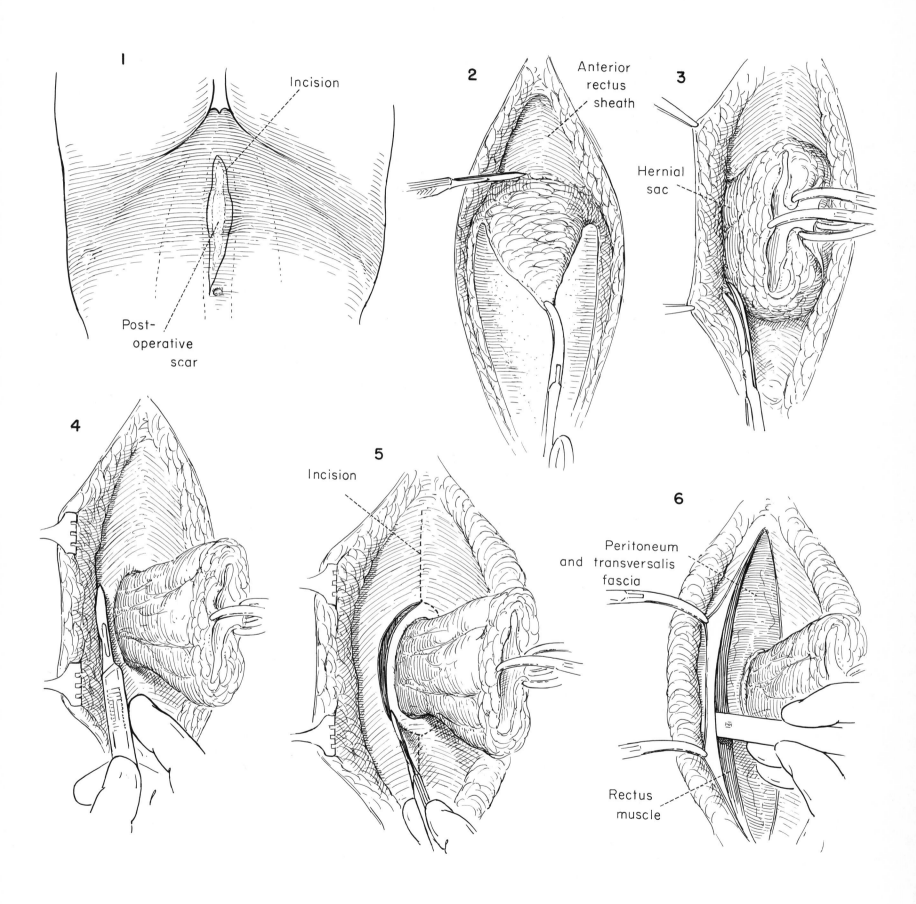

1

Incision

Post-
operative
scar

2

Anterior
rectus
sheath

3

Hernial
sac

4

5

Incision

6

Peritoneum
and transversalis
fascia

Rectus
muscle

Figure 7. The muscle edge is evident around the entire border of the central hernia. The first assistant and surgeon gently pick up the fascio-peritoneal covering in the lateral center of the hernial sac. Omentum and small bowel may be adherent to the undersurface. The incision is made through the peritoneum with great care.

Figure 8. The surgeon's forefinger is gently inserted in the peritoneal opening and any omental attachment teased off. Hemostats are placed on the cut edges to provide traction and to increase the exposure. Adherent bowel must be dissected free.

Figure 9. The hernial sac, now free of all attachments, is excised and the peritoneum opened for a short distance above and below.

Figure 10. The omentum is drawn over the small intestine to prevent adhesion to the new incision. The peritoneum and transversalis fascia are now closed with a running chromic catgut suture.

Figure 11. The rectus muscles are approximated in the midline with interrupted sutures of plain catgut.

Figures 12, 13 and 14. To strengthen the wound closure, a pulley type of catgut suture is used. In Figure 12 the suture in the fascia has been started on the right, close to the edge. It then passes beneath the fascia on the opposite side, emerging approximately ¾ inch from the edge. In Figure 13 the suture returns to the right side and enters the fascia on the superior surface at the same distance from the edge. In Figure 14 the suture emerges close to the left fascial edge. The result is a vertical figure-of-eight suture. Tying of the suture produces a stay suture effect.

Figure 15. The sutures are tied and the interstices closed with interrupted sutures.

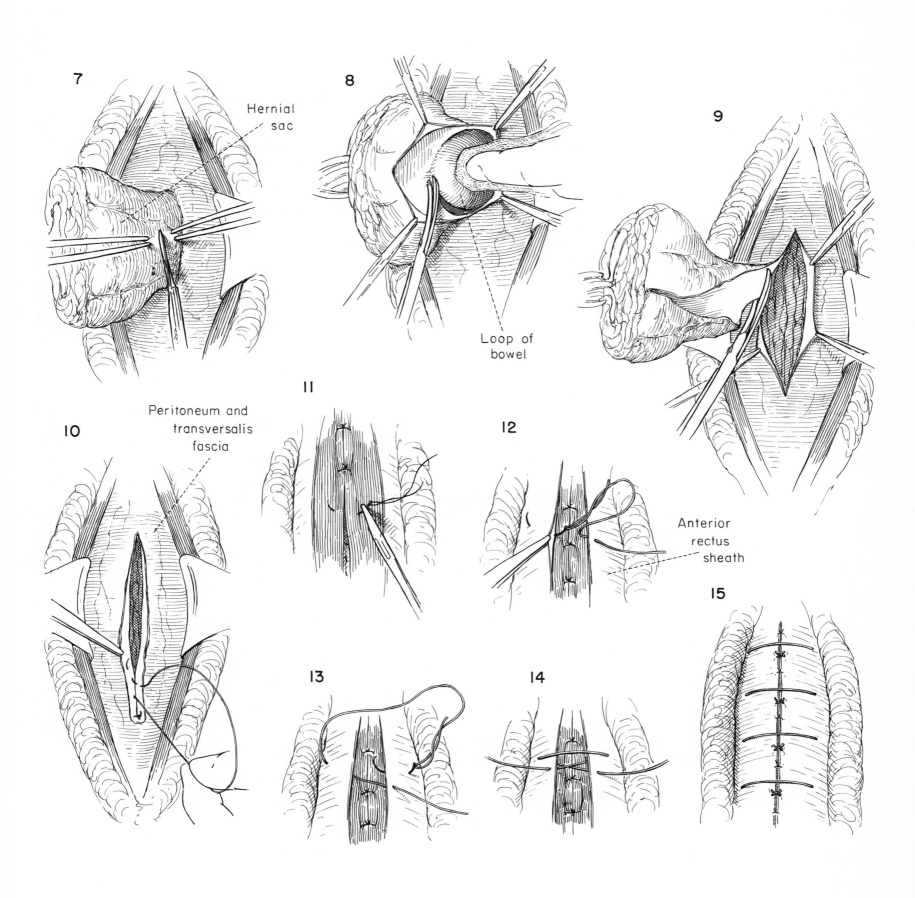

7

Hernial
sac

8

Loop of
bowel

9

Peritoneum and
transversalis
fascia

10

11

12

Anterior
rectus
sheath

15

13

14

REINFORCEMENT OF HERNIA REPAIR BY FASCIA LATA

Despite the increasing use of wire as suture material, there remains a definite place for fascial repair to reinforce a weakened abdominal wall.

Figure 1. The preliminary steps have repaired the hernia. The fascia is now being closed with interrupted sutures of silk, cotton or wire.

Figure 2. Retractors placed in a small transverse skin incision in the upper thigh provide exposure for a 1/2-inch incision in the fascia.

Figure 3. Short longitudinal incisions are made in the fascia at either end of the transverse incision.

Figure 4. The cut end of fascia is drawn through the end of a fascia stripper and grasped with a clamp.

Figure 5. The clamp is steadied as the stripper is thrust down the leg beneath the skin for its entire length. Rotation of a wheel severs the fascial strip at the distal end, and the strip is withdrawn.

Figures 6, 7 and 8. A silk suture designed to prevent fraying is placed through and around the divided end and firmly tied.

Figure 9. The prepared end is threaded on a Gallie needle, and the loose end is sutured to the long fascial strand to prevent its pulling out of the needle. The fascial strip is used as a running suture, beginning in the fascia at the lower end of the wound.

Figure 10. The needle passes through the fascial strip below the ligated end to anchor it.

Figure 11. The free end is tacked to the rectus fascia with interrupted silk sutures.

Figure 12. The continuous running suture of fascia should be applied without tension.

Figure 13. The fascial suture passes through the midportion of the strand at the upper end.

Figure 14. The fascial strip with needle attached is then divided, leaving a free end which must be anchored.

Figure 15. The free end is sutured to the underlying fascia with interrupted silk sutures.

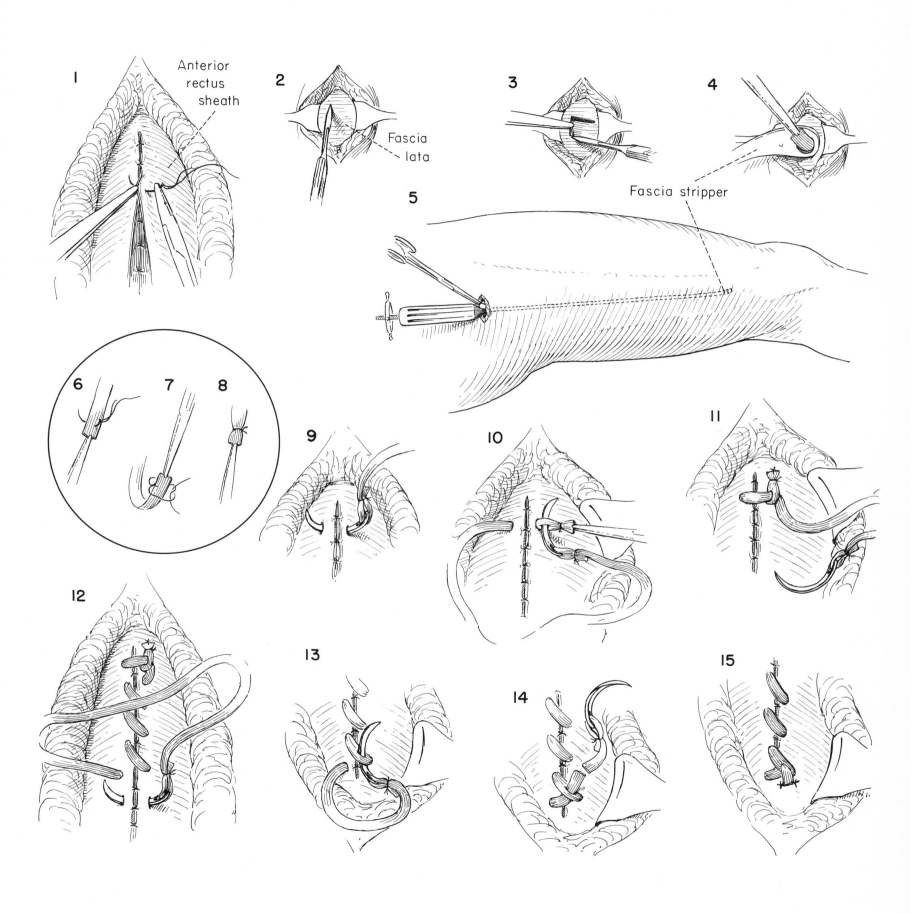

1
Anterior
rectus
sheath

2
Fascia
lata

3

4
Fascia stripper

5

6 7 8

9

10

11

12

13

14

15

INGUINAL HERNIA

An inguinal hernia in the female occurs far less often and is much easier to repair than the same abdominal wall weakness in the male. A more complete closure of the inguinal canal is possible because the surgeon does not have to contend with the spermatic cord or be concerned with the blood supply to the testis. Better approximation of the external oblique fascia to Poupart's ligament is possible. If necessary, the round ligament may be sacrificed in the interest of a stronger repair.

Should reinforcement of the tissues used in repair be necessary the surgeon may construct a flap of external oblique fascia, leaving it attached at the spine of the pubis. The free end of the fascial strip may then be used as suture material to supplement the interrupted silk sutures which have brought the conjoined tendon, muscle and fascia to Poupart's ligament. This is the so-called McArthur modification of inguinal hernia repair.

The illustrations shown here portray the simple steps of an uncomplicated inguinal hernia.

Figure 1. The skin incision parallels Poupart's ligament from the anterior superior spine of the ilium to the pubic spine and about 1 inch above it.

Figure 2. The external oblique fascia is cleaned of fat and the external ring identified. The fascia is then divided in line with its fibers, care being taken not to injure the ilio-inguinal nerve lying just beneath it.

Figure 3. The edge of the internal oblique muscle is held back to permit the surgeon to identify the sac, which is then dissected from its bed. Careful dissection will avoid injury to the deep epigastric vessels, which lie at the medial border of the internal ring. Stay sutures on the edge of the external oblique fascia keep the operative field open.

Figure 4. After assuring himself that the sac contains no bowel the surgeon opens it and explores the interior with a finger.

Figure 5. A purse-string suture is placed around the inside of the neck of the sac under direct vision and tied.

Figure 6. An outside transfixion ligature distal to the purse string ensures complete closure. The ends of this suture are left long after tying, and the sac is amputated.

Figure 7. A needle is threaded on each long end of the transfixion ligature and brought out through the internal oblique muscle. When the two ends are tied, the neck of the sac is transplanted upward.

Figure 8. Repair is effected by approximating the conjoined tendon to the pubic spine and inner aspect of Poupart's ligament with multiple interrupted silk sutures.

Figure 9. The external oblique fascia is closed with sutures of the same material.

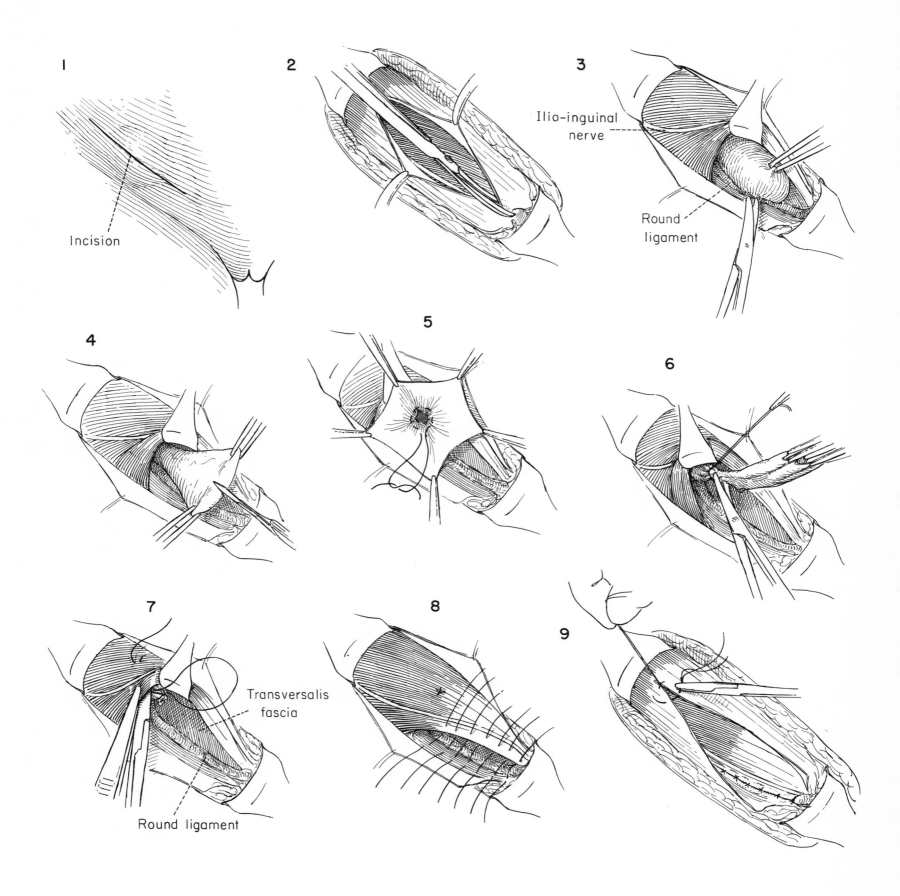

1

Incision

2

3

Ilio-inguinal nerve

Round ligament

4

5

6

7

Transversalis fascia

Round ligament

8

9

FEMORAL HERNIA

The Approach from below Poupart's Ligament

This is the most common type of hernia in the female. The repair may be accomplished in two ways: (1) The entire dissection of the sac may be carried out below the level of the inguinal ligament. The hernial sac is dissected free, the neck of the sac isolated and the opening closed. The defect beneath the inguinal ligament, medial to the femoral vessels, is then repaired by suturing Poupart's ligament to the underlying pectineus fascia. (2) The entire dissection of the hernial sac and the repair of the hernia may be carried through an incision above the inguinal ligament.

In this plate the direct approach from below Poupart's ligament will be illustrated.

Figure 1. The incision begins above Poupart's ligament and comes down into the thigh over the center of the presenting bulge. The femoral vessels are in contact with the hernia lateral to the incision.

Figure 2. The sac is encountered directly under the skin incision and is retracted with forceps and gently dissected from the medial attachment with scissors.

Figure 3. The surgeon draws the sac to the medial side and dissects along the lateral border, taking care not to damage the femoral vessels and saphenous vein.

Figure 4. The sac has been dissected free and the neck exposed. The dome is then gently incised.

Figure 5. The thin-walled sac may contain small intestine or omentum. Should the sac appear thickened, beware of a possible sliding hernia containing bladder wall or (if the hernia is on the left) large intestine. Pressure of the index finger in the sac returns the contents to the abdomen. Redundancy of omentum may be sacrificed. If the contents cannot be reduced, the operator should use the combined approach demonstrated on pages 177 and 179.

Figure 6. After identification of the neck of the sac a purse-string suture is used to close it.

Figure 7. The neck of the sac is then further closed with a transfixion suture. The femoral vessels should be retracted to prevent inadvertent damage.

Figure 8. The sac is held on traction and excised beyond the transfixing suture.

Figure 9. Retracting the femoral vessels, the surgeon now places the first suture of the repair. The interrupted sutures pass from Poupart's ligament above to the pectineus fascia below.

Figure 10. The defect in the femoral canal is now closed.

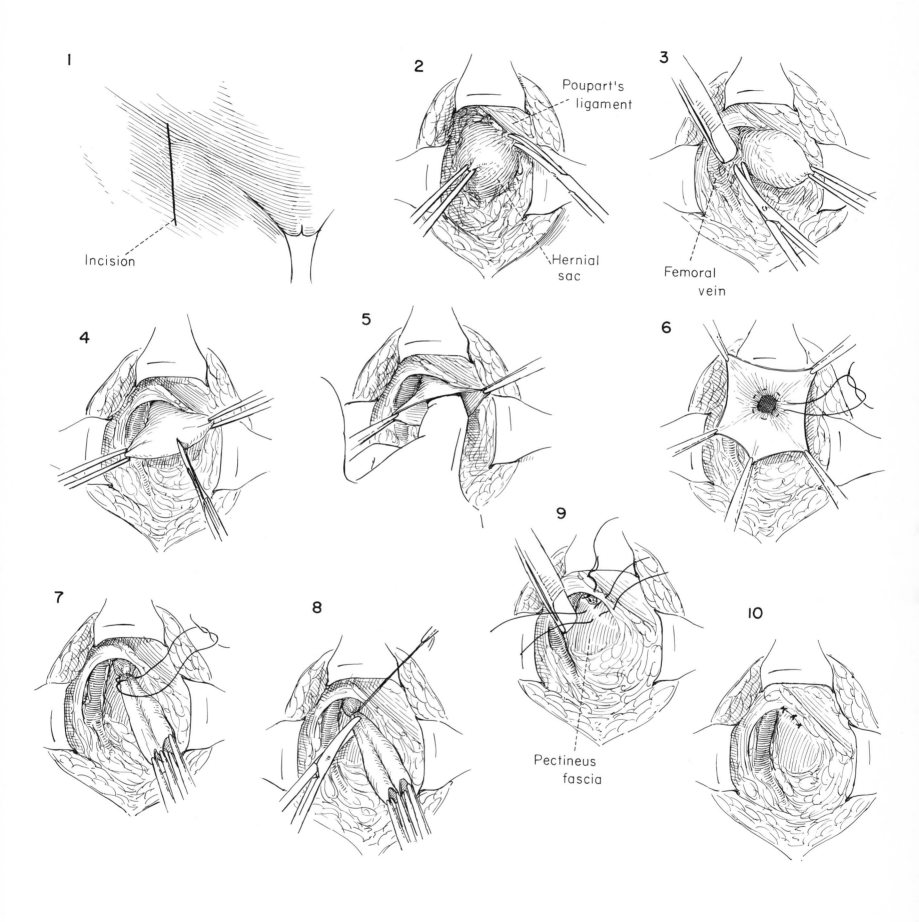

1

Incision

2

Poupart's ligament

Hernial sac

3

Femoral vein

4

5

6

7

8

9

Pectineus fascia

10

The Inguinal Approach

The best anatomical approach to the reduction and repair of a femoral hernia is made through the same incision one uses for an inguinal hernia repair. By dividing the fibers of the transversalis muscle at the base of the inguinal canal the surgeon approaches the sac at the site of its occurrence. By gentle dissection it is then possible to isolate the sac, draw it above Poupart's ligament, tie off the neck of the sac and close the incision in the manner of the repair of an inguinal hernia. In short, a femoral hernia has been converted to an inguinal hernia.

The repair is more effective because the defect in a femoral hernia is funnel shaped from above down. The attack can be made directly upon the base.

Figure 1. The incision parallels the inguinal ligament, about 1 inch above it, and runs from the spine of the pubis upward for about 3 inches.

Figure 2. The incision is carried down through the fat to the external oblique fascia. Bleeding points are controlled.

Figure 3. An incision is made through the external oblique fascia in the line of its fibers.

Figure 4. The ilio-inguinal nerve and round ligament are identified and the internal oblique muscle and conjoined tendon exposed. The round ligament is freed from the floor of the inguinal canal.

Figure 5. The internal oblique muscle and round ligament are then retracted upward. The transversalis fascia is opened in order to expose the neck of the sac.

Figure 6. By gentle traction and blunt dissection the sac may be teased into the inguinal incision.

INSET A. When it is impossible to bring the sac into the operative field because of its size or adherent content, the lower edge of the incision may be retracted downward, exposing the sac below Poupart's ligament. The femoral vessels are identified, and the dissection is carried out as on page 175.

If the sac, though freed of attachments, is too large to be reduced, it may be opened and the contents returned to the abdomen or redundant omentum excised.

Figure 7. The entire hernia has now been reduced and brought into full view above the level of Poupart's ligament. The sac is being opened.

With the dissection complete and the sac isolated the surgeon now turns his attention to the repair of what was formerly a femoral hernia but now is converted into an inguinal hernia. With all structures in view and anatomical landmarks identified, including the external iliac vessels, the reconstructive stages of the operation can be carried out with ease and without danger.

ABDOMINAL WALL PROCEDURES
FEMORAL HERNIA—INGUINAL APPROACH

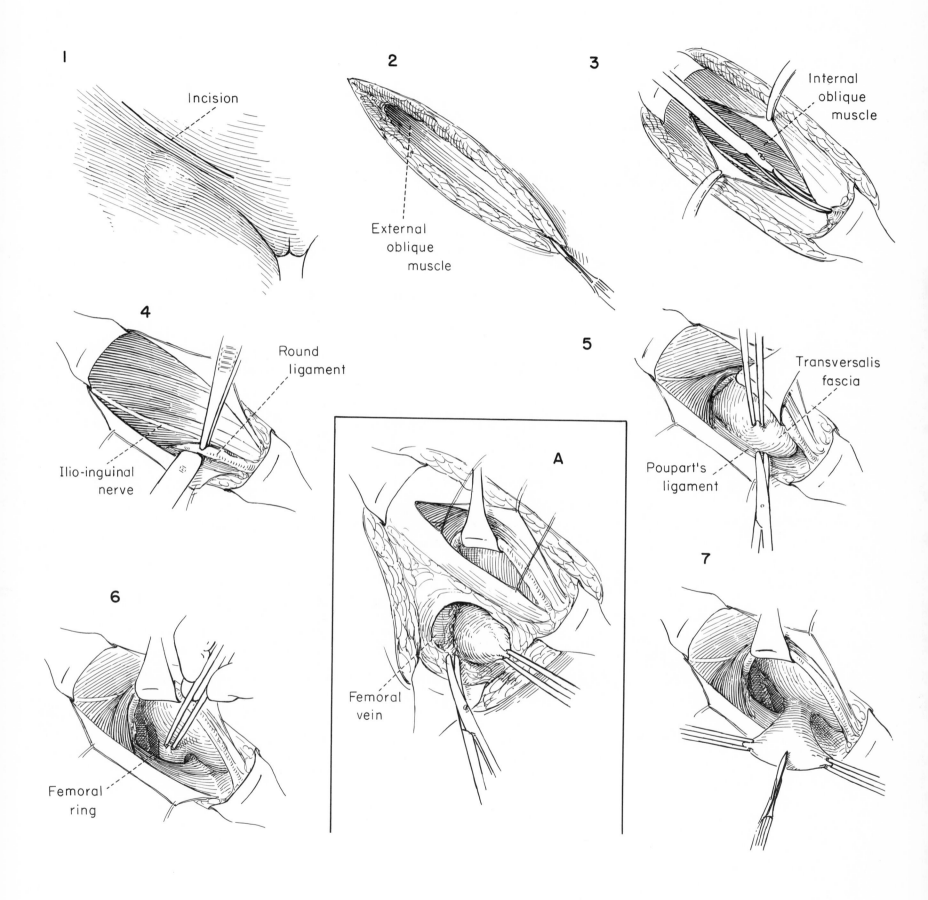

1 Incision

2 External oblique muscle

3 Internal oblique muscle

4 Round ligament / Ilio-inguinal nerve

5 Transversalis fascia / Poupart's ligament

A Femoral vein

6 Femoral ring

7

Figure 8. The interior of the sac is explored and the contents are pushed back through the broad neck into the abdomen before a purse-string suture is placed about the base.

Figure 9. With the contents out of the way the purse-string suture has been placed around the inside of the neck of the sac.

Figure 10. Because the base is broad, a simple purse-string suture will not suffice. A transfixion suture is placed outside and distal to the ligated purse-string suture. This will seal off any interstices that might remain.

Figure 11. The transfixion suture and sac are held on tension as the sac is excised.

Figure 12. The defect in the femoral canal is closed by placing interrupted silk sutures through the lacunar ligament below Poupart's and Cooper's ligaments in the medial portion of the wound. The external iliac vessels are retracted as these sutures are placed to avoid possible damage.

Figure 13. The defect in the femoral ring has been closed with interrupted silk sutures.

Figure 14. The balance of the repair now follows the steps outlined for simple inguinal herniorrhaphy. The conjoined tendon is sutured to Poupart's ligament with interrupted sutures. The deep epigastric vessels lie just medial to the point of disappearance of the round ligament and should be avoided.

Figure 15. The external oblique fascia is then closed with interrupted silk, cotton or fine wire sutures.

Figure 16. Subcutaneous fat and skin are approximated in two layers.

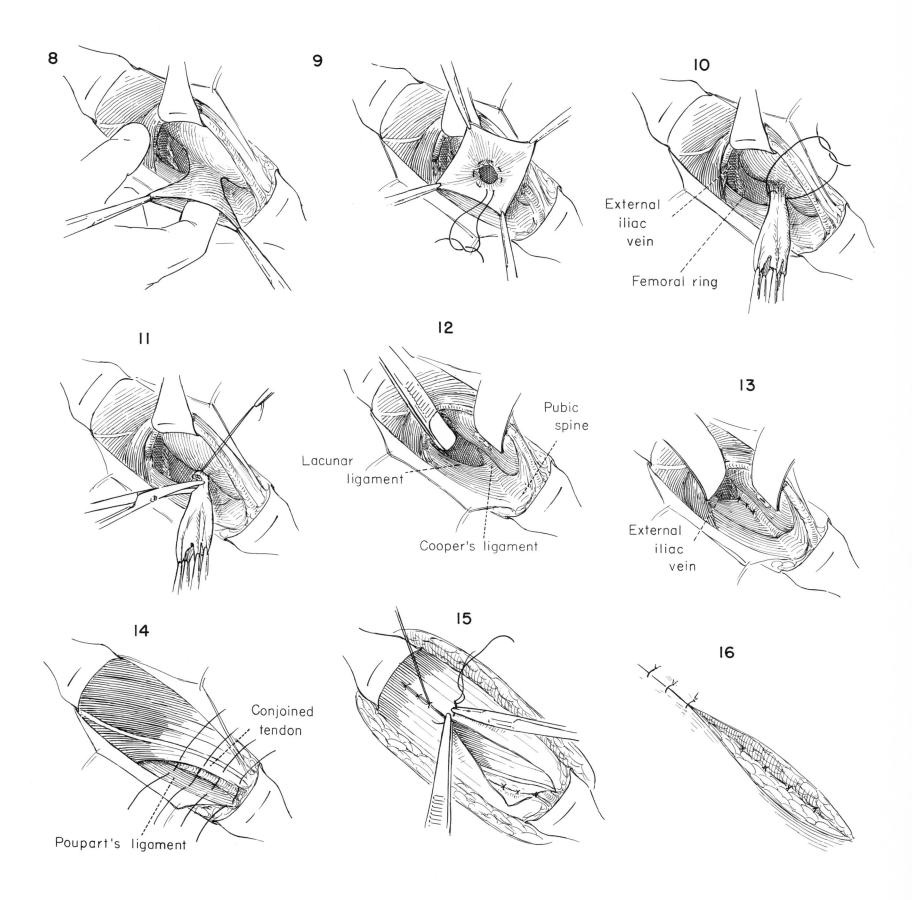

8

9

10

External
iliac
vein

Femoral ring

11

12

Lacunar
ligament

Pubic
spine

Cooper's ligament

13

External
iliac
vein

14

Conjoined
tendon

Poupart's ligament

15

16

UMBILICAL HERNIA

An umbilical hernia is a common abdominal wall defect in women. It appears as either a true hernia of the umbilicus, characterized by eversion of the navel, or more often as a para-umbilical hernia. Whatever the cause, the operative steps for its eradication and repair are identical.

The repair is accomplished by making a transverse elliptical incision to encompass the defect. Normal fascia is identified and the extent of the lateral ramifications of the hernia determined. The hernial sac is then mobilized until the edges of the fascial defect are outlined. Care must be taken in opening the sac because omentum and bowel are frequently found adherent to the inner peritoneal surface. After all adhesions have been freed the sac is closed. The diverging recti muscles are brought together after the peritoneum has been sutured. To reinforce the closure the fascia is imbricated in a transverse direction.

Figure 1. In the adult a transverse incision and repair with removal of the umbilicus is the technique least likely to result in recurrence

Figure 2. An elliptical incision is outlined extensive enough to include the umbilicus, the palpable ramifications of the sac, and the redundant overlying skin.

Figure 3. The incision is carried down to the normal fascia as the assistant retracts the skin edge. This is done over the entire area mapped out for excision.

Figure 4. With normal fascia as a landmark, the surgeon elevates the block of tissue to be removed and exposes the anterior rectus sheath by dissecting off the overlying fat. The dissection is then carried toward the midline on all sides until the fascial covering of the hernial sac is encountered.

Figure 5. The sac and defect are now completely isolated and the extent of normal fascia to be used in the repair process adequately exposed.

The surgeon then sections the anterior rectus fascia transversely on either side of the defect. The dotted line indicates the direction of the incision to be made in the fascia around the neck of the sac in the midline.

Figure 6. The incision has been carried through the fascia overlying the hernia in the midline, thus connecting the two lateral incisions. A broad flap of rectus sheath is developed for use later in the repair.

Figure 7. The assistant applies traction to the sac as the surgeon incises it at its base. Kelly clamps are applied to the cut edges to provide exposure and to avoid any damage to its contents.

ABDOMINAL WALL PROCEDURES
UMBILICAL HERNIA

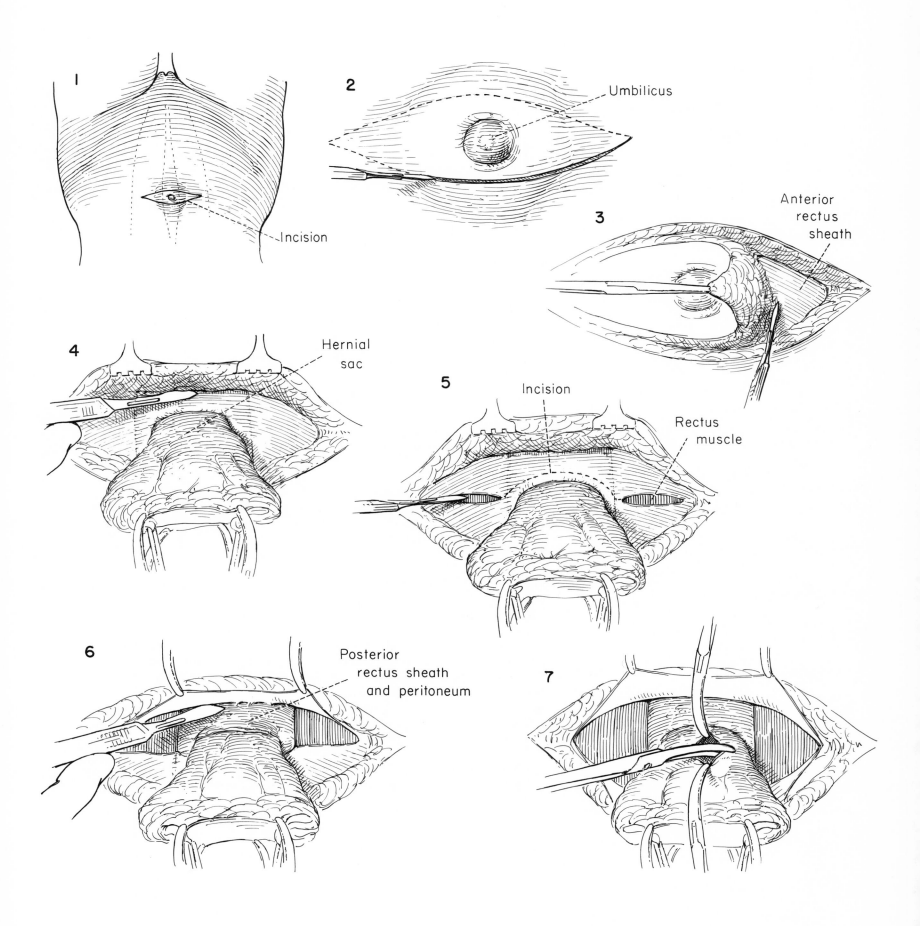

1   Incision

2   Umbilicus

3   Anterior rectus sheath

4   Hernial sac

5   Incision — Rectus muscle

6   Posterior rectus sheath and peritoneum

7

Figure 8. Invariably the omentum is adherent to the peritoneum lining the sac. This must be dissected free. Care must be taken in enlarging the opening in the sac because of the adhesions.

Figure 9. With the neck of the sac completely exposed and opened and the edges of the peritoneum held on traction with hemostats, the surgeon excises the redundant peritoneum and fascia.

Figure 10. The circular defect is converted into an ellipse by lateral traction on Kocher clamps placed on the edges of the hernial opening. The upper and lower clamps simply aid in exposure as the surgeon starts the stitch to close the peritoneum and transversalis fascia.

Figure 11. The peritoneofascial closure has been completed with a running catgut suture. A wide separation of the rectus muscles is apparent in the midline. The surgeon elevates the medial border of the right rectus and separates the muscle from its posterior sheath. This step is repeated on the opposite side.

Figure 12. After mobilizing the rectus muscles so that the opposing edges lie easily without tension, the surgeon approximates them in the midline with interrupted sutures.

Figure 13. The anterior sheath has been separated from the underlying muscle at the lower edge through its entire extent in order to form a flap. This was done deliberately in order to be able to imbricate the aponeurotic sheath and provide a stronger abdominal wall repair.

The lower edge of the sheath is held upward by the assistant as the surgeon begins a series of mattress sutures. The suture enters the lower flap approximately ¾ inch from the edge, then passes beneath it to pick up the upper edge and return through the fascia to reappear about ½ inch from the point of origin. A series of such sutures is placed through the entire transverse extent of the wound.

Figure 14. These sutures are tied, and the free edge of sheath is then tacked down with another series of interrupted sutures.

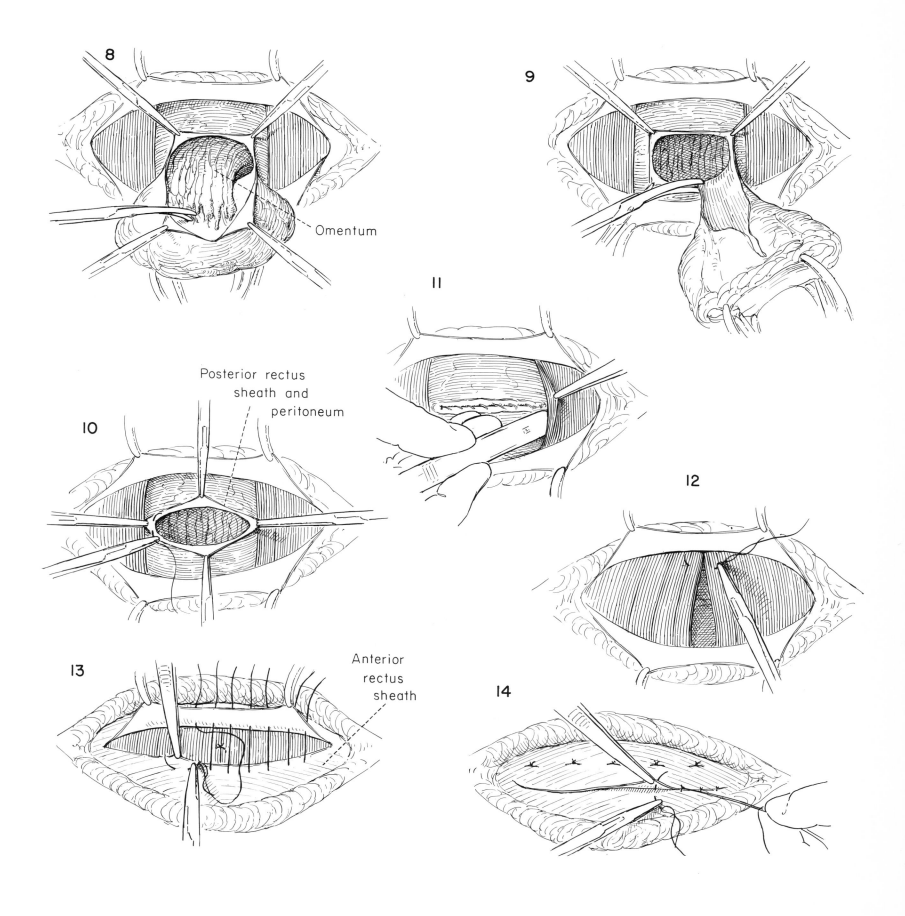

8

9

11

10

Posterior rectus
sheath and
peritoneum

12

13

Anterior
rectus
sheath

14

Omentum

DIASTASIS RECTI

As the result of repeated pregnancies the muscles of the abdominal wall may become widely separated, leaving a pronounced weakness in the midline which often extends above the level of the umbilicus. Since the separation is not confined to the lower portion of the recti muscles, it is occasionally necessary to excise the umbilicus in order that the muscles may be approximated without tension. This will make the repair much stronger. To further strengthen the wound the fascia is imbricated over the old defect.

This operation is rarely done as a sole definitive procedure, but it may be used in conjunction with others which call for abdominal intervention.

Figure 1. The umbilicus has been excised and the outline of the incision is indicated. The skin and subcutaneous fascia are dissected from the underlying rectus fascia. The limits of the lateral dissection are determined by the position of the retracted recti muscles. The extent of the separation of the two longitudinal muscles may be formidable. The defect in the peritoneum at the site of the removal of the umbilicus is closed with interrupted silk sutures.

The thinned-out medial borders of the recti are identified and the muscles laid bare in their entire extent by incision of the anterior rectus sheath.

Figure 2. The rectus muscle is elevated and the underlying peritoneum dissected free with the handle of the knife. This maneuver is carried out on both sides and over the entire extent of the muscle bundle.

Figure 3. The pelvic operation has been concluded and the peritoneum closed. The mobilized rectus muscle is then approximated in the midline with interrupted catgut sutures.

Figure 4. Because of the extent of the dead space created in the dissection it is advisable to use deep obliterating wire sutures which pass through the skin, fat and fascia.

Figure 5. When possible, the fascia should be imbricated to provide additional strength to the wound.

Figure 6. The free edge of fascia is then tacked down with interrupted sutures.

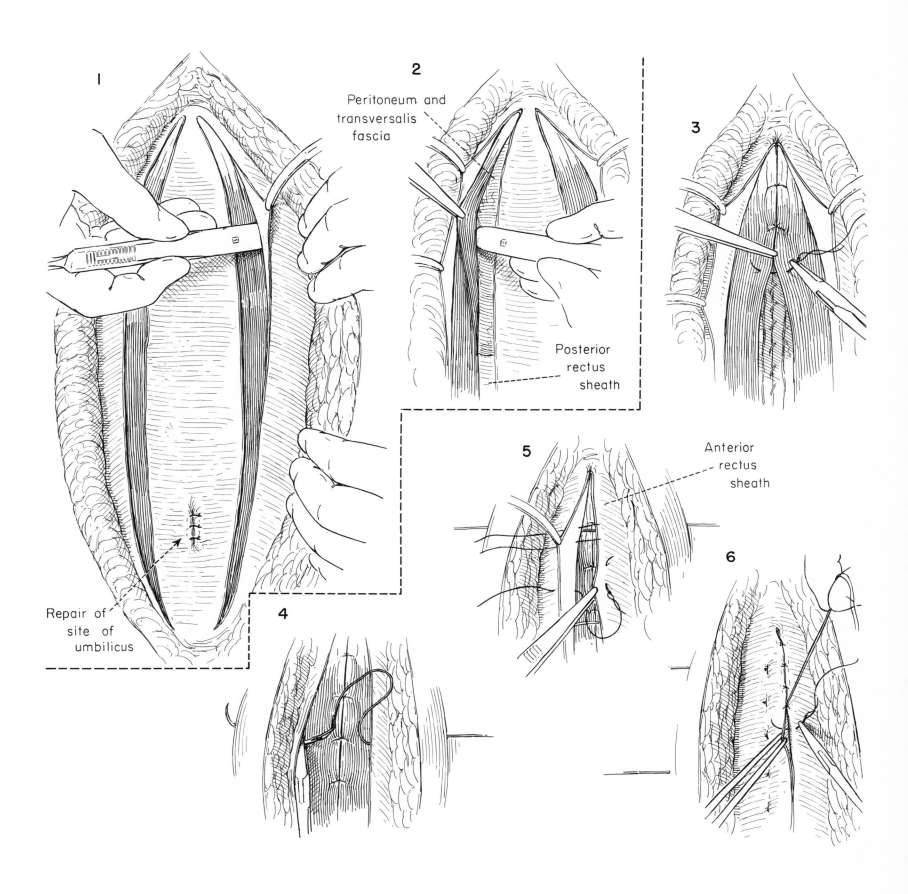

1

2

Peritoneum and
transversalis
fascia

3

Posterior
rectus
sheath

Repair of
site of
umbilicus

4

5

Anterior
rectus
sheath

6

Complications Following
Abdominal Operations

FEMORAL VEIN LIGATION

The enthusiasm for widespread use of femoral ligation has declined appreciably in recent years. The surgeon now usually prefers to institute anticoagulant therapy when the symptoms and signs suggest thrombophlebitis. However, the threat of detachment of a clot from the popliteal vein resulting in an infarct or pulmonary embolus may be avoided by ligation of the superficial femoral vein. The indications are more definite when there is evidence of an actual embolism to the lung. Ligation should be carried out bilaterally; unilateral ligations have been known to fail and the patient to succumb from an embolus from the opposite popliteal vessel. Before ligating the vein the surgeon must be sure that the clot does not extend above the point of ligation. If it does, the main trunk of the vein must be opened and the clot sucked out.

This is a simple procedure provided the surgeon establishes the normal anatomy by exposing the femoral artery as well as the femoral and profunda veins before he attempts to ligate the vein.

Figure 1. The upper portion of the body is elevated to increase venous back pressure. A longitudinal incision under local anesthesia begins at Poupart's ligament and extends down the thigh for 4 or 5 inches just medial to the pulsation of the femoral artery.

Figure 2. The skin edges are retracted and the superficial fascial layer incised in a longitudinal direction.

Figure 3. The femoral vessels are identified and their sheath exposed in the depths of the incision. The saphenous vein may be encountered and must be retracted medially.

Figure 4. The surgeon and assistant have picked up the sheath of the femoral vein to incise it longitudinally.

Figure 5. With the sheath on tension the femoral vein is exposed for about 3 inches.

Figure 6. The surgeon proceeds carefully to dissect out the femoral vein and its tributaries. It is important that the field be kept dry to aid in exposure. Any small veins must be clamped and tied. The deep femoral vein must be dissected out at the point of entry into the common femoral.

Figure 7. The assistant gently retracts the femoral artery as the surgeon passes a strand of coarse silk beneath the superficial vein just below the bifurcation of the common vessel. This suture is placed as a stay suture and is left untied.

Figure 8. A second stay suture is placed around the vein about an inch below the first. This likewise is left untied. The assistant pulls up on the upper stay suture and stands ready with a suction tip as the surgeon keeps the lower stay on traction and prepares to make a transverse incision in the anterior wall of the vein between the two sutures. Another assistant retracts the femoral artery.

Figure 9. If no free bleeding follows the introduction of a glass catheter into the lumen, venous thrombosis is present.

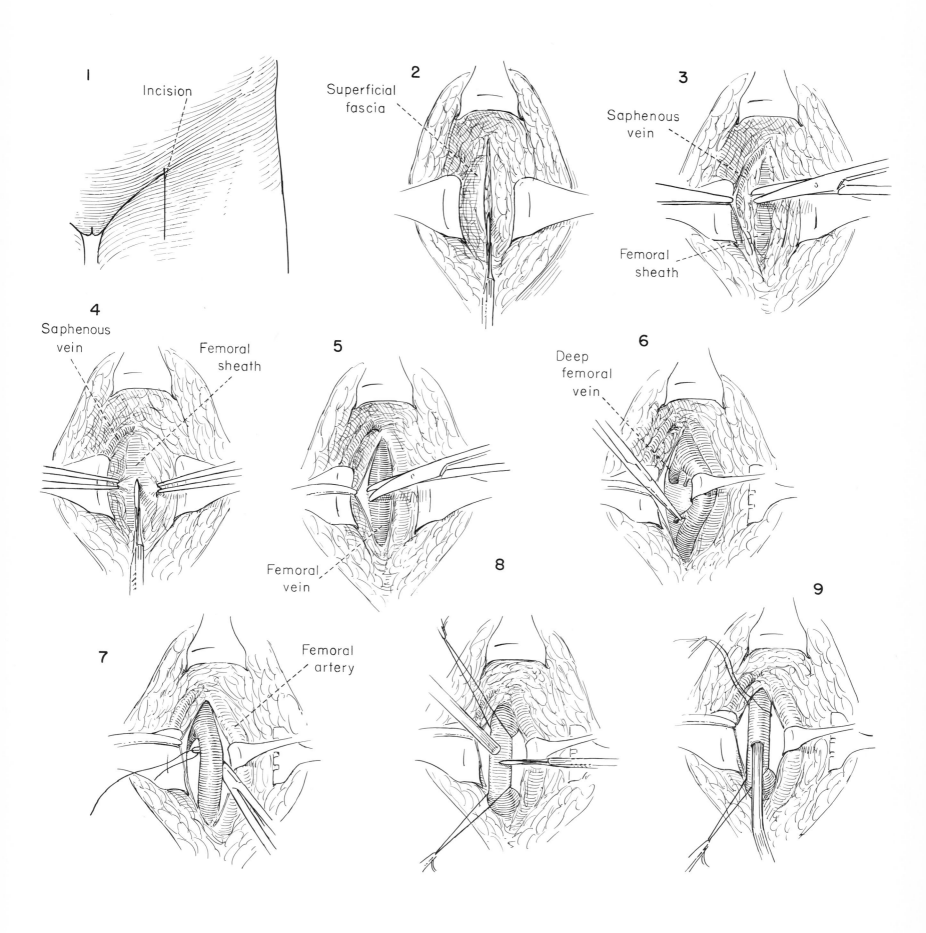

1 Incision

2 Superficial fascia

3 Saphenous vein / Femoral sheath

4 Saphenous vein / Femoral sheath

5 Femoral vein

6 Deep femoral vein

7 Femoral artery

8

9

Figure 10. The lower stay suture is held on tension to prevent bleeding and the femoral artery is retracted as the surgeon gently aspirates the clot from the upper segment of vein.

Figure 11. The lower segment of the vein must also be aspirated. Free bleeding should follow the removal of the clot. This is controlled by tension on the stay sutures whenever necessary.

Figure 12. Clamps are now placed across the main trunk of the vein below the level of the bifurcation into the deep and superficial femorals. They should be placed about ¾ inch apart to provide an adequate cuff of vein beyond the clamp on each segment, and above and below the aspiration incision.

Figure 13. The vein is then completely transected. The surgeon is preparing to ligate the upper segment of the vein exactly at the level of the junction of deep and superficial femorals. Ligation at this level is important since it eliminates a blind stump of vein where thrombosis may begin.

Figure 14. The vein has been ligated, and the surgeon now steadies the clamp on the upper divided end as he passes a transfixion suture through the cuff.

Figures 15 and 16. These figures show the ligation of the transfixed vein. The suture first passes through the walls of the vein, is tied, and then carried around the vein to be tied again.

Figure 17. The lower segment of vein has been ligated, and a transfixion stitch is being placed through the vein. This likewise will be tied first on one side and then around the entire vein.

Figure 18. The femoral sheath is then closed with interrupted silk or cotton sutures. The assistant holds up on the initial suture as the surgeon introduces the next stitch. A series of such sutures closes the defect.

Figures 19 and 20. The wound is then closed with a series of interrupted vertical mattress sutures of silk. The first stitch passes through the skin of both sides about ½ inch from the wound edge. On return the surgeon picks up the skin close to the incision.

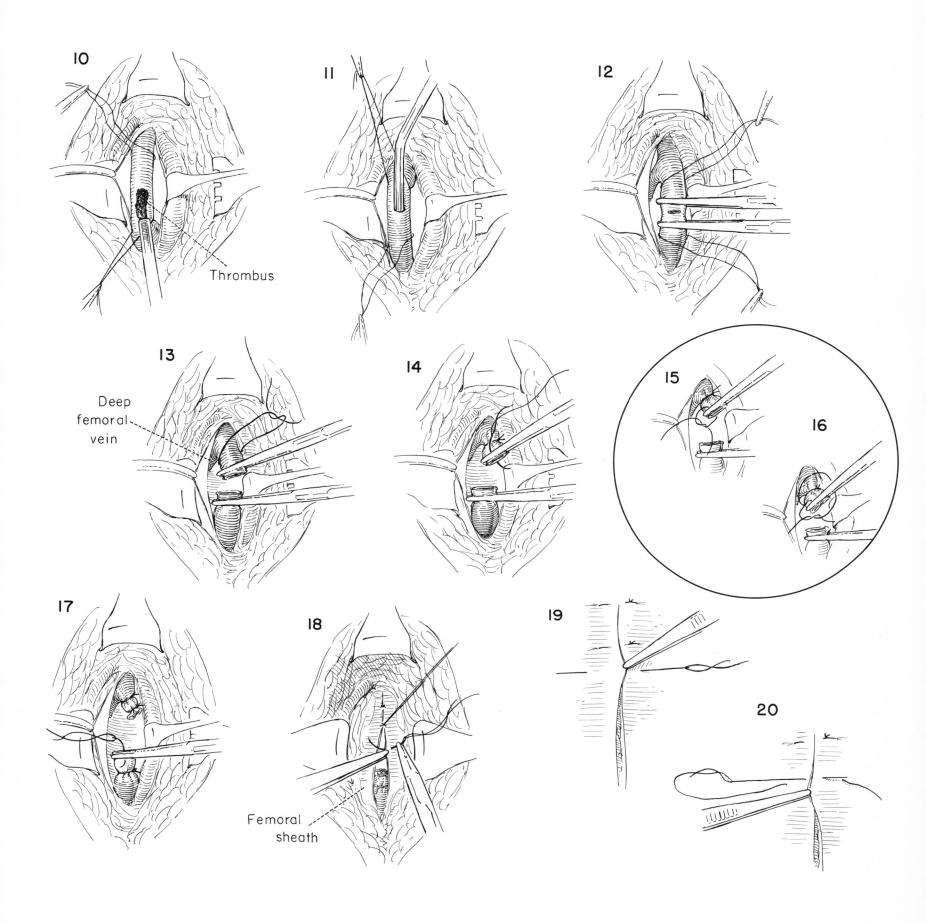

10

11

12

13

Deep
femoral
vein

14

15

16

17

18

Femoral
sheath

19

20

Thrombus

DEHISCENCE AND RESUTURE

Wound separation is a possibility in the convalescent period following any abdominal operation. It is more likely to occur following the abdominal distention that arises in association with low grade peritoneal sepsis, frank peritonitis, paralytic ileus or intestinal obstruction. The chances of wound dehiscence also increase when the primary operation has been done for pelvic inflammatory disease or malignancy, particularly if the patient is depleted or is in the older age group. Abdominal distention from whatever cause accompanied by vigorous coughing may produce wound separation. Patients who have pneumonia or atelectasis are especially susceptible.

The appearance of a serosanguineous discharge from an otherwise clean wound often heralds the dehiscence. Immediate investigation is mandatory. The inspection should be done in the operating room, not at the bedside. Although the omentum does a good job of keeping the intestine out of the wound, it may on occasion present itself. It is essential that the wound be re-explored and resutured immediately following the recognition that separation has occurred. This is the reason for inspecting the wound in the operating room. Since there is commonly an element of sepsis present, the wound should be cultured.

Time is of the essence, for these patients are usually poor risk patients. The surgeon should not attempt individual layer closure but use through and through wire sutures, passing through all layers of the abdominal wall. The end results from this type of closure are excellent, and there is little tendency to later hernia formation.

Figure 1. Omentum can be seen protruding through a disrupted wound onto the abdominal wall. The patient is anesthetized and the remaining sutures are removed and the wound inspected.

Figure 2. The peritoneum is grasped with numerous Kocher clamps. The omentum and bowel are returned to the abdominal cavity and the omentum is drawn over the intestine.

Figure 3. The quickest and safest method of resuture is to use through-and-through sutures of wire placed as interrupted sutures through all layers.

The assistant elevates the peritoneum as the surgeon places the first stitch through skin, subcutaneous fat, fascia, muscle and peritoneum. The suture is placed about 1 inch lateral to the skin incision.

To protect the underlying abdominal contents, the surgeon depresses the omentum with the left hand as he places the suture.

Figure 4. The assistant continues to elevate the peritoneum and the surgeon to depress the abdominal contents as he continues the through-and-through suture on the opposite side to emerge on the skin 1 inch lateral to the incision. A series of such sutures is placed.

Figure 5. The wires are drawn taut, but without undue tension, and secured, either by tying them or by twisting the ends. They are left in place at least two weeks.

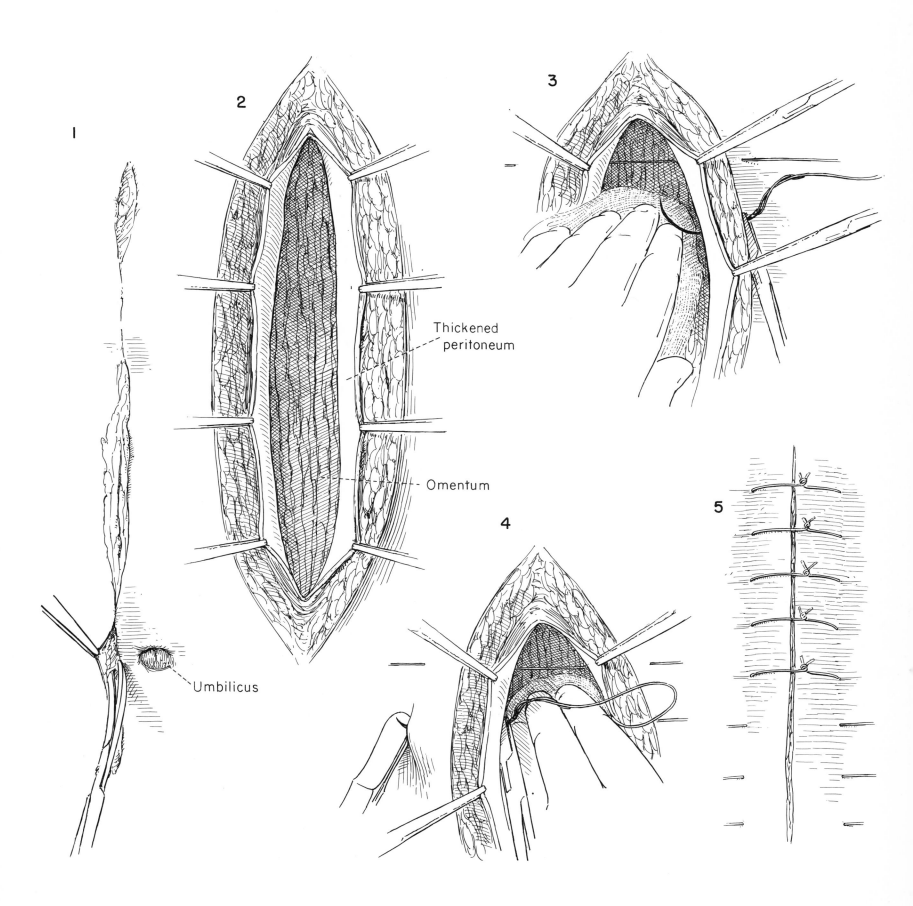

1

2

Thickened
peritoneum

Omentum

Umbilicus

3

4

5

RETROPERITONEAL DRAINAGE OF PELVIC ABSCESS

Despite the success achieved by intensive antibiotic therapy in the control of pelvic sepsis, abscess formation may appear in the broad ligament or cul de sac and require surgical drainage. It may occur after abdominal or surgical procedures or be the natural development of pelvic disease in the absence of any operative interference.

The location of the pelvic abscess will depend on the site of the original infection and will tend to follow normal tissue planes. The point of election for drainage will depend on the localization. The timing of the drainage is also of great importance. To this end the surgeon should look at the patient as well as the chart. He must assure himself that he will make the incision into an abscess cavity and not an area of porky induration. The palpation of soft tender areas in an otherwise firm mass is a fair indication that pus is present.

An abscess localizing in the upper levels of the broad ligament may point above Poupart's ligament and be palpated there. Drainage may then be established by an incision in the inguinal region which permits exploration of the retroperitoneal space and avoids the danger of contaminating the abdominal cavity. The primary exploration, following the incision, should be made with a syringe and needle. The presence of pus in the aspirate provides ample indication for continuing to establish drainage through the extraperitoneal approach.

Figure 1. The localization of the abscess in relation to the skin incision is shown.

Figure 2. The skin and fat are incised and retracted. The fibers of the external oblique are split in the long axis.

Figure 3. The retractors are introduced below the external oblique muscle on either side of the muscle incision and the wound converted into a transverse field. The internal oblique is then divided in the line of its fibers.

Figure 4. Retractors are placed beneath the muscle on the lower edge as the surgeon gently separates the transversalis fascia and retracts the peritoneum with the palm of the hand and extended fingers.

Figure 5. The indurated wall of the abscess cavity is palpated in the deep recesses of the wound at its base. The peritoneum is held back by a Deaver retractor. Before attempting to incise the abscess cavity, the surgeon should try to aspirate pus by exploring with a needle and syringe.

Figure 6. With presence of pus established and suction tip available to control spillage, the tip of a Kelly clamp is thrust into the abscess and the jaws spread.

Figure 7. The cavity is then aspirated with the suction tip.

Figure 8. The finger then explores the cavity to break up any compartments which might contain pus.

Figure 9. A gauze-filled drain is introduced into the cavity and another into the retroperitoneal space.

Figure 10. The muscle is loosely closed around the drains.

Figure 11. The fascia is also loosely approximated with interrupted catgut. A word of caution is necessary: At no point in the drainage tract should the drains be constricted; looseness of closure is emphasized.

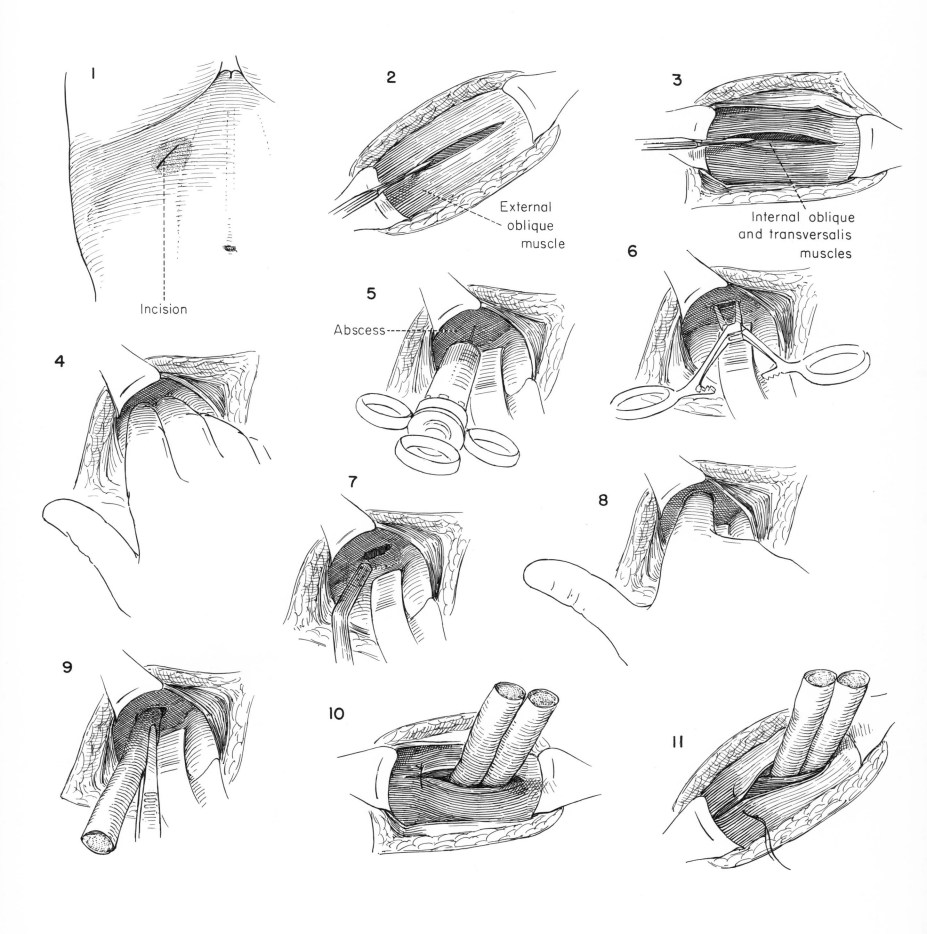

INCISION AND DRAINAGE OF PELVIC ABSCESS
THROUGH THE VAGINA

Whenever possible a pelvic abscess should be drained through the vagina. Fortunately, the majority of abscesses in the female, regardless of cause, will tend to localize in the cul de sac at the base of the broad ligament. Timing of the drainage is of basic importance. The surgeon must be sure that the abscess cavity is fixed to the vaginal wall and that pus is present and not brawny indurated tissue. If it is not fixed, an ill-advised attempt to drain the abscess may result in damage to bowel and the possibility of contaminating the general peritoneal cavity. The surgeon will accomplish little if the drainage is made into an area of porky induration. If there is any doubt about the fixation or the presence of pus the operation should be delayed until these two criteria are thoroughly established.

A soft, tender bulging mass behind the cervix which is fixed to the vaginal epithelium may be drained without danger.

Figure 1. The patient is placed in the lithotomy position, the cervix exposed and traction applied to it with a tenaculum. Note the fixation of the abscess to the vaginal wall. In all probability the uterus will not descend into the vaginal canal to any extent because of the fixation. The abscess cavity is shown in relation to other anatomical landmarks.

Figure 2. The cervix is elevated toward the urethra and the bulge of the abscess is apparent in the posterior fornix. An incision is made in the vaginal epithelium in the midline over the abscess cavity at the point of maximum fluctuation.

Figure 3. Maintaining the cervix on upward traction with the tenaculum, the surgeon thrusts a Kelly clamp into the abscess cavity.

Figure 4. An exploratory finger is introduced into the opening and the incision widened by blunt dissection.

Figure 5. The cervix is maintained on traction while the assistant steadies the lower edge of the incision with forceps. The surgeon then aspirates the cavity with a suction tip.

Figures 6 and 7. Gauze-filled drains are introduced into the cavity and sutured to the vaginal epithelium.

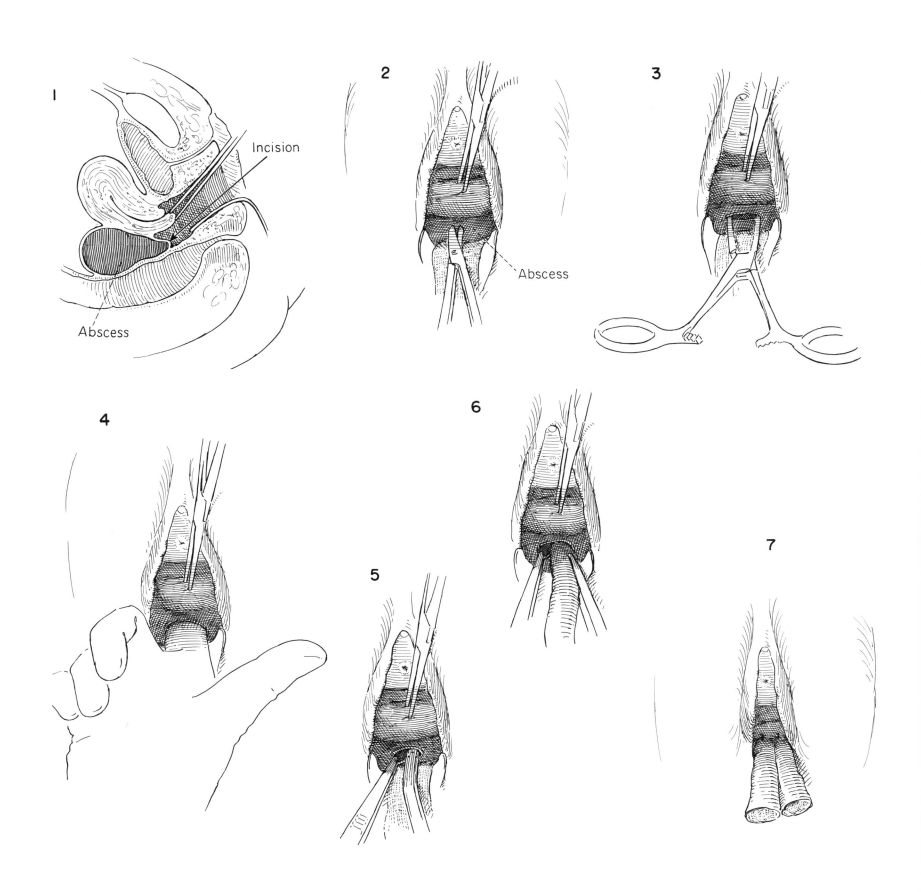

1

Incision

Abscess

2

Abscess

3

4

5

6

7

DRAINAGE OF PELVIC ABSCESS THROUGH THE RECTUM

Although the ideal place to drain a deep pelvic abscess is through the vagina, it may develop in the cul de sac and present as a bulging mass in the rectal lumen rather than in the vagina.

Drainage through the rectum may be readily accomplished provided the surgeon can be certain that the abscess cavity is fixed to the rectal wall. The incision should be made under direct vision with the anal sphincter sufficiently dilated to permit introduction of retractors to expose the most dependent fixed point.

Figure 1. The uterus is absent. The abscess is shown dissecting below the pelvic floor to bulge on the rectal side. The arrow points to the optimum drainage site.

Figure 2. The patient is placed in the lithotomy position. When the patient has been anesthetized, the anus is dilated. The surgeon's two index fingers apply gradual pressure to stretch the anal sphincter. This maneuver should not be hurried or forced if damage to the sphincter is to be prevented.

Figure 3. Narrow blade Richardson retractors should be introduced into the rectum and traction applied to either side.

Figure 4. Allis clamps grasp the rectal mucosa at the point of greatest fixation to the underlying abscess. The surgeon then divides the mucosa in the long axis.

Figure 5. The blunt end of a Kelly clamp is forced into the abscess cavity and the jaws of the clamp are spread.

Figure 6. An exploratory finger bluntly widens the opening and explores the cavity.

Figure 7. The surgeon steadies the lower edge of the incision as he introduces a suction tip to aspirate the cavity. The assistants maintain exposure with the retractors.

Figure 8. The interior of the rectum is shown in relation to the opening into the abscess. No drains are necessary.

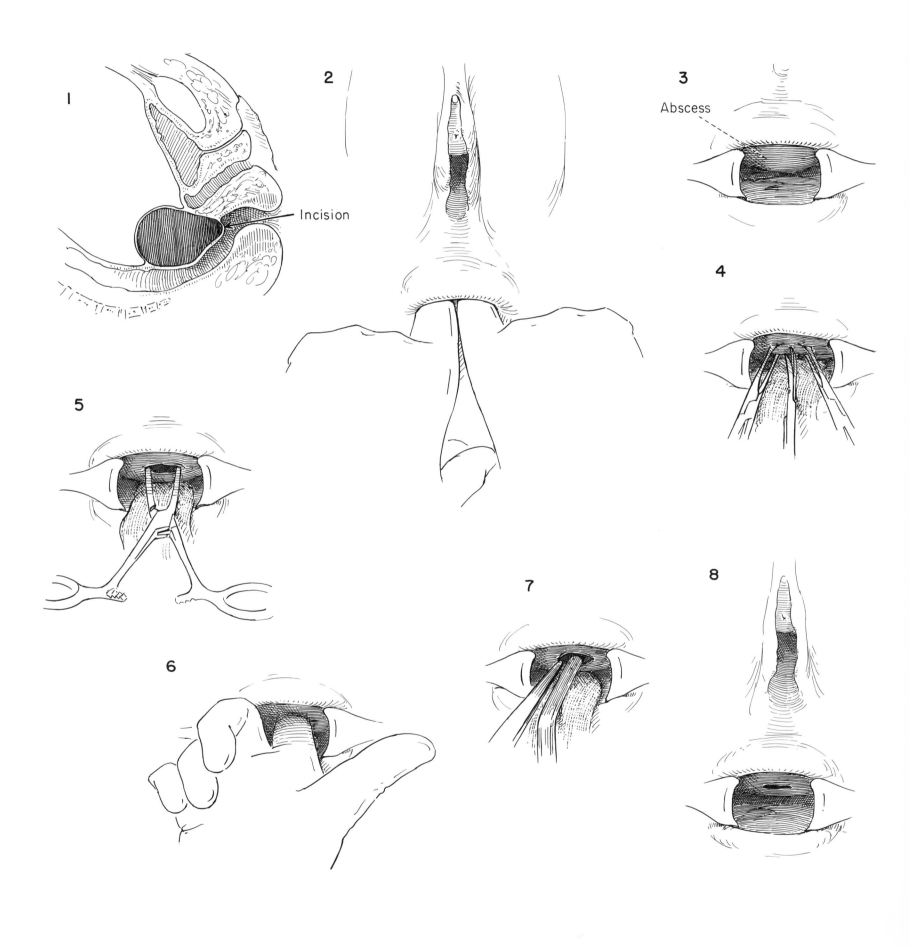

Section II

Vaginal and Perineal Operations

EXAMINATION UNDER ANESTHESIA

Before being operated on for disease within the uterus, anatomic derangement or dysfunction, the patient should have a pelvic examination under anesthesia whether the surgery is to be done through the abdomen or by the vaginal approach.

This permits the surgeon to check his preoperative office findings and allows him to re-evaluate the condition for which he is operating in relation to the other lesions which may be present in either the uterus or adnexa. An empty bladder makes the examination more meaningful. Pelvic relaxations which were moderate during the office examination may be quite pronounced when the patient is relaxed under anesthesia. When a tumor exists in the presence of an overlarge uterus, or when adnexal disease is present, the surgeon must decide whether the vaginal or abdominal approach will best answer the patient's needs.

Except for minor procedures, a dilatation and curettage must precede any operation performed in the vagina when there is a uterus present, just as it must be done as a preliminary step in all pelvic operations performed from the abdominal side. It would also be advisable to stain the cervix and upper vagina with Schiller's solution.

Figure 1. The patient is in the lithotomy position with the feet held by ankle straps which suspend the legs within the upright bars of the wide-angled stirrups. Note that there is no pressure on the calves of the leg.

Figure 2. The vulva and perineum are prepared with soap and water followed by one of the antiseptic solutions. The vaginal canal is similarly prepared.

The bladder should then be completely emptied by catheter. The entire area is now draped with protective linen.

Figure 3. As a check on the findings of the preoperative office or clinic examination the pelvis should again be palpated. If there has been any question in the surgeon's mind whether the operation should be done from above or below, the examination at this time should crystallize the decision. Unexpected fixation of the uterus due to pathologic processes in the adnexa or overenlargement of the uterus may influence the surgeon in performing an abdominal rather than a vaginal operation.

Figure 4. Following the vaginal examination, the surgeon also carries out a rectal examination and then concludes the draping. In this illustration a commercial plastic towel with adherent selvage at one edge is being used, thus avoiding the need for clips to the skin.

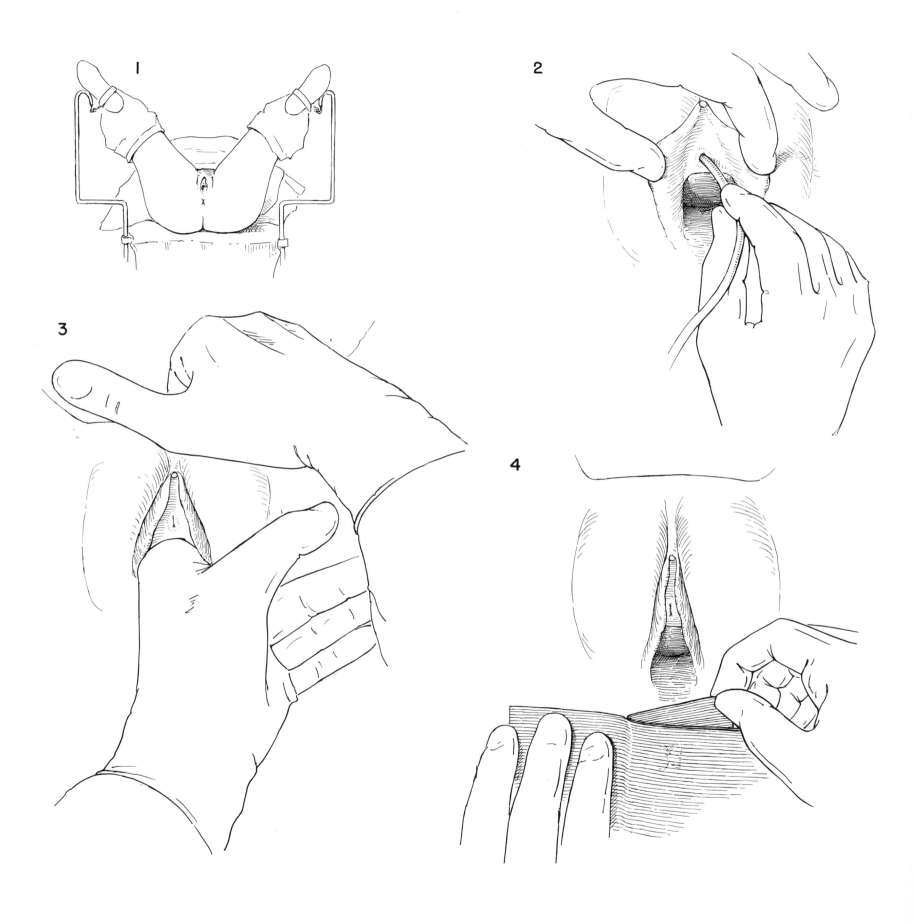

DILATATION AND CURETTAGE

The surgeon must be absolutely certain that no malignant disease is present in the external portion of the cervix, within the endocervical canal or in the uterine cavity itself. To supplement the clinical observations and increase the accuracy in interpretation of what is seen and felt in the cervix and upper vagina the surgeon will be well advised to paint them with Schiller's solution. A biopsy should be taken of any suspicious areas and a frozen section performed on the specimen. The endocervical canal must be curetted as a separate maneuver independent of the curettement of the endometrial cavity. In curetting the endometrial cavity special attention should be paid to the cornua. This area is easy to bypass and diseased tissue may be missed if no sample is taken. A curettage, however well performed, is never 100 per cent accurate; frequently an endometrial polyp is missed. In the interest of thoroughness the surgeon should explore the uterine cavity, after curettement, with a blunt grasping instrument such as the common stone searcher.

All tissue, however small in amount, should be preserved. Any suspicious material should be given to the pathologist for immediate examination. If there is any question about the benign nature of the curettings, the operation should be deferred to wait the report of the permanent pathologic sections.

Figure 5. The upper portions of the vagina and the cervix are exposed by inserting a Sims speculum into the vagina and exerting downward pressure on the posterior vaginal wall. The vaginal epithelium of the upper vagina and cervix are then painted with a gauze sponge saturated with Schiller's solution. It is important to view both areas so that the contrast between their appearance before and after the stain was applied can be properly evaluated.

Figure 6. Normal vaginal epithelium and that of the portio of the cervix will stain a deep mahogany brown because of the affinity of glycogen for iodine. Abnormal epithelium contains no glycogen and will remain the same or appear as a white area.

Figure 7. If a redundant anterior vaginal wall obscures the cervix, it may be brought into view by applying the thumb of the left hand against the bulging anterior vaginal wall. As upward pressure is exerted the cervix is exposed and the tenaculum may be safely applied to the upper lip.

Figure 8. A second tenaculum should be placed on the cervix because of the likelihood that one will tear out and produce a laceration and troublesome bleeding.

Figure 9. The tenacula are drawn toward the symphysis and a probe is gently introduced into the uterine cavity to measure its depth. This must be done with care to avoid the danger of perforation. This is particularly true if there has been a recent pregnancy or the uterus is in the atrophic state of the menopause.

If perforation occurs, exploration of the uterine canal should be discontinued. Abdominal intervention is required only when there are signs suggesting internal bleeding.

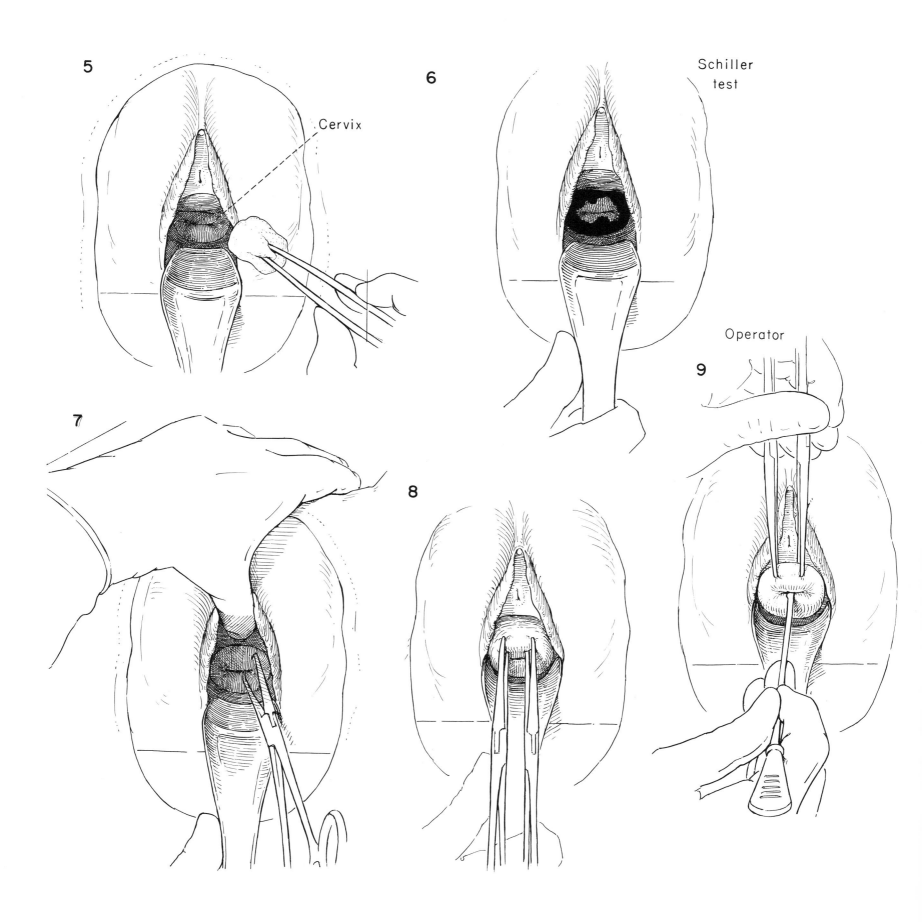

5

Cervix

6

Schiller test

7

8

9

Operator

The figures on this plate illustrate a useful maneuver that may be done when the pelvic examination under anesthesia has not been completely satisfactory either because of obesity or the extent of the uterine disease. In many instances the size, contour and position of the uterus or adnexa are inadequately outlined.

The use of a dilator in the uterine cavity held firmly in position will serve as a lever and will frequently bring the uterus into a position where it can be easily palpated. It is also possible to move the uterus to one side or the other away from any diseased tissue palpated in the adnexal area. In this fashion it may be possible to determine whether a mass is primary in the ovary or tube or whether it is connected with the uterus.

Figure 10. The actual maneuver suggested is simply an adjunct to the routine dilatation of the cervix customarily performed in any curettage.

The first of a series of dilators graduated in size is introduced into the uterine canal. This must be done easily in order to avoid a plunger-like action which may force endometrial contents out through the open fallopian tubes into the peritoneal cavity. The possibility of introducing implants of endometriosis or perhaps malignant tissues onto the pelvic peritoneum is thus avoided.

Figure 11. The dilators are serially introduced into the cervical canal and the cavity gradually stretched until the largest of the dilators has been passed.

To better evaluate the position and size of the uterus the largest of the dilators is retained in the uterine cavity. The surgeon pulls down firmly on the tenacula while at the same time thrusting upward on the dilator. All instruments are firmly grasped at the level of the cervix with the left index finger supporting the cervix from behind.

By this maneuver a lever has been provided which will permit the uterus to be moved in any direction desired. A posteriorly placed uterus can be brought into a position in which it can be more readily palpated or directed to one side or the other in order to better evaluate the state of the adnexa. This procedure should never be carried out with force.

INSET A. The anatomic figure shows the manner of fixation of the instruments by the left hand, the dilator in the uterine cavity and the palpation of the uterus in its new position by the right hand of the operator.

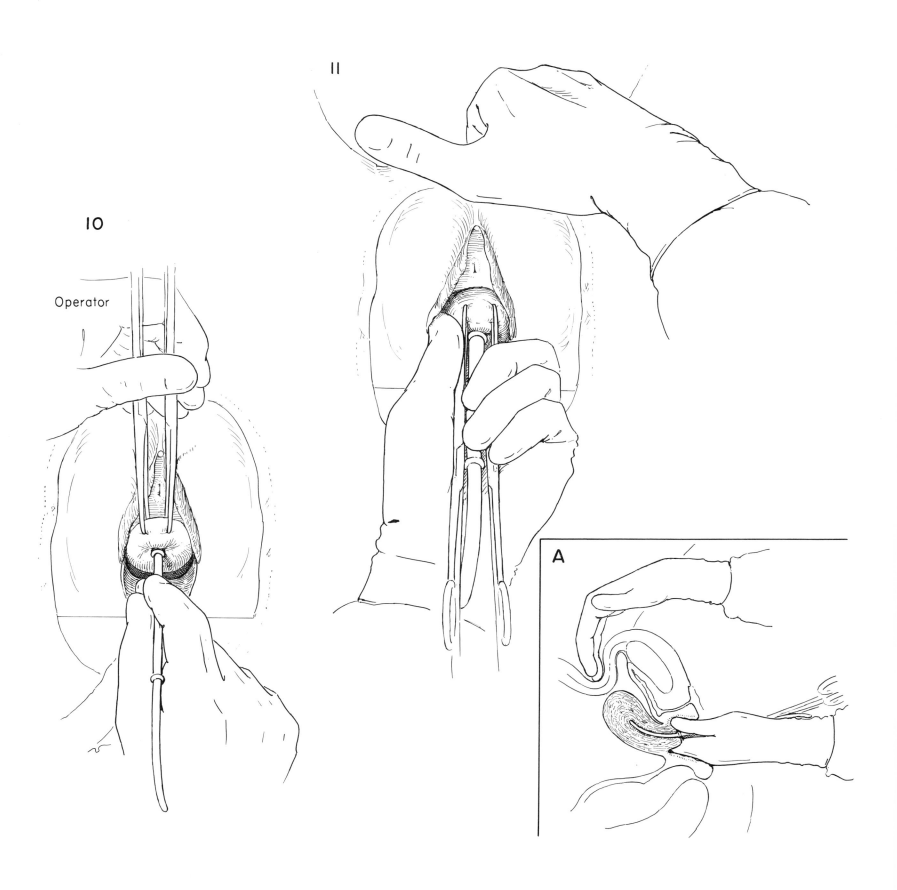

10

Operator

11

A

Figure 12. A biopsy should be taken of any suspicious area on the portio of the cervix that feels indurated or abnormally hard, is ulcerated or fails to take the stain with Schiller's solution. This is true whether or not the uterus or cervix is to be removed and is best done with a knife blade rather than a cautery. The latter tends to coagulate the tissue because of the heat, making it practically impossible for the pathologist to make an accurate evaluation.

Figure 13. The specimen removed should be presented to the pathologist for frozen section examination.

Figure 14. The dilatation of the cervical canal is now complete, and the surgeon is ready for curettage.

Figure 15. Because endometrial polyps on a stalk are able to move freely, they may be completely missed with the curette. To avoid this, and in the interest of complete evacuation of the endometrial contents, a common duct forceps or any similar blunt grasping forceps is inserted and the cavity further explored by successive and systematic grasping movements of the forceps.

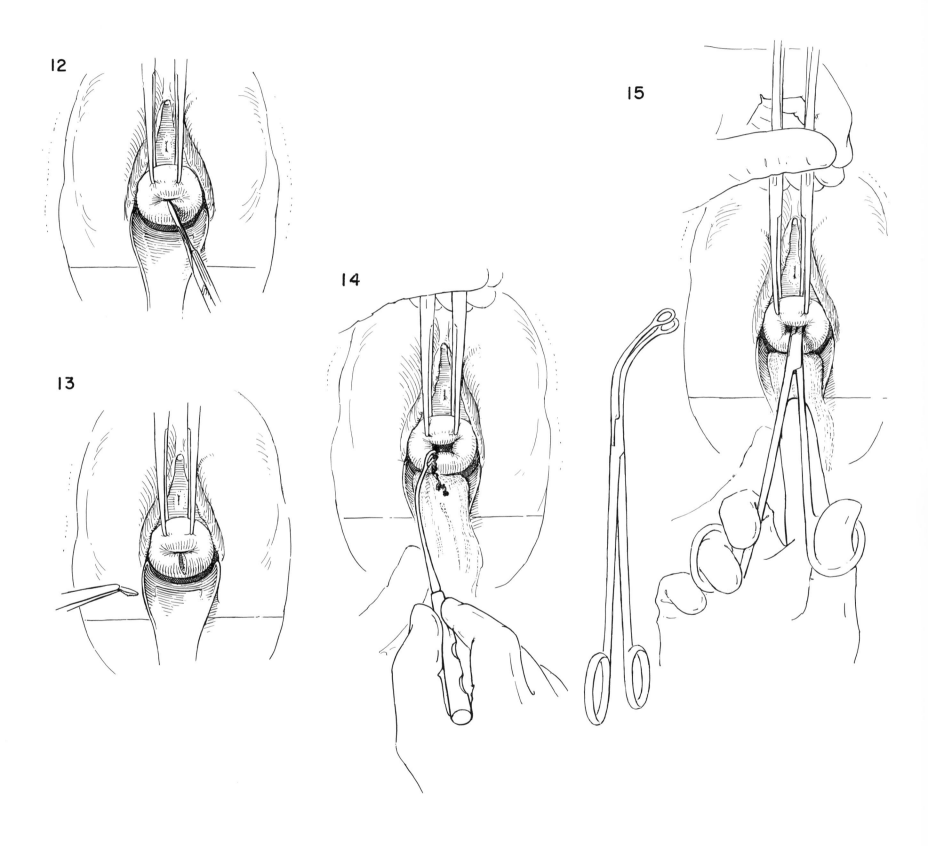

ADVANCEMENT OF THE BLADDER

The figures outlined in the next few plates present the basic steps taken in the majority of operations performed through the vagina whether the primary purpose is to remove a diseased uterus or to correct the various manifestations of prolapse. They apply equally well to the problems involved when the surgeon wishes to repair vesicovaginal fistula, obliterate the vagina for prolapse after the uterus has been removed or for urethrovesical neck suspensions for stress incontinence.

These moves can be carried out in a relatively bloodless field when proper attention is paid to the existing cleavage planes. It is not necessary to inject saline with adrenaline to establish them. The basic concept for establishing these planes rests in the fact that the blood vessels do not invade the vaginal wall at right angles but are held against it by fine fibrous bands. Separation of these attachments will free the vessels without damaging them. The trick is to leave the vessels on the bladder side. If the vessels are detached in this manner, the so-called bloody angle near the urethra can be avoided.

Although lesser degrees of descensus lend themselves to this procedure, for sake of clarity in outlining the individual moves, the operation will be shown as it is performed in a case of procidentia.

Figure 1. To provide better exposure, four interrupted catgut sutures through skin and labia place the latter on tension. The cervix is held on traction away from the symphysis.

Figure 2. The surgeon notes the last transverse fold of vaginal epithelium and divides it transversely just above this landmark.

Figure 3. Kelly clamps grasp the full thickness of the vaginal wall and keep it on tension. The open tips of the scissors keep constant pressure against the undersurface of the vaginal wall away from the bladder as they are advanced toward the urethra. The bladder is thus separated from the vaginal wall in a bloodless field.

Figure 4. With the uterus and vaginal wall held on tension the surgeon incises it in the midline as far as the urethra.

Figure 5. The divided edges of the vaginal wall are placed on tension by wide blade Allis-Adair clamps.

Figure 6. This is the most important of all the steps. The secret of bloodless separation of the bladder lies in the recognition of the fact that the small vessels and their supporting fibrous strands which bind the bladder to the vaginal wall lie on rather than penetrate the vaginal wall. They are exposed by traction.

The assistant elevates and separates the Allis forceps while the surgeon draws the bladder to the opposite side with the flat portion of the fingers laid over gauze placed on the bladder.

The surgeon then lightly separates with a knife blade the fine fascial attachments above each of the small vessels as they are encountered along the lateral vaginal wall.

VAGINAL SURGERY
ADVANCEMENT OF THE BLADDER

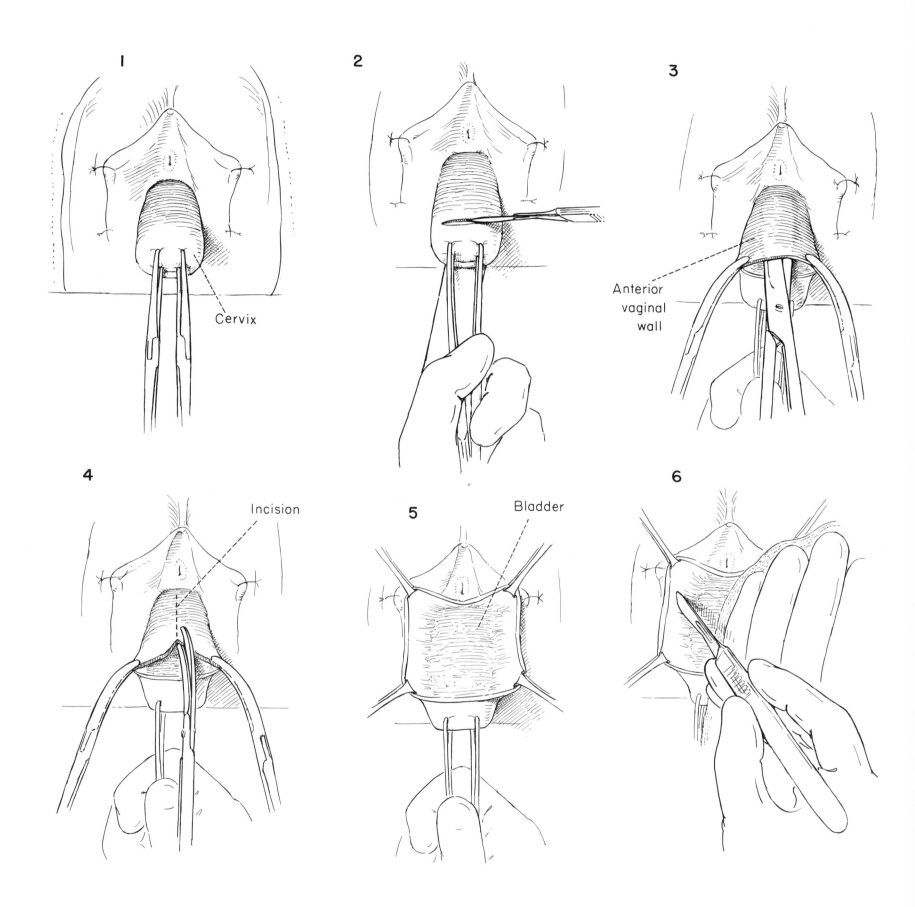

1

Cervix

2

3

Anterior
vaginal
wall

4

Incision

5

Bladder

6

Figure 7. Once the fibrous strands holding the vessels have been divided, the bloodless plane of cleavage can be further developed with the handle of the knife, gently pushing the bladder with the vessels lying on it toward the midline. Traction and countertraction make this possible.

Figure 8. The dissection is extended in this same avascular plane in order to completely separate the bladder from the vaginal wall. Note the angle of the knife handle. The proper cleavage plane is at a 45 degree angle, with the operator's hand retracting the bladder to the midline. The assistant exerts countertraction on the clamps.

Figure 9. This is the so-called bloody angle. By using the same principle of traction, counter-traction and division of the fibrous strands above the vessels, this portion of the operation may be made bloodless.

Figure 10. After division of the attachments of the vessels the knife handle may again be used to bring the cleavage plane into view. This dissection is then carried up along the underside of the symphysis, freeing the urethra laterally.

Figure 11. If the separation is properly developed, the index finger may be inserted into the sulcus formed by the bladder, urethra and lateral vaginal wall without producing any bleeding.

Figure 12. The same steps are repeated on the opposite side. The urethra has been freed from the pubic rami in such a manner that the paraurethral tissue at the bladder neck can be approximated in the midline without tension. This is a necessary step when there is any element of stress incontinence.

Figure 13. At times the most distal portion of the bladder is not easily identified. To bring this out more clearly and to avoid injury to the bladder, the surgeon may elect to introduce a uterine probe into the urethra, advancing it into the bladder until the lower border becomes obvious in its relation to the cervix.

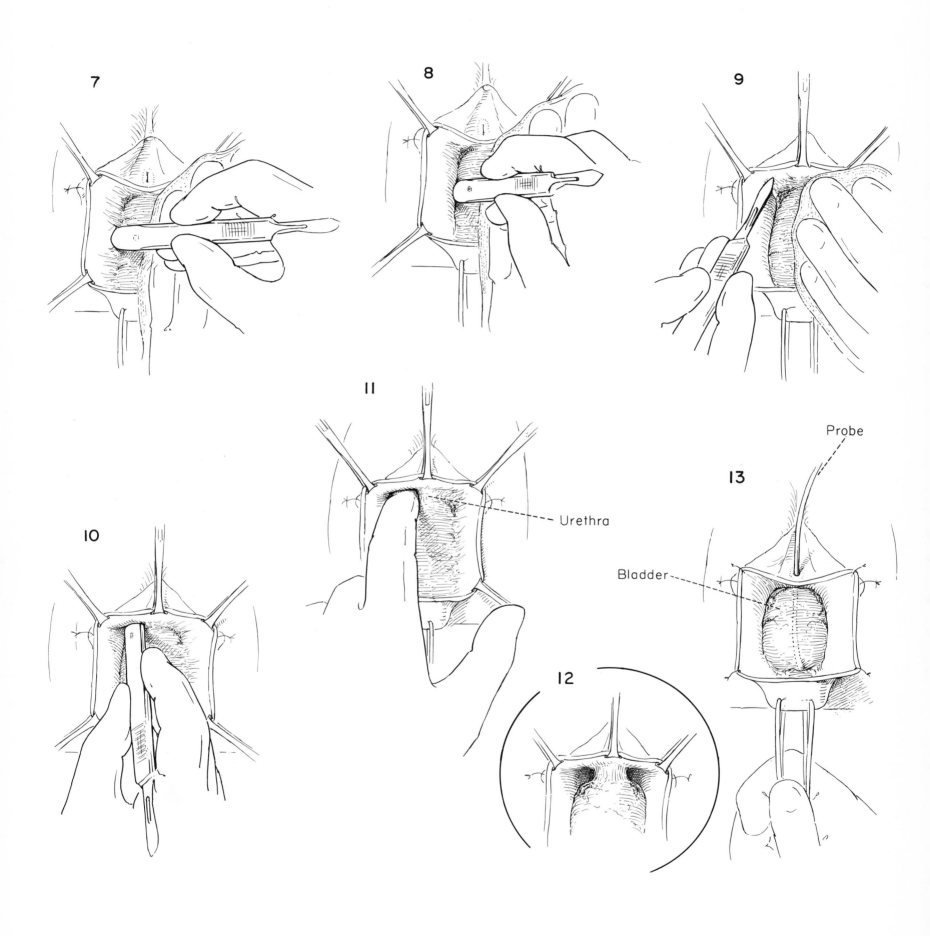

7

8

9

11

Urethra

10

13

Probe

Bladder

12

Figure 14. Though the bladder and urethra are now free of all lateral attachments to the vaginal wall, the bladder is still attached to the cervix and must be separated.

To increase the exposure the clamps on the vaginal wall are removed and the edges sutured to the skin with four to six interrupted catgut sutures.

The assistant holds the uterus downward on traction as the surgeon picks up the lowermost portion of the bladder in the midline above the cervix.

Figure 15. The assistant maintains downward traction on the cervix while the surgeon elevates the bladder in the midline and gently separates the undersurface from the cervix for a short distance with the index finger. The attachments at this point are areolar, and a bloodless plane of cleavage should be present. The lateral attachment of the bladder to the cervical vessels is evident on the left side.

Figure 16. In order to advance the bladder this attachment must be divided. The plane of cleavage between bladder and cervix is gently developed laterally. This can be done with the blunt end of the Kelly clamps. The cervical branch of the uterine vessels lies lateral to the cervix and on a plane parallel to it and must be avoided. It can easily be seen.

Figure 17. Two Kelly clamps are placed across the lateral attachment, avoiding the bladder above and the uterine vessels below. The surgeon then divides the fascia between the clamps. The assistant applies counter-traction to the tenacula on the cervix.

Figure 18. The bladder with clamps on the lateral attachment is elevated as the surgeon places a stitch ligature around the lower clamp and ties it.

Figure 19. The clamp on the bladder side is similarly treated.

Figure 20. The same procedures are carried out on the opposite side.

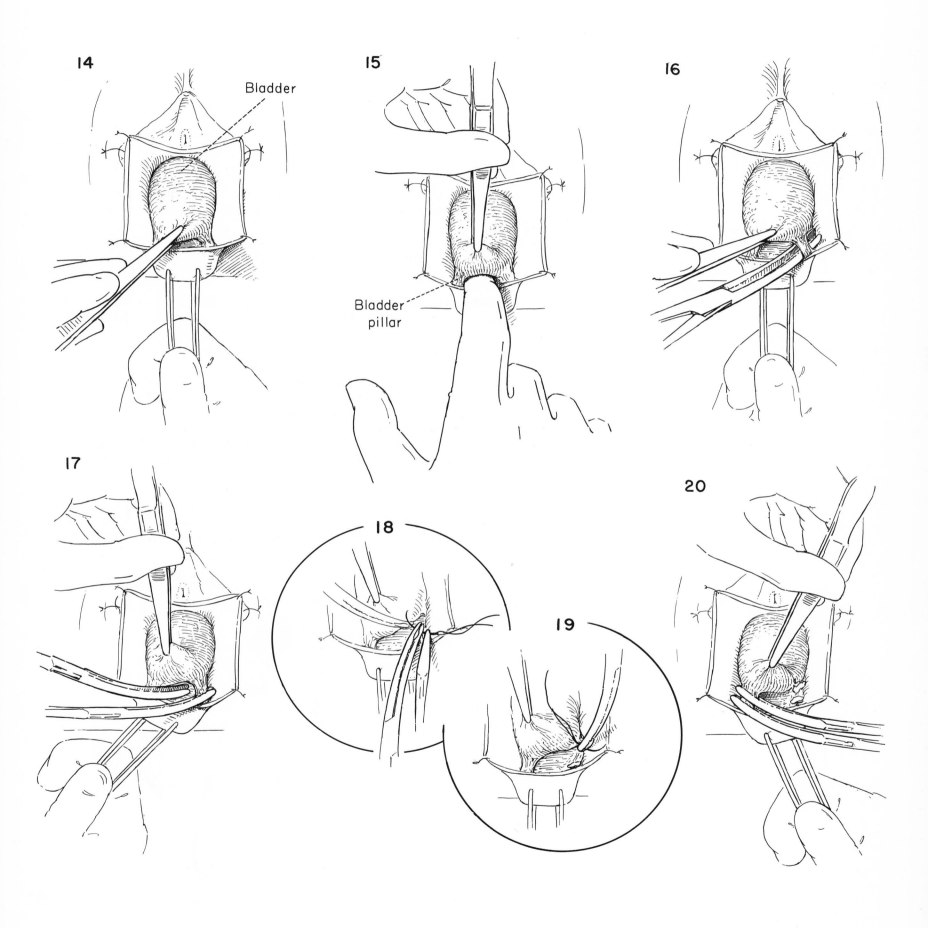

14

Bladder

15

Bladder pillar

16

17

18

19

20

Figure 21. The surgeon now elevates the bladder in the midline with smooth thumb forceps and further dissects the areolar attachments of the bladder from the underlying cervix in the midline. The tips of the scissors point toward the cervix away from the bladder. The assistant pulls downward on the tenacula to provide better exposure.

Figure 22. The assistant continues the traction on the cervical tenacula as the operator elevates the bladder with smooth forceps and completes its separation from the cervix in the midline with the index finger.

Figure 23. The bladder is still attached to the cervix laterally and cannot be sufficiently advanced until the attachments are divided.

There is real danger of damaging the ureter at this point. Before applying Kelly clamps to this point of fixation the surgeon would do well to palpate the ureter between the thumb and forefinger on both sides. Its presence is detected by a snapping sensation as it is rolled between the fingers.

Figure 24. With the position of the ureter identified, a Kelly clamp may be safely applied by staying on a plane superior to the underlying uterine vessels. The tissue between the clamp and the bladder is then divided.

Figure 25. The bladder is retracted medially and the clamp on the lateral side enclosed in a stitch ligature and tied.

Figure 26. With the bladder completely free of attachment to vaginal wall and uterus, it may easily be displaced upward off the cervix and uterus.

Figure 27. This figure shows the bladder completely detached. The vesicouterine fold of peritoneum can often be seen beneath the bladder.

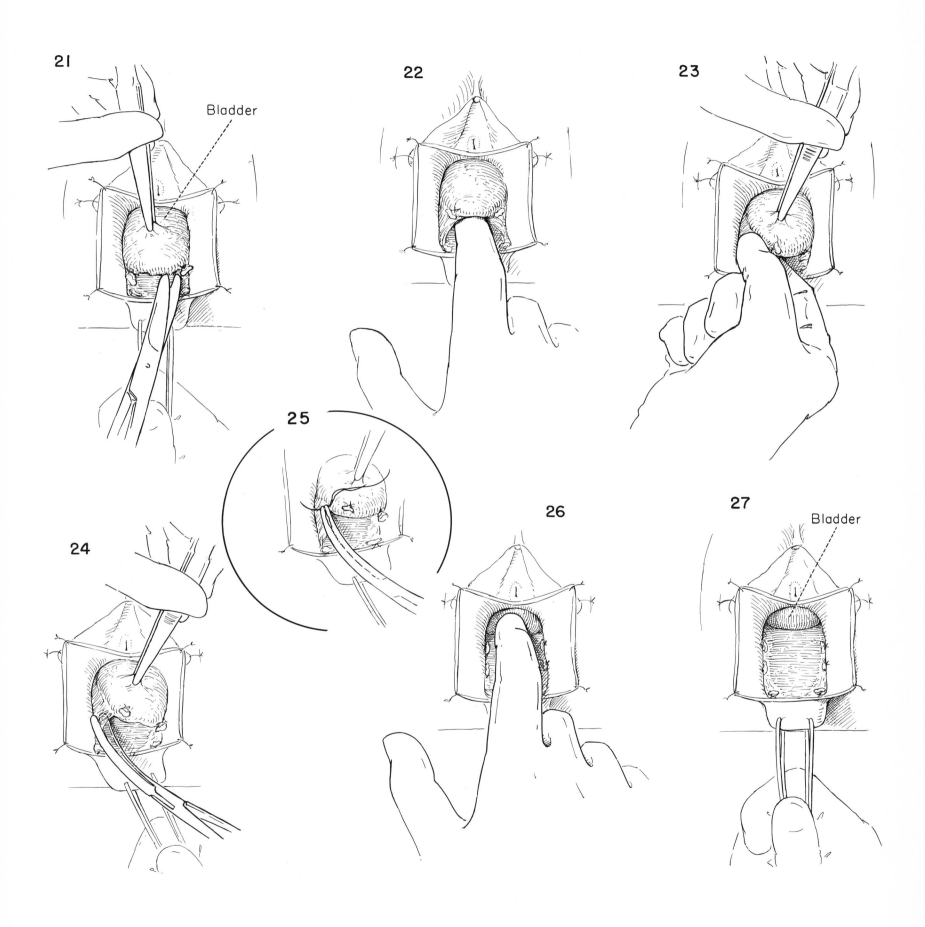

21

Bladder

22

23

25

24

26

27

Bladder

CYSTOCELE REPAIR

As in any hernia repair the cardinal principle is to have tissues approximated without tension. This is the reason it is advisable to advance the bladder off the cervix as the primary step in the cystocele repair. To secure proper infolding of the redundant bladder wall in the repair of the cystocele it must be separated from the vaginal wall and from the uterine vessels and their cervical branches. The dissection must be carried out far enough laterally so that the reparative sutures will correct the anatomic defect without being left on undue tension.

The sutures are placed in the musculofascial layer which completely envelops the bladder. They should not be introduced so deeply that they enter the interior of the bladder nor so widely that they include the intravesical portion of the ureter. A word of caution is offered. Once the initial sutures are placed and tied it is unwise to place a second series of sutures beyond the original line. There is real danger of including the ureter when this is done. The position of the ureter can often be determined by rolling the lateral bladder wall between the thumb and forefinger.

In this plate the bladder has been advanced off the cervix. The surgeon must now decide whether the anatomic findings call for a simple cystocele repair or whether a Manchester operation or vaginal hysterectomy is indicated.

In these illustrations the technique of cystocele repair will be shown.

Figure 1. An Allis-Adair clamp is placed on the incised edge of the vaginal wall in the midline. The assistant applies downward countertraction on the tenacula as the surgeon draws the bladder down into the field with smooth forceps.

Figure 2. The assistant lifts upward on the Allis forceps while the surgeon retracts the bladder downward with the index finger placed over gauze on the bladder wall. This brings the urethra into view in relation to the bladder. A small curved needle with an atraumatic catgut suture is placed lateral to the urethra, passing into the fascial envelope covering the neck of the bladder.

Figure 3. The same stitch continues across the bladder neck and is passed from below upward in the corresponding position on the other side of the urethra.

Figure 4. The assistant elevates the clamp on the initial untied suture and pulls down on the cervix with the tenacula. The surgeon then retracts the bladder to the right and places another suture into the bladder wall well out laterally on the left side.

Figure 5. The bladder is then drawn to the left, and a parallel suture is placed in the right lateral wall again from below upward. The assistant continues the traction and countertraction.

Figure 6. A third suture similar to the previous sutures is placed in the anterior wall of the bladder. All are clamped and left untied. All these sutures must carefully avoid penetrating too deeply in order not to enter the interior of the bladder or catch the transvesical portion of the ureter.

CYSTOCELE REPAIR

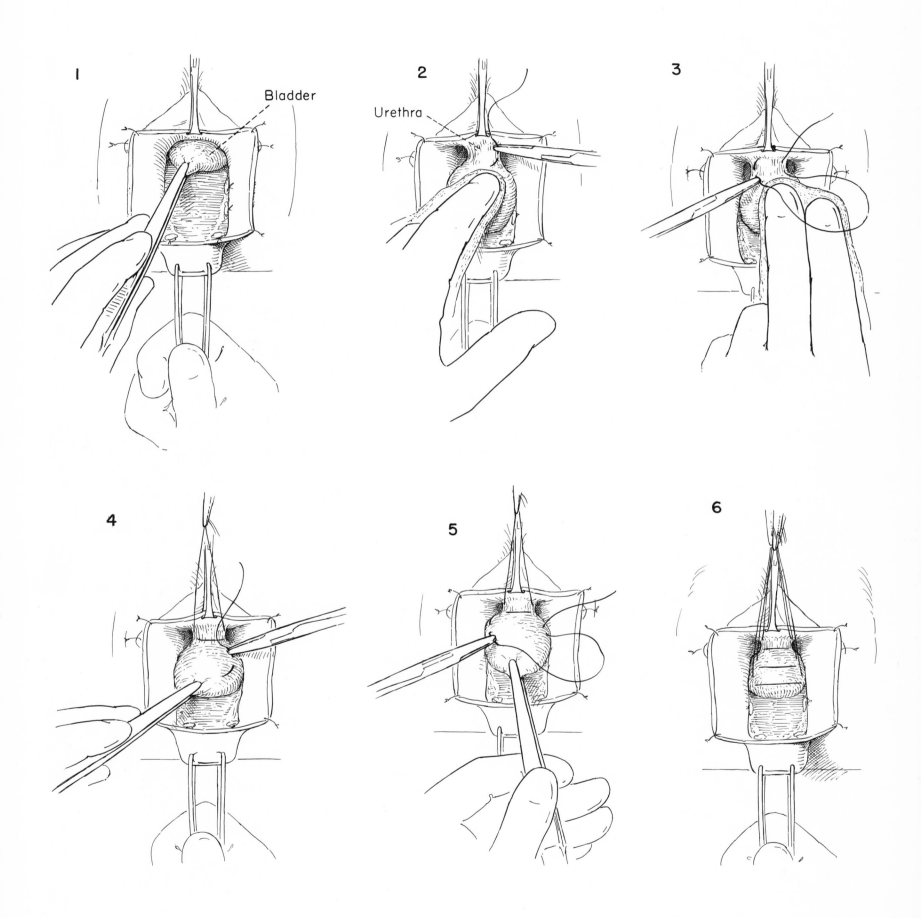

Figure 7. The sutures are now tied, beginning at the urethra and descending toward the cervix. The sutures are not divided until the surgeon assures himself that a sufficient number have been placed to satisfactorily infold the redundant bladder; more sutures may be needed. The operator should be cautioned against placing another row of sutures lateral to the initial row. There is great danger of including the ureter in a stitch if this is attempted. In this illustration the last suture is being tied.

Figure 8. The midline Allis clamp is removed and the stitches holding the cut edges of vagina to the skin are cut. Kelly clamps are placed on the vaginal wall on both sides opposite one another both above and below. The excess is then cut away. It may be ill advised to sacrifice too much tissue lest narrowing of the vaginal canal result.

Figure 9. The assistant places an Allis clamp at the upper limits of the midline defect. This clamp is held upward while the cervix is held down as the surgeon places the first of the interrupted catgut sutures which will close the vaginal wall.

Figure 10. A series of interrupted sutures of catgut reapproximates the edges of the incision in the vaginal wall. Each suture is held up before being divided to aid the surgeon in the placing of the next stitch.

Figure 11. The longitudinal portion of the incision has been finished. Further interrupted sutures close the transverse defect. Clamps on the incised edges of the vaginal wall provide exposure.

Figure 12. The closure is now complete and the tenacula are removed.

Figure 13. The cervix has returned to its normal position. Only the sutures in the anterior vaginal wall can be seen. An indwelling catheter is left in the bladder for constant drainage.

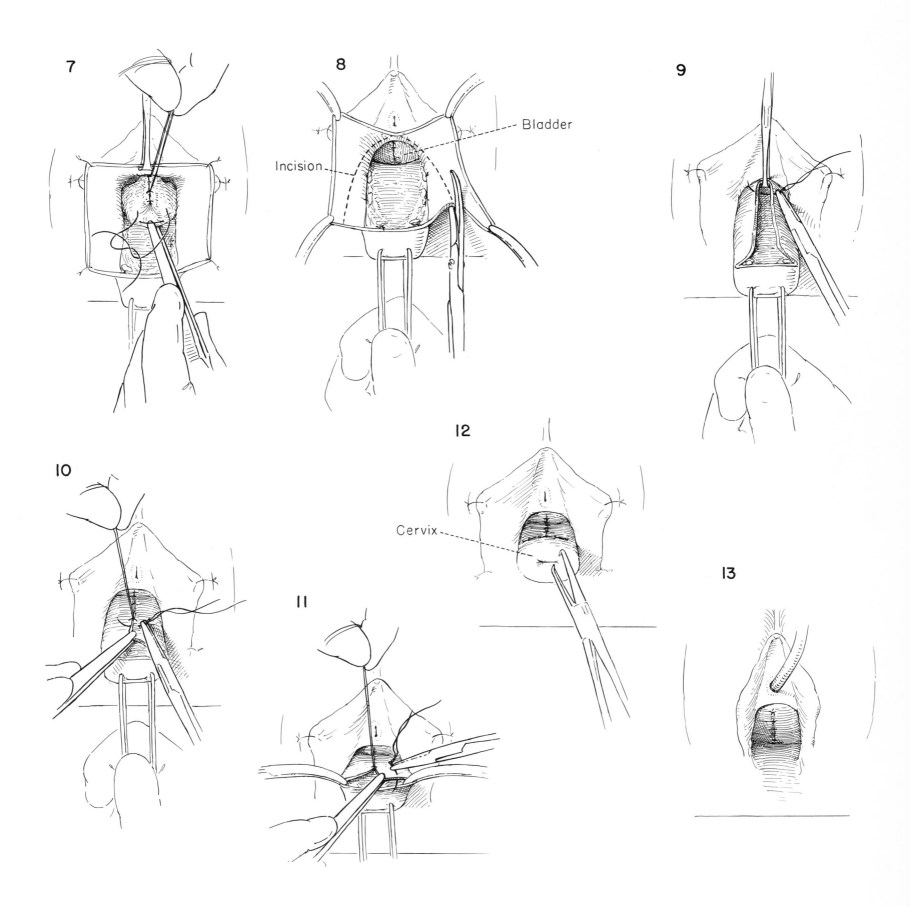

THE MANCHESTER (DONALD OR FOTHERGILL) OPERATION

A moderate degree of prolapse of both bladder and uterus can be effectively handled by the Manchester (Donald or Fothergill) operation. If there is a tendency for the uterus to prolapse and the bladder is advanced off the cervix in the repair of a cystocele, a long cervix extends into the vaginal canal. Amputation of the cervix is a part of the Fothergill procedure. It is useful in this situation and has particular application when the patient is in the reproductive age group with her family not yet complete. The uterus is preserved for any subsequent pregnancy which may follow.

The effectiveness of the operation revolves around the approximation of the cardinal ligament in front of the cervix. The elongated cervix, common to uterine prolapse, is amputated.

The major support of the uterus rests with the cardinal ligaments. Normally they adhere closely to the side wall of the cervix, but in the relaxed state they may drift laterally, forming a V with the cervix. The operation brings the arms of the V together to form a Y-shaped support; this is accomplished by use of interrupted sutures on either side of the amputated cervix which are tied in the midline.

Figure 1. After the cervix has been dilated and the bladder advanced, the reparative steps begin. The cardinal ligaments, consisting of the uterine vessels and fascial sheaths, can be seen coming in on either side of the cervix.

Figure 2. The bladder is kept out of the field by a small Deaver retractor placed over gauze. The key to the support of the uterus in this operation is the shortening of the cardinal ligaments. This is accomplished by suturing them to the amputated cervix. Strong traction of the uterus to the patient's right exposes the left arm of the cardinal ligament, and the first Fothergill suture is placed through the fascial bundle.

Figure 3. The uterus is now pulled to the patient's left as the surgeon continues to stitch across the surface of the cervix into the fascial sheath of the opposite side.

Figure 4. Two more such sutures are placed. Traction on the lowermost suture serves to expose the upper and more lateral portion of the ligament. The untied sutures are held in a clamp while the operator proceeds with the amputation of the cervix.

Figure 5. The cervix is held upward and the posterior vaginal wall is incised at the level of the original anterior incision.

Figure 6. The vaginal wall is stripped from the posterior wall of the cervix for an appreciable distance.

MANCHESTER (DONALD OR FOTHERGILL) OPERATION

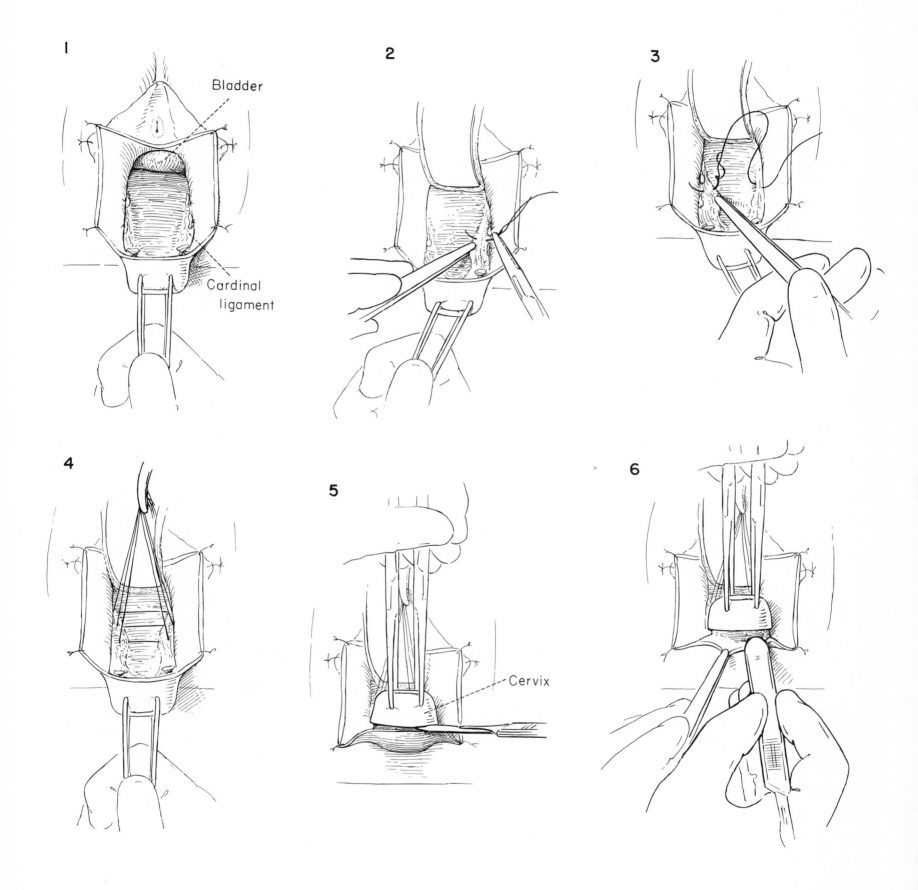

Page 221

Figure 7. A Kelly clamp grasps the cervix at the level where amputation is to be done. It should be allowed to slip off the cervix to ensure that it includes all the tissue lateral to the cervix. The tissue in the clamp is then cut.

Figure 8. The tissue in the clamp is secured with a stitch ligature. These steps are repeated on the opposite side.

Figure 9. A final Fothergill stitch is placed through the stump of the cardinal ligament, and the ends are added to the group held long in the clamp.

Figure 10. The untied sutures are held taut, and countertraction is applied on the tenaculum as the surgeon begins to amputate the cervix just below the position of the last suture.

Figure 11. The amputation continues, with slight bevelling of the cervix toward the canal. In order to continue traction after the cervix has been amputated it is necessary to replace the tenacula on the lateral sides of the uterus just below the ties on the cardinal ligament before the final division is made.

Figure 12. Both the tenacula and the long ties on the cardinal ligament are held downward as the surgeon removes the retractor and pulls the bladder into view with smooth forceps.

Figure 13. The cystocele must now be repaired. The assistant applies traction to the tenaculum as the surgeon places the bladder neck on tension with the index finger laid over gauze on the bladder wall. The first of the reparative sutures is then placed in the paraurethral tissue to the left of the urethra.

Figure 14. This suture on a small curved needle is carried across the face of the bladder to enter the paraurethral and bladder tissue directly parallel to the suture on the left.

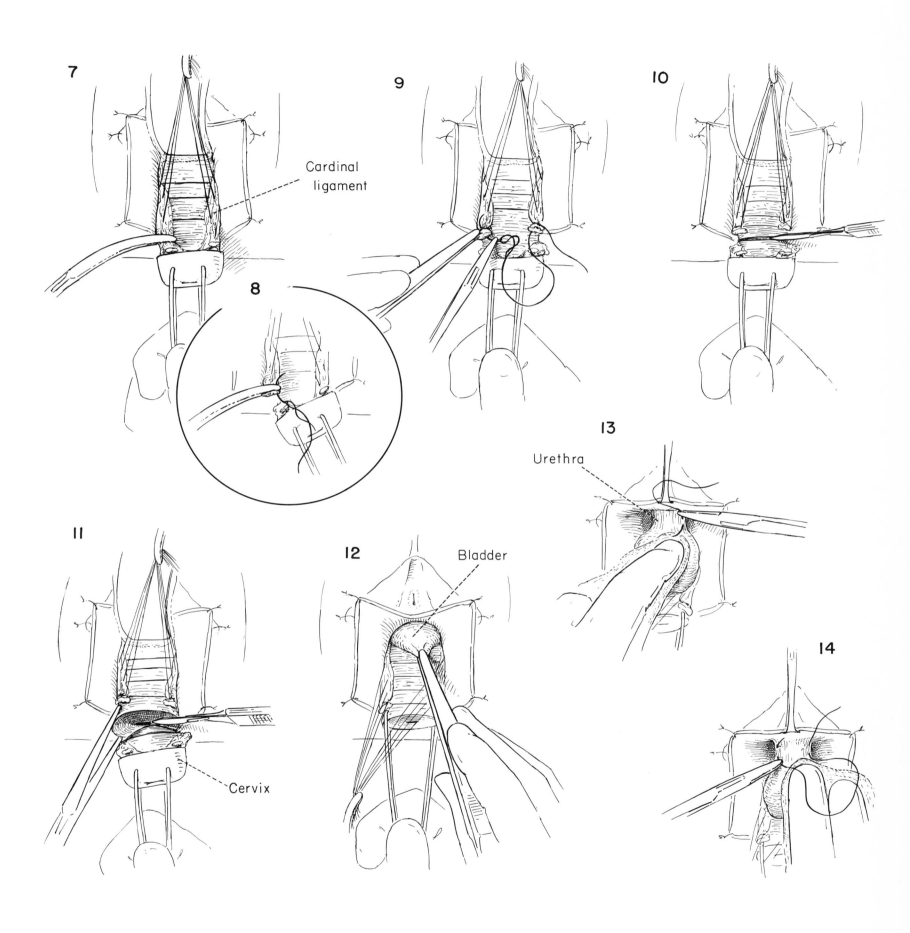

7

9

Cardinal
ligament

8

10

13

Urethra

11

12   Bladder

Cervix

14

Figure 15. A series of interrupted sutures beginning at the urethra and descending toward the cervix has been placed in the anterior bladder wall. Enough sutures are placed to satisfactorily infold the redundant bladder. The assistants hold the bladder sutures upward and the long ties on the cardinal ligaments down.

Figure 16. Each of the series of sutures is tied and held long. The assistant dunks the redundant bladder wall as the last suture is tied.

Figure 17. After the sutures have been tied and cut, the bladder retracts upward in normal position. The retraction sutures holding the cut edges of vagina have been divided and replaced with clamps.

Attention now turns to the amputated cervix, which must be covered by the vaginal wall. A Sturmdorf stitch will be used to draw the wall into its final position, where it should lie without tension. A catgut suture on a cutting needle picks up the posterior vaginal wall in the midline about 1/8 inch from the incised edge.

Figure 18. Half of a complete tie is made with this suture. The cervix is then held upward as the surgeon introduces the cutting needle into the cervical canal and brings it out through the cervical muscle and vaginal wall just lateral to the midline.

Figure 19. As the assistant holds up the posterior vaginal wall, the other end, also on a cutting point needle, is placed in the cervical canal and brought through muscle and vaginal wall to emerge parallel to the first suture approximatley 1/4 inch from it.

Figure 20. The suture is pulled taut, thereby drawing the vaginal wall over the raw surface of the cervical stump up into the canal. The tenacula are removed. Control over the position of the cervix can now be maintained by a clamp on the long ends of the Sturmdorf stitch.

Figure 21. Each of the sutures in the cardinal ligament beginning from below upward is now serially tied.

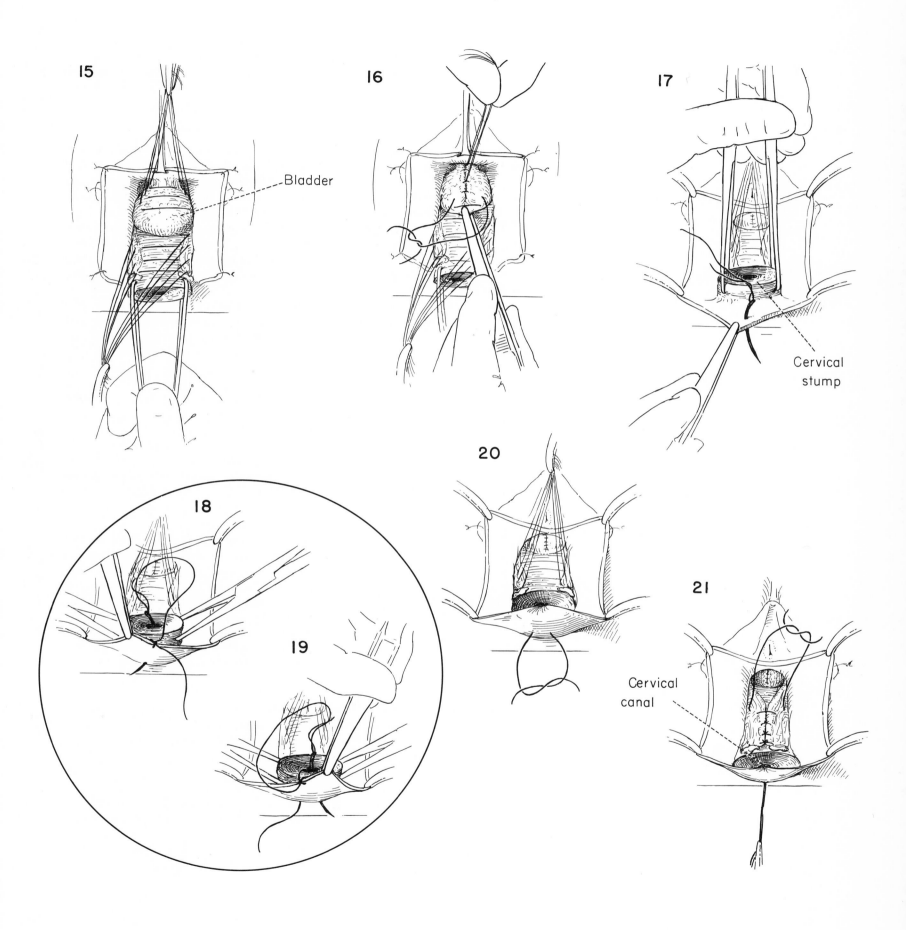

15

16

17 Cervical stump

Bladder

18

19

20

21 Cervical canal

Figure 22. The cystocele has been repaired, and the cardinal ligaments are approximated in front of the amputated cervix. The vaginal wall has also been drawn into the cervical canal. The excess vaginal wall on the anterior flaps is now excised.

Figure 23. The success or failure of the operation may depend on how well the following steps are carried out. Despite the fact that the amputated cervix has been dilated, there is always the chance that cervical stenosis may occur in the convalescent phase. Great care must be taken in the proper coverage of the raw edges of the amputated cervix by the vaginal wall flaps.

The surgeon must carefully estimate the amount of vaginal wall necessary to cover the anterior half of the cervix. It must lie easily in position within the new cervical canal. The Sturmdorf stitch is very useful in drawing the mobile vaginal edges across the amputated cervix and into the cervical canal; it should rest without tension.

The assistant places the left anterior flap on tension as the surgeon passes a curved cutting point needle with catgut suture through the vaginal wall at the point selected. The suture passes through the vaginal wall and cervix to emerge in the canal.

Figure 24. With the vaginal wall on tension the needle returns through the wall from below upward about $1/8$ inch from the corner.

Figure 25. The stitch continues through the opposite leaf of vaginal wall at the same relative position, the suture being introduced from above downward.

Figure 26. The position of the needle is reversed and enters the cervical canal to emerge through muscle and vaginal wall opposite the point of origin.

Figure 27. Downward traction is exerted on the cervix. To exert counter-traction an Allis clamp is placed in the midline at the upper limit of the anterior vaginal wall incision as the surgeon places the first of a series of interrupted sutures on the incised vaginal edges. The anterior Sturmdorf stitch is in place but has not yet been tied. It is clamped and held downward.

Figure 28. The Allis clamp is removed as the first of a series of vaginal wall sutures is tied. As each suture is placed and tied, the previous suture is cut. The anterior Sturmdorf suture, which pulls the vaginal wall over the raw cervix and into the canal, is now tied.

Figure 29. The anterior vaginal wall defect is now closed. The assistants steady the last sutures on each corner as the surgeon introduces a dilator into the canal to ensure the patency.

During the convalescent phase, periodic dilation of the canal should be carried out as an office procedure until healing is established.

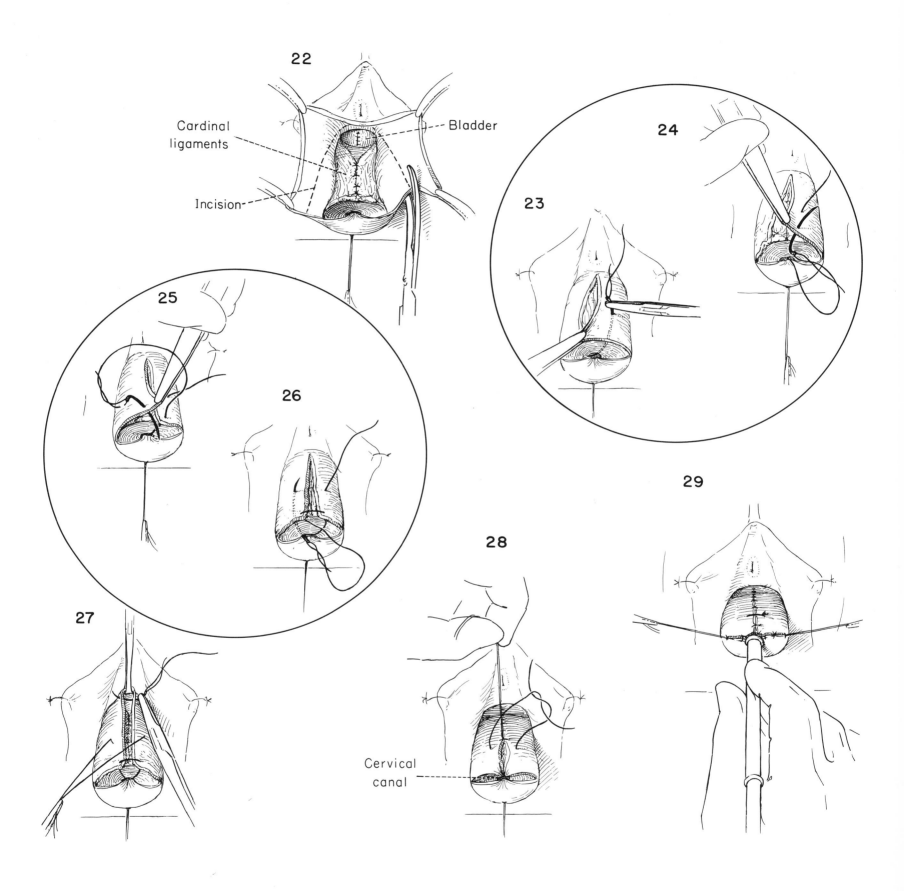

22

Cardinal ligaments

Bladder

Incision

23

24

25

26

27

28

Cervical canal

29

VAGINAL HYSTERECTOMY

When procidentia or moderate relaxation of the pelvic floor exists, the surgeon may elect to remove the uterus in the interest of a more satisfactory repair. Moreover, the vaginal approach may be selected deliberately for removal of the uterus in older patients when the risk of abdominal surgery is significant. The risk, however, must be balanced against the technical difficulty of performing this operation in the presence of a fixed uterus or one containing a sizable tumor. Safety and comfort of the patient rather than the operator's technical facility should be the guiding principle in the choice of the vaginal rather than the abdominal approach. Finally, if any suspicion of malignant disease has been raised, vaginal hysterectomy should not be performed. As in abdominal hysterectomy, dilatation and curettage are the first step.

The decision for or against removal of the uterus is made after the bladder has been advanced off the cervix. In most instances the anterior peritoneal reflection can be seen beneath the bladder, lying on the anterior wall of the uterus. It is possible to enter the abdominal cavity by incising the flap. The fundus can then be drawn out through the opening. The removal of the uterus can be accomplished from the adnexa downward as in an abdominal hysterectomy. As a result of the local findings, the surgeon may elect to proceed entirely along one side of the uterus before turning attention to the opposite side, or he may alternate from side to side as the operation progresses.

When the uterus is somewhat fixed and cannot be brought out easily through the opening in the anterior peritoneum, greater mobility can be obtained by starting from below, stripping back the posterior vaginal wall off the cervix and dividing the uterosacral and cardinal ligaments. At times the fixation may be such that it will be necessary to remove the uterus entirely from below upward.

The main principles involved are those of continued traction in order that the individual structures may be identified. No tissue is divided before being first clamped and secured with a stitch ligature. The emphasis is on a bloodless field.

Figure 1. The uterus has been curetted and the bladder advanced. The cystocele is not repaired until the reconstructive phase of the operation is begun.

Figure 2. The cervix is held upward toward the symphysis, exposing the posterior wall of the cervix and vagina. The surgeon then transects the vaginal wall on the back of the cervix with a knife at the level of the initial anterior incision.

Figure 3. With the uterus on tension the vaginal wall is stripped off the cervix. Bleeding is minimal in the proper cleavage plane.

Figure 4. The vaginal wall is separated from the posterior cervix until the uterosacral ligaments stand out on either side and the peritoneum of the posterior cul-de-sac appears between them.

Figure 5. Upward traction on the uterus continues as the surgeon picks up the posterior peritoneum and incises it, thus entering the peritoneal cavity.

Figure 6. If the bleeding from the incised vaginal edge is troublesome, it may be controlled by placing an interrupted suture through the wall and peritoneal edge and tying it. This will be removed later.

VAGINAL HYSTERECTOMY

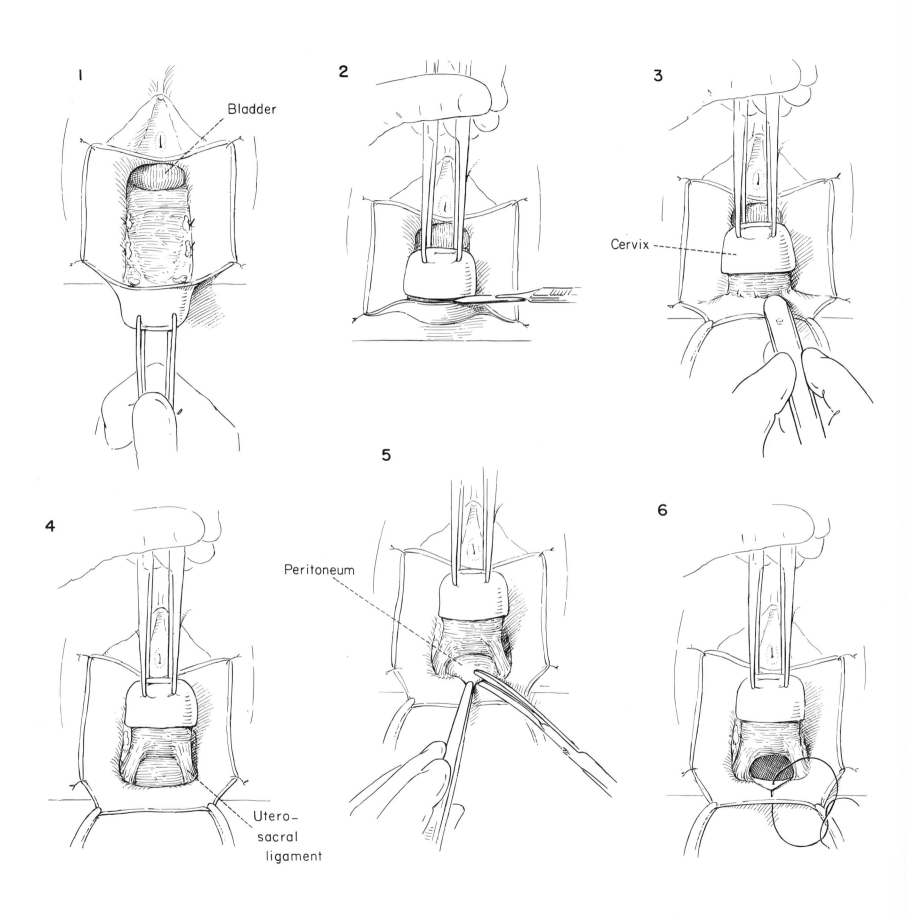

Figure 7. The index finger is then inserted into the peritoneal cavity and the cul-de-sac explored to be sure that nothing is adherent to the uterosacral ligament.

Figure 8. The cervix is placed on traction in the upward direction while the uterosacral ligament is clamped and the tissue intervening between it and the uterus is sectioned with the knife.

Figure 9. The tissue held in the clamp is secured with a stitch ligature and tied, but not cut. The ties are left long and clamped. They will be used later in the subsequent repair. The same steps are repeated on the opposite side.

Figure 10. The assistant draws the uterus sharply downward and to the patient's left as the surgeon places a Kelly clamp on the lower end of the cardinal ligament on the right side at the point of its attachment to the cervix. The clamp grasps the cervix and is allowed to slide off it to ensure that all tissue is included. Another clamp is placed below it on the uterine side.

Figure 11. The tissue between the clamps is then divided and a stitch ligature placed around the upper clamp and tied.

Figure 12. A second stitch ligature secures the pedicle on the uterine side. The cardinal ligament on the other side is similarly treated.

Figure 13. The uterus is held on traction and the index finger of the right hand inserted in the peritoneal cavity and around anterior to the uterus to identify the anterior peritoneal fold.

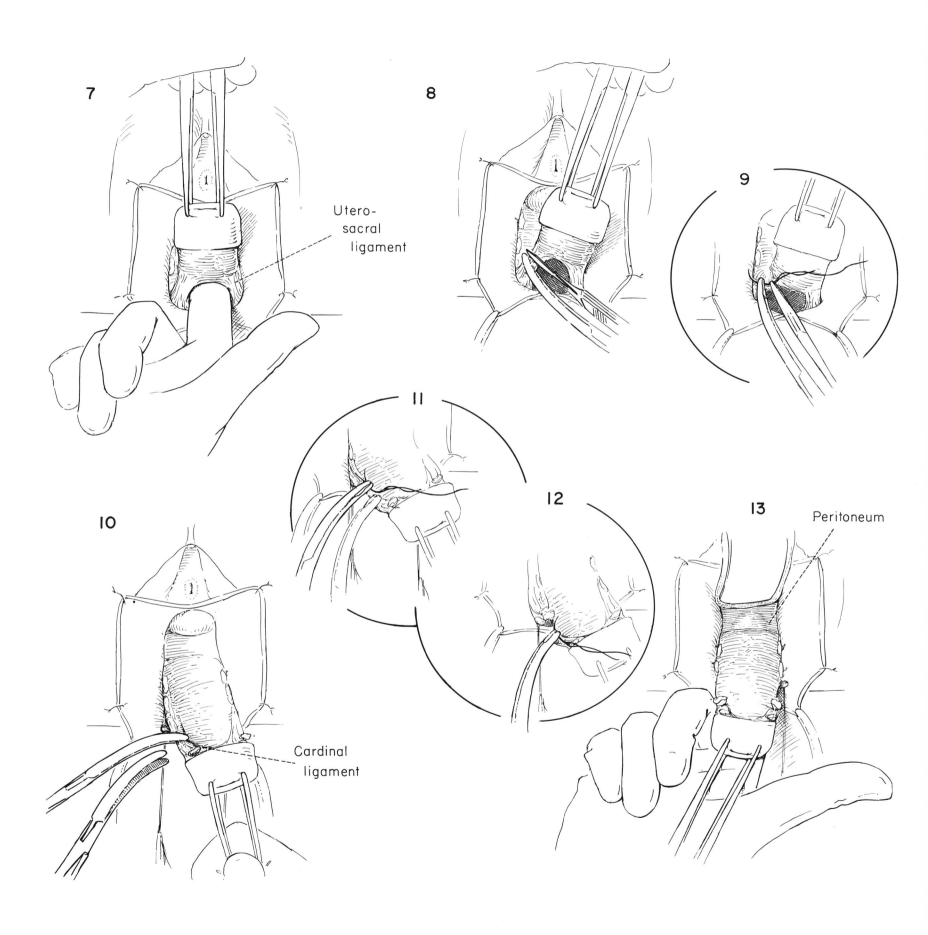

7

8

9

Utero-
sacral
ligament

11

10

12

13   Peritoneum

Cardinal
ligament

Figure 14. A small Deaver retractor is used to retract the bladder while the uterus is placed on downward traction. The operator then picks up the anterior peritoneal fold and divides it with scissors.

Figure 15. To aid in subsequent identification of the anterior leaf of peritoneum, a stitch ligature is placed through it and tied. The ends are left longer than usual after section so that it can easily be found when the time arrives for peritoneal closure.

Figure 16. The surgeon then inserts the fingers of the right hand into the peritoneal cavity to palpate the posterior uterine surface and adnexa for possible tubo-ovarian disease. A retractor now holds back both peritoneum and bladder.

Figure 17. As the hand is withdrawn the fundus of the uterus is pulled outward through the opening into the operative field, and a double hook is applied to the fundus. A retractor anteriorly protects the bladder and aids in exposure.

Figure 18. The fundus is sharply angulated downward in order to expose the adnexa on the left side.

The operator inserts the index finger of the left hand below the adnexa to ward off possible descent of small intestine and places the first stitch around the fallopian tube and ovarian vessels. This stitch is then tied and held long.

Figure 19. A Kelly clamp is placed across the ovarian ligament and fallopian tube on the uterine side as the assistant holds the initial suture on tension and prepares to clamp the cut end of the stump.

Figure 20. The operator places another stitch ligature around the clamp and ties it, thus placing two ties on the ovarian vessels. Both ties are then cut.

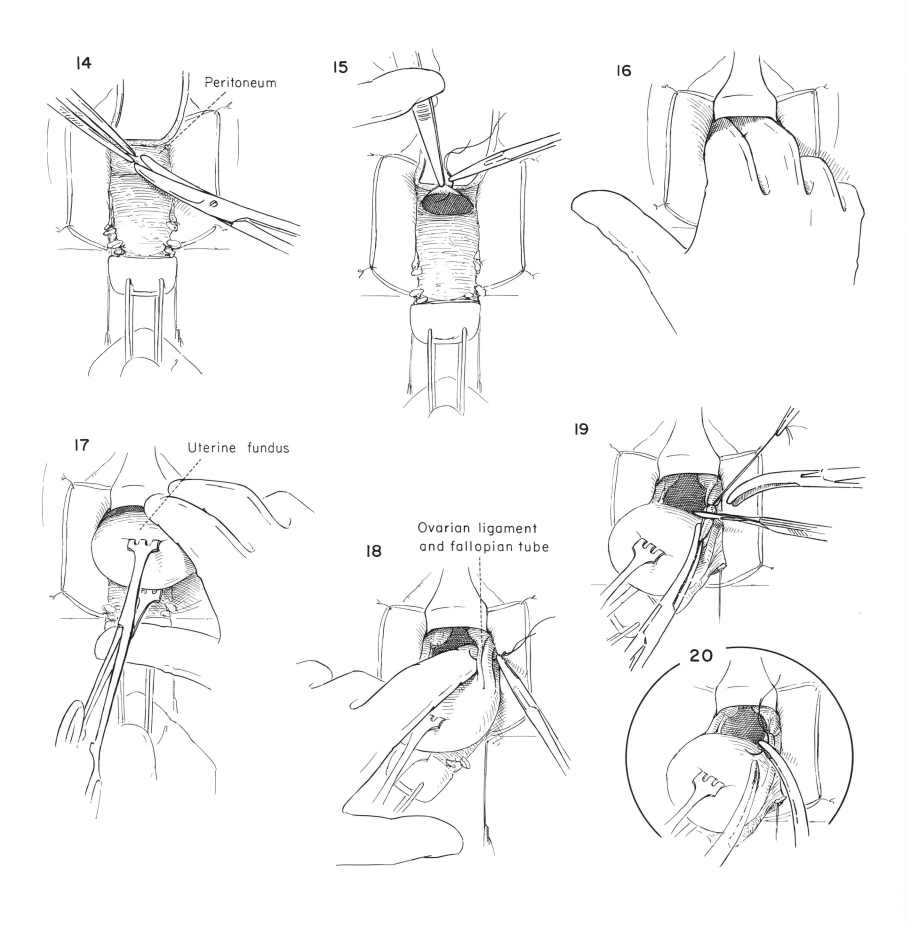

14

Peritoneum

15

16

17

Uterine fundus

18

Ovarian ligament
and fallopian tube

19

20

Figure 21. The operator pulls the uterus to the patient's right, removes the clamp on the proximal stump of the ovarian ligament and tube, and reapplies it to include the round ligament as well.

Figure 22. A stitch ligature is applied around the round ligament and tied. The ends are clamped and left long. The round ligament will be used in subsequent reconstruction of the pelvic floor.

Figure 23. The uterus continues to be drawn to the patient's right side as the assistant applies traction on the round ligament to the left. The surgeon then divides the ligament between the clamp on the uterine side and the long tie on the round ligament.

Figure 24. Whenever possible, the authors choose to continue to remove the uterus from above downward as in the abdominal hysterectomy. At times because of the fixation produced by associated disease it may be necessary to approach the uterine vessels from below. The operator may elect to repeat each step on both sides as he goes along or free the uterus entirely on one side, identifying and securing the vessels before turning his attention to the opposite side. These are the steps described here.

Whatever method is chosen, adequate exposure must be obtained, since the ureter is in close proximity. By stripping back the vaginal wall the broad ligament is brought into view. This move has the double advantage of producing lateral retraction of the ureter as well as exposing the uterine vessels in their relation to it.

A single clamp has been placed across the broad ligament close to the uterus in order to control the ovarian branch of the uterine artery. The tissue between the uterus and clamp is then divided.

Figure 25. A stitch ligature secures and ties the tissue in the clamp.

Figure 26. The uterine vessels are now isolated from the surrounding tissue.

Figure 27. Two clamps are placed on the uterine vessels, and the operator divides between them, leaving a cuff projecting from the lateral clamp.

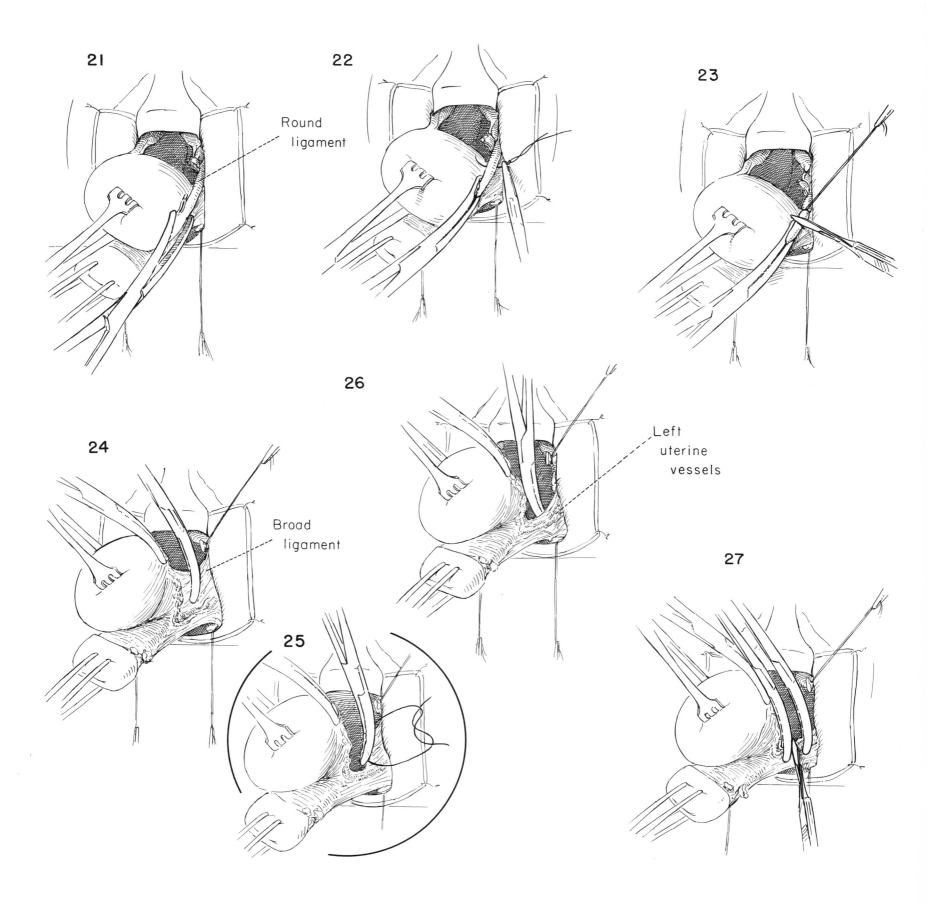

21

22 Round ligament

23

24 Broad ligament

25

26 Left uterine vessels

27

Figure 28. The uterus continues to be drawn to the right as a second clamp is placed on the cuff of the sectioned uterine vessels.

Figure 29. A stitch ligature is placed around the vessels lateral to the clamps.

Figure 30. The operator now prepares to tie this stitch as the first of the clamps is removed, leaving the second clamp to control the vessels if the primary tie should break.

Figure 31. The stitch is now tied and a second stitch is placed around the remaining clamp.

Figure 32. A final strand of tissue still holds the uterus on the left side. This contains the cervical branch of the uterine artery and must be clamped.

Figure 33. The tissue in the clamp is then tied and cut. This is in keeping with the principle that no attachment to the uterus should be cut without previously clamping it, since these supports will always retract, carrying bleeding vessels with them.

Figure 34. All steps are repeated on the right side.

Figure 35. The uterus has been removed. The identifying tie originally placed on the posterior peritoneal edge is removed, and closure of the peritoneal opening is begun in the center with a fine atraumatic catgut suture.

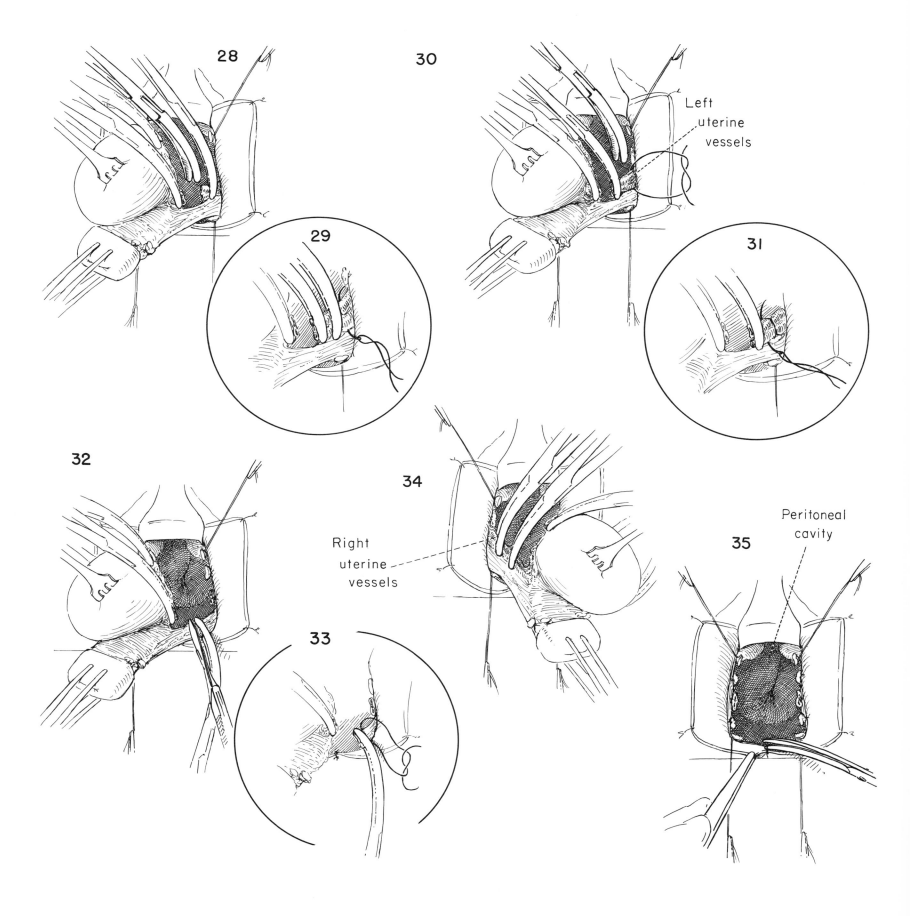

28

30

Left
uterine
vessels

29

31

32

34

Right
uterine
vessels

33

35

Peritoneal
cavity

The reconstructive phase is as important as that of the removal. In most instances the choice of the vaginal procedure will have been made because of an element of prolapse or vaginal relaxation. The reparative steps must be well conceived and executed if prolapse of the vaginal apex is to be avoided. An excellent support to the upper part of the vagina will result if the round and uterosacral ligaments are first sutured together and then attached to the vaginal wall at the apex of the vagina on either side. As the ligaments retract, the vagina is drawn upward. An adequate vaginal canal is obtained in this way. It is better than bringing the broad ligaments together in the midline in front of the bladder. When this type of repair is done there tends to be foreshortening of the vagina.

Figure 36. The first step in the reconstructive phase calls for closure of the peritoneum. The simplest method is to employ a purse-string type of suture. The anterior leaf of the peritoneal reflexion is identified by the suture placed on it at the time the peritoneal cavity was opened. The purse-string suture begins at this point.

Figure 37. The exposure is made easier when traction is made on the long sutures which were placed at the time the round cardinal and uterosacral ligaments were divided and secured. A series of bites are taken, with the stitch ligature beginning on the anterior peritoneum and continuing in circular fashion to include that of the broad ligament at the lateral extensions of the opening. The stitch continues in the peritoneum in the posterior margins of the opening on to the right side and again embodies the peritoneum on the inner side of the broad ligament. The stitch continues into the anterior peritoneum until it meets the original suture. Note that the stumps of the round and uterosacral ligaments are outside the area of the defect which has been sutured.

Figure 38. The two ends of the suture are then placed on traction. This will bring the tissues together in purse-string fashion, closing off the abdominal cavity from the rest of the wound. Note again that the round and uterosacral ligaments with their long sutures attached lie outside the abdominal cavity.

Figure 39. Holding the long sutures and the round and uterosacral ligaments on tension, the surgeon now places a figure-of-eight suture to include both ligaments in one stitch. This is tied and the suture clamped and left long. The same thing is done on the opposite side.

Figure 40. The bladder is now brought into view with smooth thumb forceps.

Figure 41. An Allis-Adair clamp is placed on the edge of the vaginal wall in the midline and drawn upward. The surgeon pulls down on the bladder and places the stitches to repair the cystocele. They are clamped and left long.

Figure 42. The last of the interrupted sutures for correction of the cystocele is being tied.

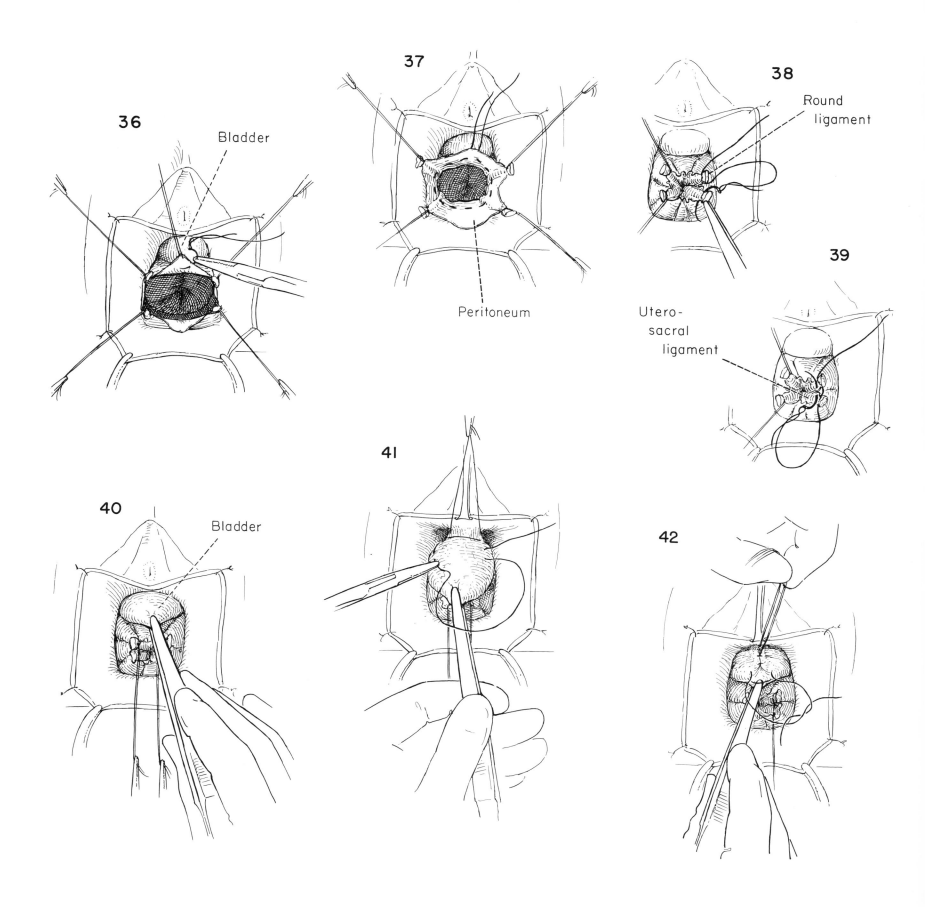

36

Bladder

37

Peritoneum

38

Round
ligament

39

Utero-
sacral
ligament

40

Bladder

41

42

Figure 43. The surgeon removes some of the excess anterior vaginal wall.

Figure 44. A needle is threaded on one end of the suture which brought the left uterosacral and round ligaments together. This is then carried through the posterior vaginal wall about ½ inch from the cut edge. The same maneuver is carried out on the other loose end of the suture. Again these sutures are left untied and clamped. The same thing has been done on the right side.

Figure 45. An Allis clamp pulls the upper end of the anterior vaginal wall incision toward the symphysis while Kelly clamps draw down at each angle of the vaginal wall defect as the first interrupted suture closing the defect in the vaginal wall is placed.

Figure 46. A series of interrupted sutures approximate the vaginal edges. The untied sutures on the uterosacral and round ligaments are now tied. As the ligaments retract, the apex of the vagina is drawn upward and becomes suspended, thus minimizing the risk of subsequent prolapse.

Figure 47. The uterus has been removed, the cystocele repaired, and the apex of the vagina suspended. To complete the operation the surgeon should do a perineorrhaphy.

Figure 48. After removal of the interrupted sutures holding back the labia, a transverse incision is made at the junction of skin and vaginal wall at the fourchette. By using Kelly clamps as traction, the tips of the scissors are advanced upward, staying close to the undersurface of the posterior vaginal wall.

Figure 49. The rectum is separated from the posterior lateral vaginal wall.

Figure 50. Separation of the rectum from the vaginal wall exposes the levator muscles. A series of interrupted sutures approximates them in front of the rectum.

Figure 51. These sutures are tied. The first interrupted suture to approximate the vaginal edges is being placed at the apex.

Figure 52. A few final stitches have been placed in the skin to complete the operation.

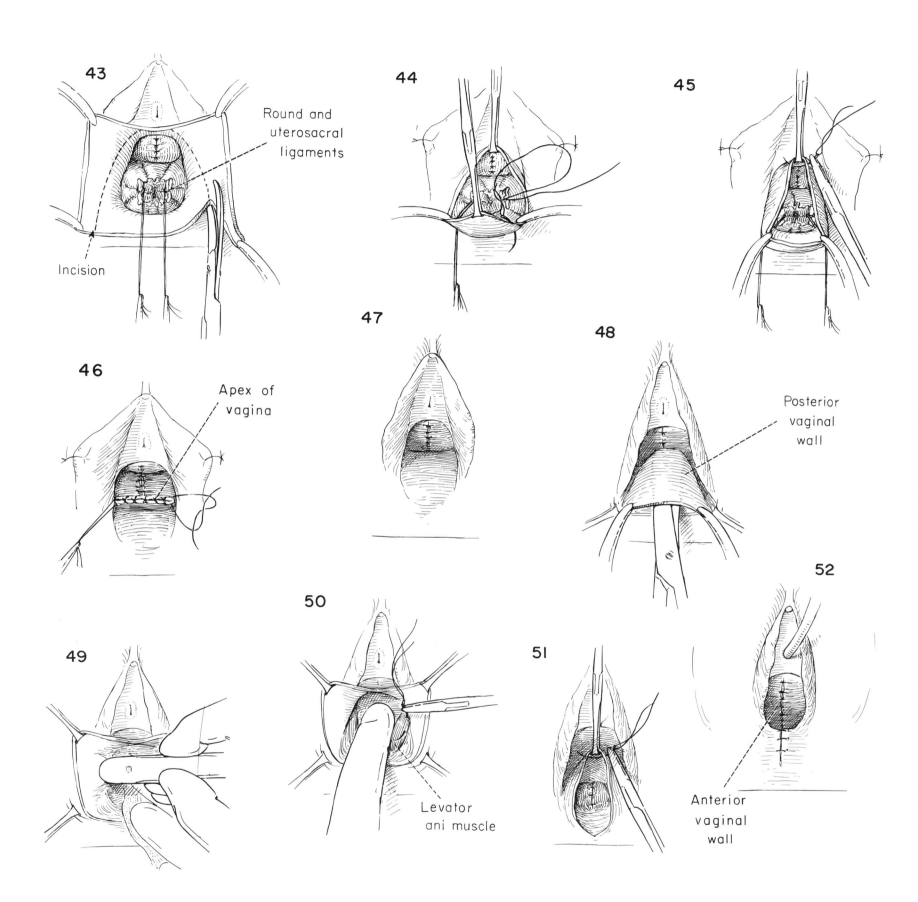

43

Round and
uterosacral
ligaments

Incision

44

45

46

Apex of
vagina

47

48

Posterior
vaginal
wall

49

50

Levator
ani muscle

51

52

Anterior
vaginal
wall

THE LE FORT OPERATION

Procidentia may occur in an elderly poor risk patient who may not be able to withstand the strain of a vaginal hysterectomy. Preservation of a normal vaginal canal is no longer a consideration. The Le Fort procedure is technically simple and can be performed with a minimal amount of shock to the patient. There is little blood loss. If necessary, the procedure can be done under a local anesthesic.

The anterior and posterior vaginal walls are denuded, leaving a cuff of normal epithelium around the cervix. A series of purse-string-like sutures brings the anterior and posterior walls together. Successive layers are placed until the denuded area is completely closed. On completion of the operation the uterus is completely invaginated. A gutter covered with normal vaginal epithelium is left on each side. The net result of the completed procedure is an obliteration of the vagina.

Since the uterus is to be retained it is important to do a preliminary curettage and cervical biopsy. If there is any reason to believe the uterus is not healthy, this operation should not be done. Similarly, this type of operation would not be suitable for a patient with symptoms of stress incontinence, since the repeated infolding of the vaginal walls advancing the uterus upward will place too great a strain on the bladder neck, thereby worsening the stress incontinence.

Figure 1. The prolapsed uterus is placed on downward traction and the portion of the anterior vaginal wall to be removed is outlined. A transverse incision is made through the vaginal folds above the cervix, leaving enough vaginal wall to be brought together over the cervix without tension later in the reconstructive phase.

Figure 2. The edges of the flap thus started are grasped with Kelly clamps, held upward on tension and stripped away with scissor dissection.

Figure 3. The cervix is held upward toward the symphysis. The surgeon outlines the area of posterior vaginal wall to be denuded. Care should be taken that this is not too extensive. Bringing the raw surfaces of anterior and posterior vaginal wall together may produce tension on the bladder neck and create stress incontinence.

The lines of incision flare outward on each side as they approach the fourchette, where they are connected by a transverse cut.

Figure 4. The posterior flap is held upward and stripped away over the area outlined.

Figure 5. The surgeon picks up the edge of the vaginal wall cuff on the left side of the cervix and passes a curved needle with catgut suture through the lateral corner of the anterior vaginal wall.

Figure 6. This suture passes across the face of the upturned cervix and enters the posterior vaginal wall at a point directly opposite the origin of the suture on the anterior wall.

Figure 7. This suture is tied. The anterior and posterior edges of the vaginal cuff are thus approximated in front of the cervix.

LE FORT OPERATION

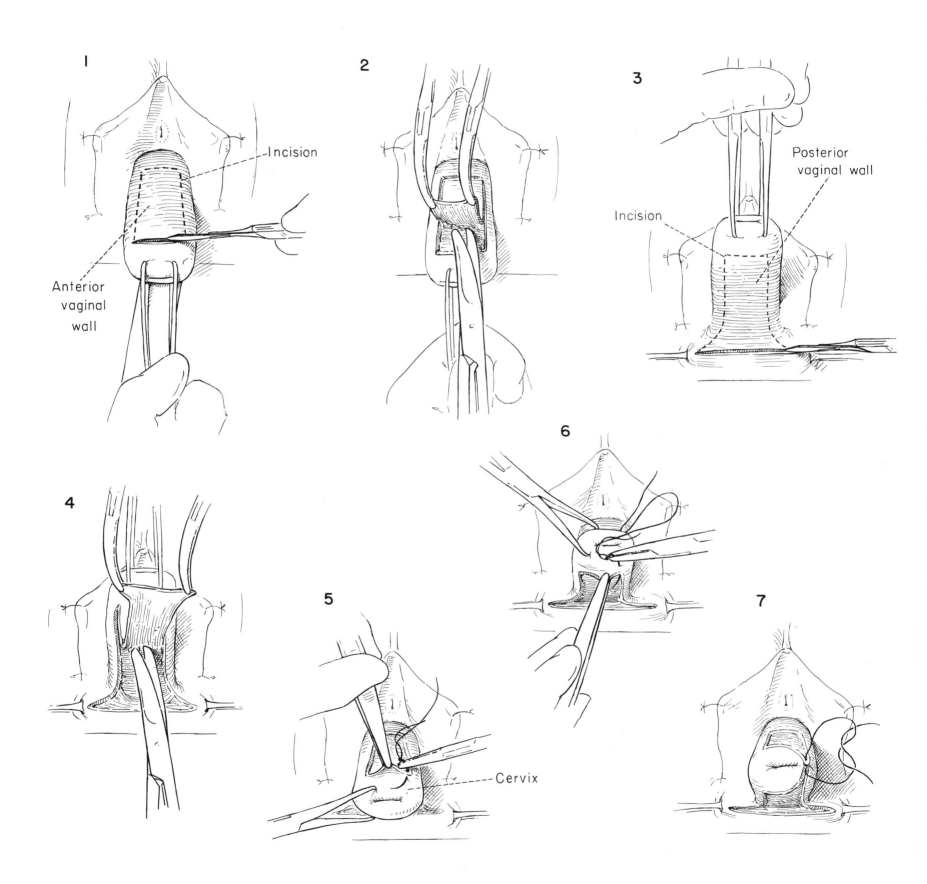

Figure 8. A series of interrupted sutures bring the raw edges of the vaginal wall cuff together, front to back. The cervix disappears behind this barrier. The last of the primary row of sutures is being tied.

Figure 9. A second row of interrupted sutures buries the first layer. These sutures are begun laterally and are placed progressively across the face of the buried cervix. The first suture in this series is being introduced. This one approximates the cut edge of vagina as a horizontal mattress suture.

Figure 10. Additional vertical mattress sutures are laid in across the raw surfaces. These are not tied until all are properly in position.

Figure 11. Successive layers are placed, tied and cut in this manner. As each layer is completed, the uterus is advanced farther upward.

Figure 12. Note that the vaginal wall defect gradually closes as each of the inverting layers of sutures is placed. The defect at the fourchette also narrows down toward the midline.

Figure 13. The anterior closure is complete and the uterus displaced upward. Interrupted sutures are now placed in the levator ani muscles and held long until all are placed. They are then tied and cut, thereby approximating the levator ani muscles in front of the rectum.

Figure 14. Before completion of the closure of the vaginal wall, interrupted catgut sutures are placed in the perineal body. These are then tied and cut.

Figure 15. The remaining raw edges of the vaginal wall are approximated in the midline with interrupted sutures.

Figure 16. The vaginal wall closure is now complete. The opening of one of the two lateral wall canals left along the side of the closed vagina is indicated by the tip of a Kelly clamp. These canals allow for drainage. An inlying catheter is left in the bladder.

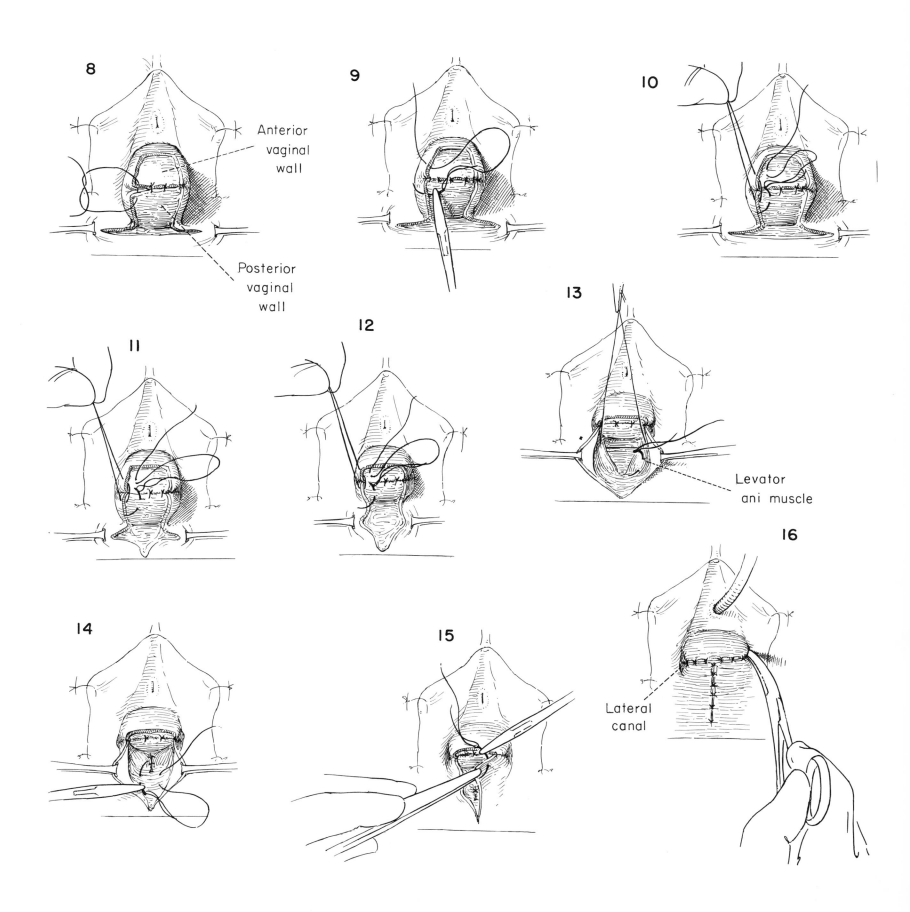

8

Anterior
vaginal
wall

Posterior
vaginal
wall

9

10

11

12

13

Levator
ani muscle

14

15

16

Lateral
canal

TOTAL COLPECTOMY

After total removal of the uterus, the support of the apex of the vaginal wall may become so enfeebled that varying degrees of prolapse may result. When the patient is in the age group in which marital relations are important, the surgeon turns to the various types of operations which are designed to support the vagina while maintaining patency of the canal.

In the older age group, when marital relations are no longer a consideration, the surgeon may elect to obliterate the vagina. If the uterus is present, this can be accomplished by the Le Fort procedure previously described. When it is absent, obliteration of the vagina can be satisfactorily accomplished when the vagina is denuded of all epithelium and the pubococcygeus muscles are approximated and sutured in the midline.

The redundant vaginal wall is placed on tension and incised at the apex in the usual way. The bladder is advanced and the cystocele repaired. The peritoneal reflection and abdominal cavity are identified; after trimming of the excess peritoneum, the defect is closed, thereby sealing off the abdominal cavity. The pubococcygeus muscles are identified on either side of the vaginal canal. They are usually relaxed and can easily be brought together in the midline. If they are not relaxed, they can be freed up by making an incision at their point of attachment along the ascending ramus of the pubis. When freed, the muscles fall medially; they are then sutured. What remains of the vaginal wall is approximated and the operation completed by a perineorrhaphy.

Figure 1. The prolapsed apical portion of the vaginal wall is held on tension in exactly the same manner one would grasp the cervix if the uterus were present. A transverse incision is made in the anterior vaginal wall. The lateral corners are placed on traction, and the bladder is separated from the vaginal wall by advancing the tips of the scissors upward toward the urethra as pressure is applied to the undersurface.

Figure 2. The anterior vaginal wall is divided in the midline.

Figure 3. The loose areolar attachments of the bladder wall are gently separated from vaginal wall and peritoneum with the thumb.

Figure 4. The posterior vaginal wall is exposed by traction upward on the vaginal apex, and an incision is made at the fourchette.

Figure 5. The apex of the vagina is held upward and the lower corners downward as the surgeon advances the tips of the scissors along the under-surface of the vaginal wall.

Figure 6. The vaginal wall is split in the midline.

Figure 7. The vaginal wall is then peeled off the rectum.

Figure 8. The vaginal apex is turned downward and traction applied as the anterior lateral wall is incised transversely at the apex.

Figure 9. The anterolateral walls are then stripped from the underlying peritoneal cover of the vaginal hernia with the handle of the knife.

TOTAL EXCISION OF THE VAGINA

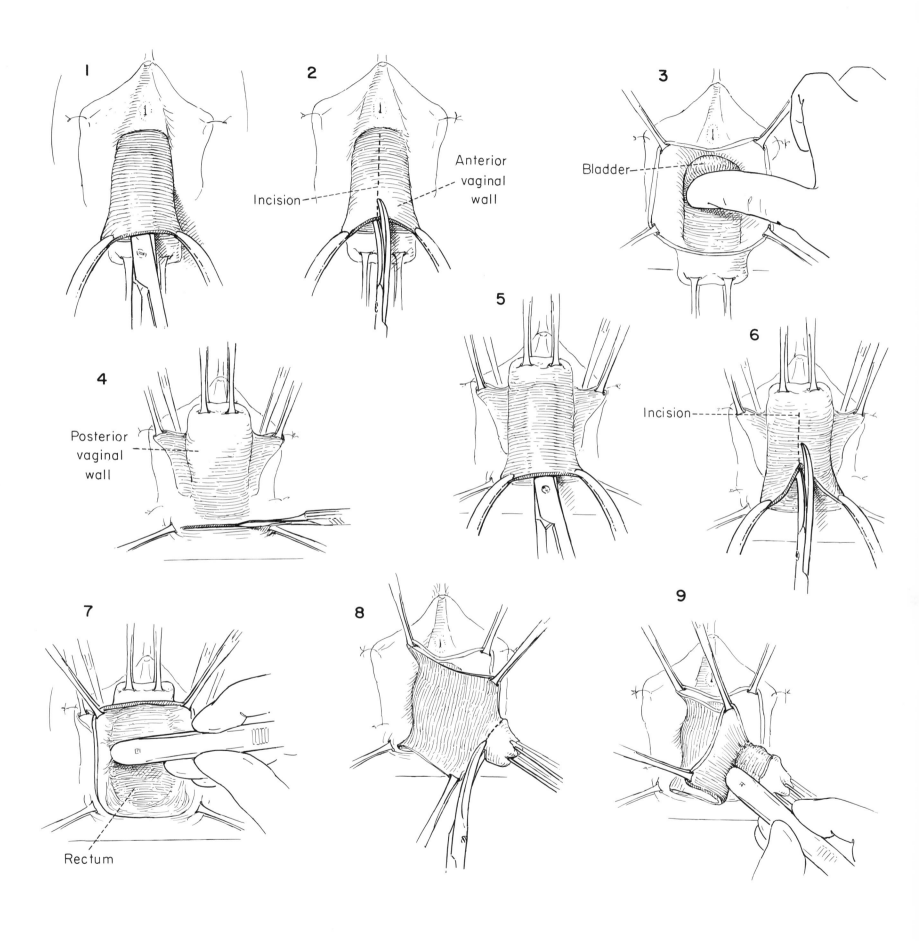

Figure 10. The vaginal apex and peritoneal herniation, completely denuded of vaginal wall, are placed on traction as the excess of vaginal wall is excised.

Figure 11. The anterior fold of peritoneum is identified, picked up with forceps and incised.

Figure 12. Stay sutures are placed on the upper edge of peritoneum and the excess of peritoneum representing the hernial sac is excised as it is placed on tension.

Figure 13. The peritoneal cavity is then closed with interrupted catgut sutures.

Figure 14. The cystocele is repaired in the usual fashion.

Figure 15. The remaining vaginal wall is placed on tension as the surgeon develops the edge of the pubococcygeus muscle with the knife handle, gently separating the muscle so that it can be mobilized medially. This is done on both sides.

Figure 16. The peritoneum is protected with the index finger as the surgeon places a catgut suture on a curved needle into the muscle bundle on the left from above downward. This is carried across the face of the bulging peritoneum and enters the muscle bundle on the opposite side and is passed from below upward.
A series of such sutures are so placed.

Figure 17. The pubococcygeus has been approximated in the midline by interrupted sutures which have been tied and cut. The opposing surfaces of the levator muscles will be brought together to strengthen the support. The initial suture enters the muscle from above downward, passes across the rectum, which is protected by the index finger, and enters the right levator in the same corresponding position.

Figure 18. A series of such interrupted sutures are placed, tied and cut. The apex of the vaginal wall incision is held upward as the first of a series of interrupted catgut sutures is introduced. Each suture is held until the next one is in position and is then cut.
Because of a tendency to form hematoma and abcess deep to the muscle closure, it is our custom to drain this space for three days with a short segment of rubber tubing split at the inner end.

Figure 19. The vaginal wall has been closed and the vagina obliterated. An inlying catheter is placed in the bladder.

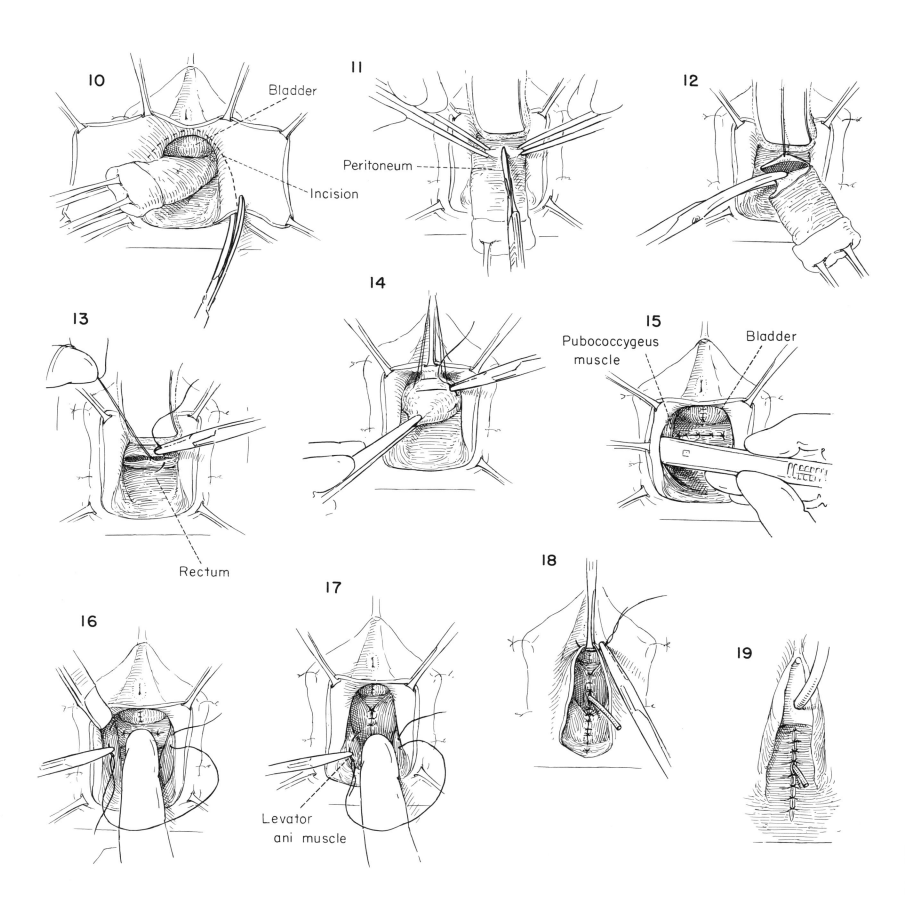

EXCISION OF CERVICAL STUMP

After supracervical hysterectomy the remaining cervix may exhibit a variety of lesions of precancerous connotation; it may be the source of chronic infection; it may descend from its normal position at the apex of the vagina. All such conditions would call for its removal.

The secret of excision of the cervical stump rests in the application of constant traction while the operation is being done. The vaginal epithelium is stripped back from the cervix, which provides exposure to the lower end of the cardinal ligaments containing the cervical branches of the uterine cavity. These are then clamped, sectioned and ligated. The only remaining supports for the stump are the round ligaments which have been attached to it at the previous operation. These are similarly secured and divided. Occasionally, the stump can be removed without entering the abdominal cavity.

Figure 1. The labia are tacked to the skin with interrupted sutures. Tenacula on the cervical stump are placed on downward tension as the surgeon makes an incision in the vaginal wall below the transverse folds.

Figure 2. The tenacula are held upward toward the symphysis and the posterior vaginal wall is incised at the same level, completing the circumcision of the stump.

Figure 3. With the vaginal wall and tenacula on tension the surgeon dissects the flap away from the anterior wall of the cervix with the tips of the scissors held downward. The secret of this procedure is to stay on the cervix at all times.

Figure 4. The cervix is retracted upward and the posterior surface similarly freed.

Figure 5. With the cervix denuded of vaginal wall on all sides, the attachments of the cardinal ligaments containing the cervical branches of the uterine artery come into view on the lateral side. The cervix is drawn to the patient's right and a clamp applied to the ligament before dividing it.

Figure 6. The tissue in the clamp is secured with a stitch ligature.

Figure 7. The peritoneum is gently pushed back off the cervix with the handle of the knife, the round ligament attachments are clamped and divided, and a stitch ligature is placed around the clamp and tied. The same steps are repeated on the opposite side.

Figure 8. The assistant exerts countertraction on the vaginal wall as the surgeon pulls down on the tenacula and teases the peritoneum off the upper end of the cervical stump.

Figure 9. The cervix can usually be removed without entering the peritoneal cavity. Any rent in the peritoneum must be closed.

Figure 10. The vaginal opening is closed transversely.

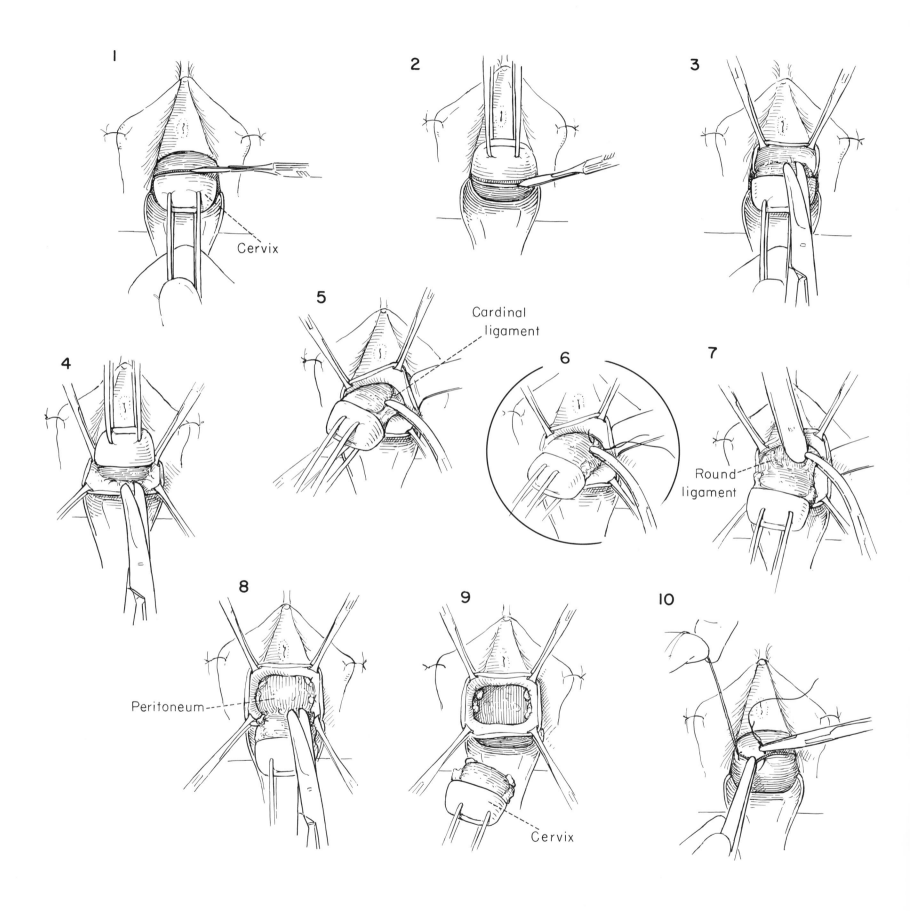

SIMPLE PERINEAL REPAIR

In many instances, particularly in association with an abdominal hysterectomy, a simple perineal repair gives added pelvic support and an increased sense of well-being by reconstructing the perineal body.

Figure 1. Allis clamps are placed on the lateral sides of the vagina opposite one another at the point indicated by the hymeneal remnants. These clamps are placed on tension, and a transverse incision is made across the vaginal wall just above the fourchette.

Figure 2. Traction continues as the surgeon elevates the upper edge of the posterior vaginal wall and gently separates it from the underlying muscles of the perineal body.

Figure 3. The apex of the triangular flap of vaginal epithelium is then pulled downward and the excess removed with a V incision.

Figure 4. The levator muscles come into view on either side. A stitch is placed in the muscle on the left.

Figure 5. This is carried across the front of the rectum and inserted in the levator ani muscle on the right in the same relative position.

Figure 6. The first stitch has been laid in and is being held as the second stitch is placed.

Figure 7. The sutures are tied, bringing the muscle bundles together, and then cut. Additional sutures are used to approximate the structures which form the perineal body, thus raising the fourchette and re-establishing the normal relationship between anus and vagina.

Figure 8. The vaginal wall is now closed with interrupted catgut sutures loosely tied.

Figure 9. The Allis forceps is removed after the first stitch has been introduced and each stitch held long as the next one is placed.

Figure 10. The vaginal wall has been closed. There is still a defect in the skin of the perineum. The skin edges are brought together without tension by interrupted sutures.

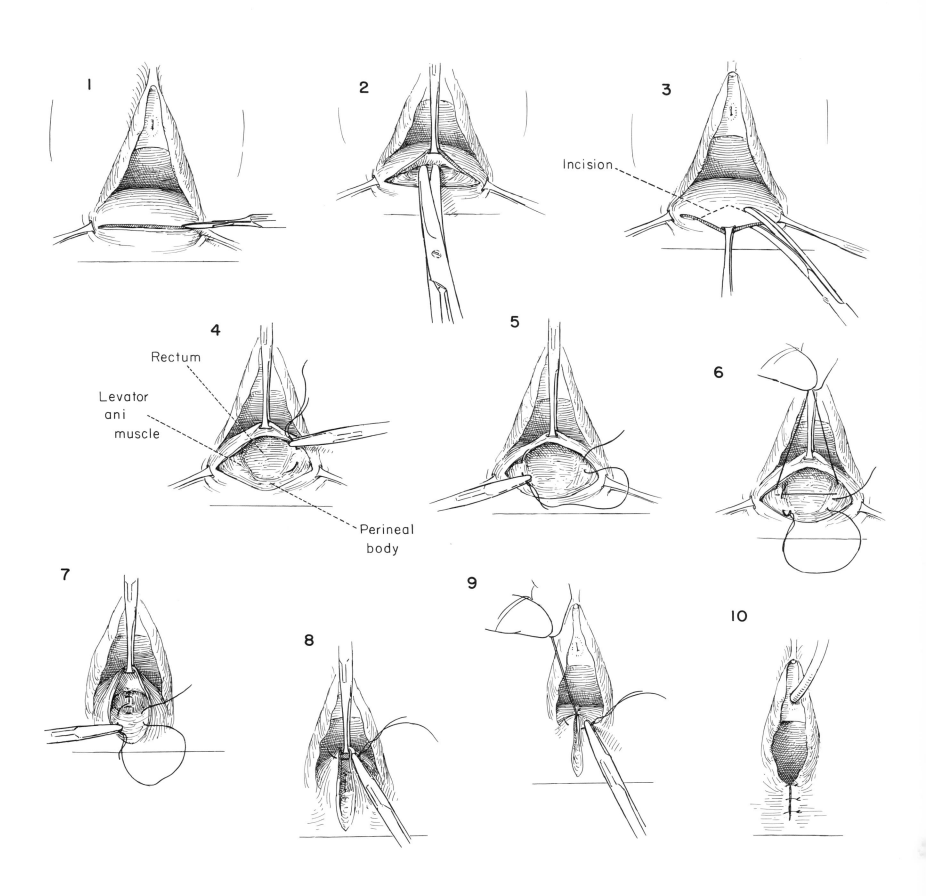

RECTOCELE REPAIR

When the separation of the levator ani muscles has been extensive, the posterior vaginal wall in its upper portion bulges out over the relaxed perineal body. Repair of this defect is rarely carried out as the sole definitive vaginal procedure, for posterior vaginal wall defects infrequently give rise to symptoms. It is commonly employed in combination with other procedures performed through the vagina. Occasionally, it is performed as the only vaginal procedure other than curettage when an abdominal hysterectomy is done. Replacement of the levator ani muscles in their normal position after reducing the rectocele does contribute to pelvic floor support.

Identification of the rectum follows the same principles previously outlined for separation of the bladder from the anterior vaginal wall, since the same relation of small vessels to the posterior vaginal wall and rectum applies. Careful dissection will minimize the blood loss.

To make sure that the upper portion of the rectum does not roll out over the reconstructed perineal body the fascial envelope which surrounds it must be approximated in front of the bowel.

Figure 1. Allis clamps are so placed that when they are brought together in the midline a normal vaginal outlet results.

Figure 2. These clamps are used to hold the posterior vagina on tension as the surgeon incises the vaginal wall transversely between the clamps.

Figure 3. Kelly clamps are placed on the upper edge and pulled downward as the surgeon advances the scissors with the tips upward, staying close to the vaginal wall in the midline.

Figure 4. With the edges still on traction the surgeon divides the elevated vaginal wall in the midline.

Figure 5. The upper edges of the vaginal flap are grasped with Allis forceps on either side. The traction is maintained on the lower clamps throughout the procedure to the final steps.

Figure 6. The edges of the right flap are held on traction to the patient's right as the surgeon pulls the rectum medially with gauze laid over the rectal wall for increased purchase. He then begins to dissect the fibrous strands, holding the small vessels free from the undersurface of the vaginal flap.

Figure 7. Once the cleavage plane is established the rest of the separation is readily accomplished by using the knife handle.

Figure 8. The levator ani muscle on both sides is freed from the bulging rectum to permit careful placing of the sutures.

Figure 9. The upper and lower clamps are held on tension as the surgeon places a mattress stitch in either levator ani muscle bundle. As each suture is placed the rectum is pushed back with the left index finger to avoid injury to it.

RECTOCELE REPAIR

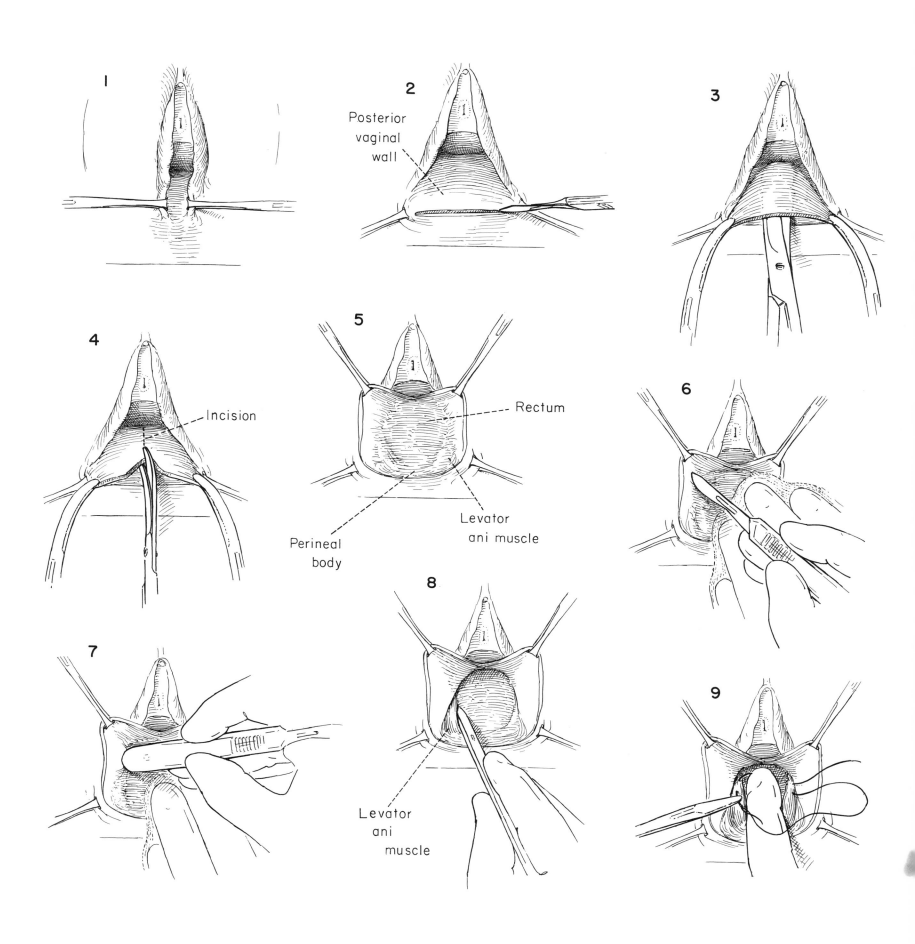

1

2 Posterior vaginal wall

3

4 Incision

5 Rectum
Perineal body
Levator ani muscle

6

7

8 Levator ani muscle

9

Figure 10. Each suture is clamped and held long on tension as the next muscle suture is laid in, clamped and held. Three or four such sutures are used.

Figure 11. The clamped sutures are then pulled down to expose the thin edges of the fascia above the point of divergence of the levators. An atraumatic catgut stitch on a small curved needle inserted on either side reduces the bulging rectum in the midline.

Figure 12. Several sutures are placed, tied and cut.

Figure 13. The sutures in the levators are then elevated and snugly tied from above downward.

Figure 14. Excess vaginal wall is trimmed away on both sides.

Figure 15. The closure is begun at the apex with interrupted catgut sutures loosely tied.

Figure 16. Several additional sutures are used to reconstruct the perineal body.

Figure 17. When the new fourchette is reached, the closure is continued, bringing together the skin edges of the perineum.

Figure 18. This figure shows the completed closure. An inlying catheter is placed in the bladder.

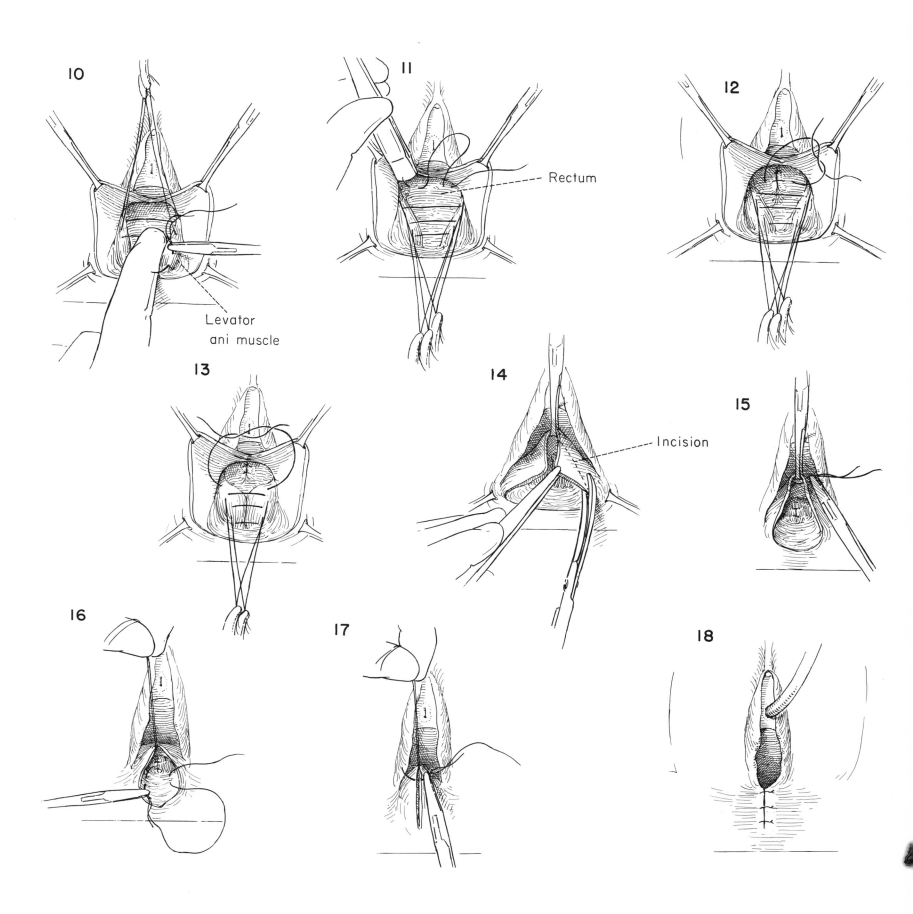

10

11 — Rectum

12

Levator
ani muscle

13

14 — Incision

15

16

17

18

REPAIR OF THIRD DEGREE TEAR

The ultimate in posterior lacerations sustained during childbirth is a tear which extends through the anal sphincter into the rectum. This complication is usually successfully repaired when it occurs. Occasionally, however, the injury is not recognized or the immediate repair fails and incontinence of feces results. The problem of late repair involves separate closure of the bowel wall and vagina with careful reconstruction of the perineum and the anal sphincter mechanism.

Figure 1. This figure shows the everting mucosa of the bowel in the position formerly occupied by the perineal body. An incision is made around the exposed mucous membrane through the full thickness of skin or vaginal wall.

Figure 2. Allis clamps are applied, and the vaginal wall is gently separated from the rectum with scissor dissection.

Figure 3. With the vaginal wall on tension the dissection is carried laterally, freeing the rectum anteriorly and on both sides.

Figure 4. Kelly clamps are applied to the cut vaginal edges and held downward. The surgeon extends the dissection upward in the cleavage plane between rectum and vagina with the tips of the scissors held upward and against the posterior vaginal wall.

Figure 5. The vaginal wall is incised in the midline.

Figure 6. The operative field has been completely developed.

Figure 7. The usual plane of cleavage between the vaginal flap and the rectal wall has been developed on both sides. The rectum is held medially to provide exposure as further separation is accomplished with the knife handle. Complete mobilization of the rectum permits closure of the bowel wall without tension.

Figure 8. The surgeon now trims any remaining scar from the edges of the exposed rectal mucosa.

Figure 9. The upper edge of the torn rectum is held by an Allis clamp. A row of fine atraumatic catgut sutures in the rectal wall inverts the mucosa and closes the defect. This is continued until the mucocutaneous margin of the anal opening is reached. A normal anal opening is recreated.

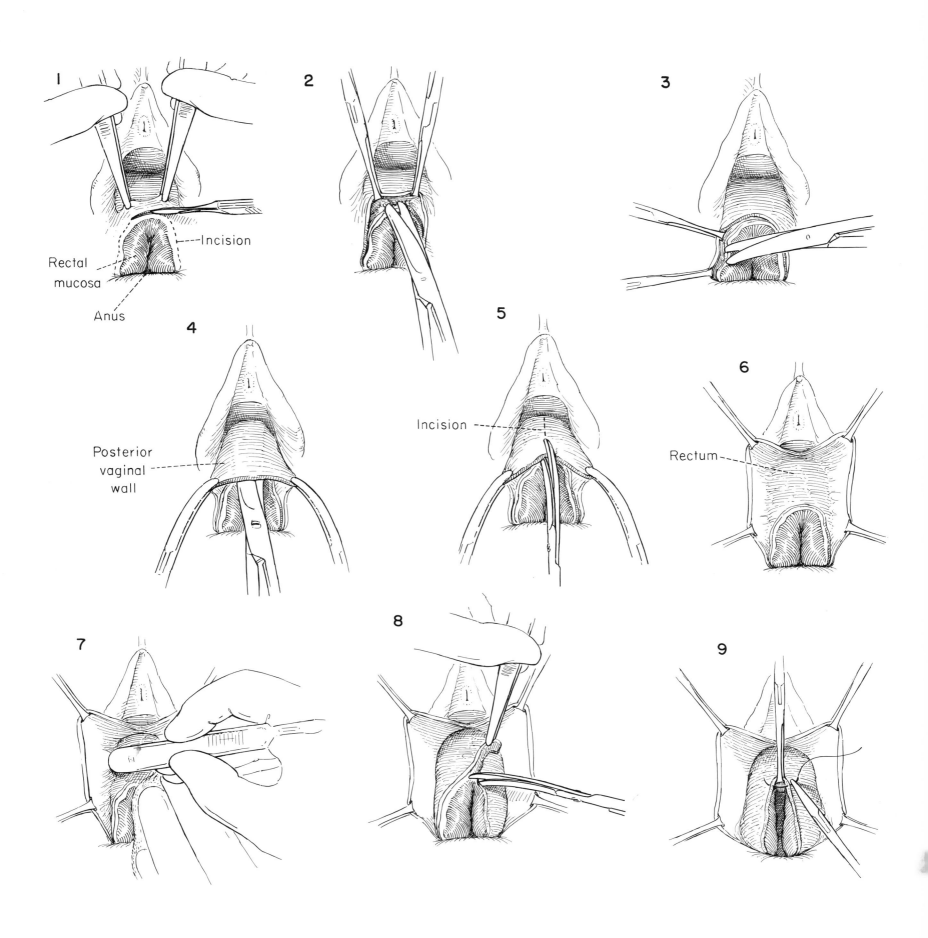

1

Rectal
mucosa

Incision

Anus

2

3

4

Posterior
vaginal
wall

5

Incision

6

Rectum

7

8

9

Figure 10. A second layer of closure is mandatory. These sutures reinforce, infold and bury the first line of sutures. Although the caliber of the anal opening appears to be reduced, it will prove to be functionally adequate.

Figure 11. A deliberate attempt is now made to secure and approximate the retracted ends of the sphincter ani muscles. Their location will be indicated by dimples on either side of the rectum at the point of the old perineal body. A nerve hook is introduced into the tissues at this point on either side.

Figure 12. With the two hooks held upward a finger in the anal opening will demonstrate to the surgeon whether the sphincter has been secured. The tissues can then be approximated in the midline with several strong catgut sutures.

Figure 13. Several additional sutures are used to strengthen the sphincter repair. If the hooks are crossed and held on tension, the sutures can be tied without difficulty.

Figure 14. The steps now proceed as in the repair of a rectocele. A series of interrupted sutures in the levator muscles is being placed in position.

Figure 15. All the levator sutures have been introduced and the ends held in clamps downward. Such traction allows the surgeon to place several interrupted sutures in the fascia above the divergence of the levator muscles.

Figure 16. All the levator sutures are then tied and cut. Any redundancy of the lateral vaginal flaps is excised.

Figure 17. The raw edges of vaginal wall are brought together with interrupted catgut sutures.

Figure 18. Each suture is held until the next is in position and then cut. Additional interrupted stitches are used to reconstruct the perineal body.

Figure 19. When the vaginal wall is closed, the skin defect below is similarly treated. An inlying catheter is inserted in the bladder.

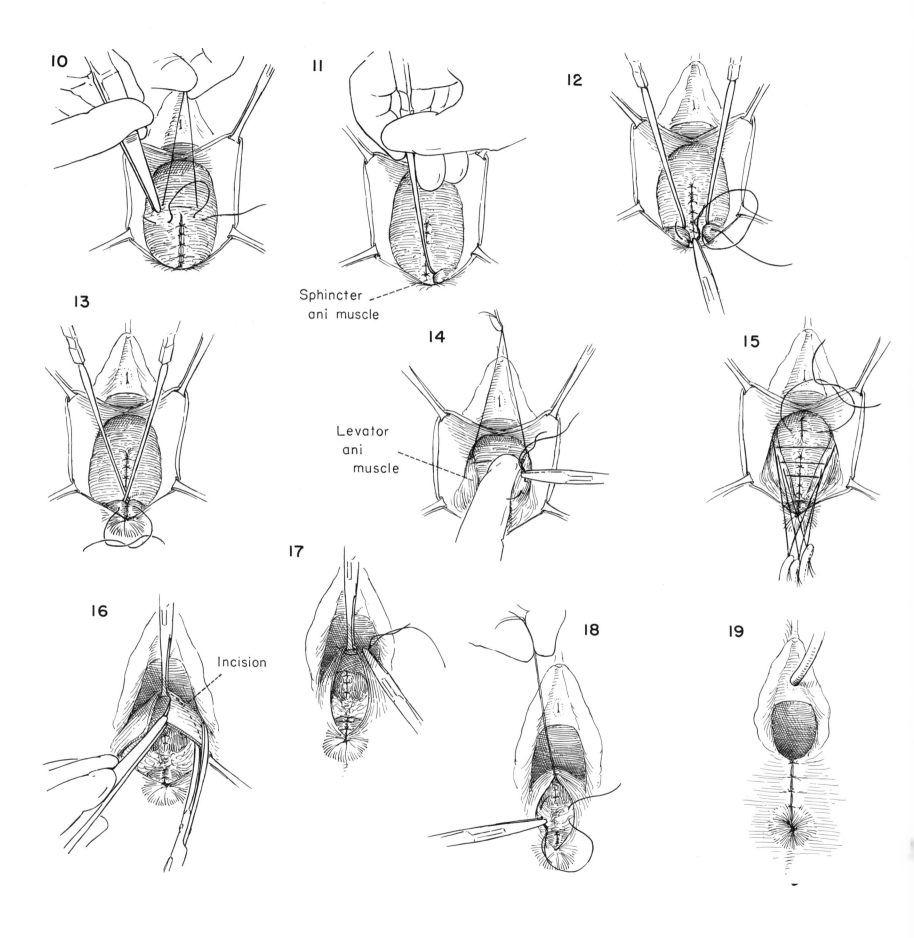

10

11

Sphincter
ani muscle

12

13

14

Levator
ani
muscle

15

16

Incision

17

18

19

VAGINAL REPAIR OF ENTEROCELE

An enterocele is a true hernia of the posterior vaginal wall which always contains a complete peritoneal sac. It seems to arise from the anterior wall of the pouch of Douglas between the uterosacral ligaments below the level of the cervix and may extend down to the introitus. It is often mistakenly called a high rectocele. Although it commonly occurs with a rectocele, it is actually a true hernia with its own peritoneal sac which often includes small intestine and omentum but never rectum; it lies on top of the rectum but has no connection with it. One should be on the alert to the possible presence of an enterocele when the rectocele seems to include the upper portion of the vaginal wall.

Failure of recognition of its presence undoubtedly explains occasional dissatisfaction following vaginal hysterectomy and rectocele repair.

Its presence may be noted on rectal examination. If one finger is placed in the rectum and the thumb in the posterior wall of the vagina, a bulging sac can often be felt above the rectal finger. If the finger in the rectum does not enter this sac, an enterocele is present and must be dealt with independently since the routine perineorrhaphy will not correct the defect. A hernial sac containing bowel can be both felt and heard as pressure is applied to the sac with the examining fingers and gas or fluid is forced out. The enterocele can be repaired from the vaginal side, but in some instances it is necessary to dissect out the sac from the vaginal side and correct the hernia by a concomitant abdominal operation designed to obliterate the anatomic defect between the uterosacral ligaments.

In the accompanying illustrations the enterocele is repaired from the vaginal side. The levator ani muscles are developed and the hernial sac dissected free of the rectum lying beneath it. It is dissected upward toward the cervix as far as possible and then opened. The neck of the sac is closed with a purse-string suture and the redundant peritoneum excised after reinforcement of the closure with a second layer of sutures. The neck of the sac is then sutured to the posterior wall of the cervix between the uterosacral ligaments if the uterus is present, or to the round and uterosacral ligaments if a vaginal hysterectomy has been done. A perineorrhaphy completes the operation.

Figure 1. A transverse incision is made in the vaginal wall as in a rectocele repair.

Figure 2. The edges are held down and the scissors separate the vaginal wall from the underlying rectum.

Figure 3. The vaginal wall is then divided in the midline.

Figure 4. The incision is carried higher than the usual incision for rectocele repair. With the vaginal wall on tension the tips of the scissors are held upward against the posterior vaginal wall as they are advanced.

Figure 5. The lateral separation of the rectum from the vaginal wall is made with the knife handle after the proper cleavage plane has been established.

Figure 6. The two distinct bulges consisting of the rectum and the peritoneal cover of the enterocele are apparent after dissection of the vaginal wall.

Figure 7. The surgeon picks up the superior surface of the enterocele and elevates it while he gently separates the sac from the rectum lying below it.

Figure 8. With the sac completely separated from the rectum, the edges of the enterocele are picked up at two points while the surgeon incises it with a knife.

Figure 9. The peritoneal cavity is now open.

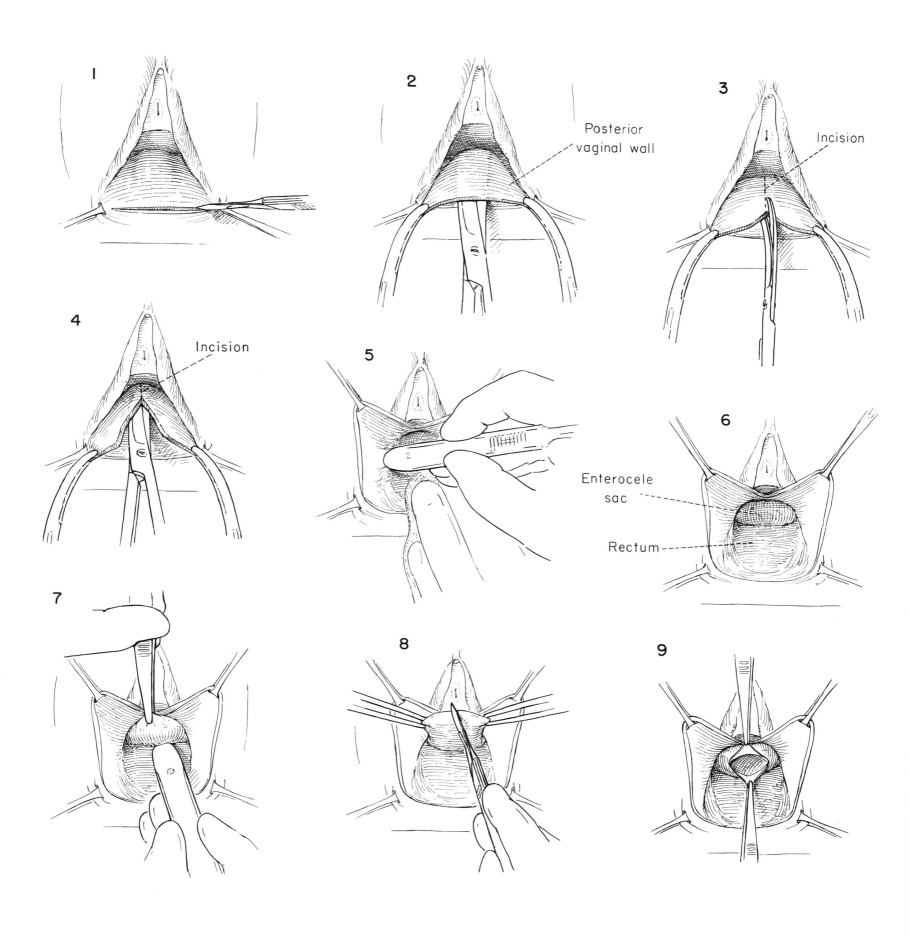

1

2 Posterior vaginal wall

3 Incision

4 Incision

5

6 Enterocele sac — Rectum —

7

8

9

Figure 10. Since the uterus is present and the hernial sac must be attached to the cervix between the two uterosacral ligaments, tenacula are applied to the cervix for the purposes of traction and consequent exposure of the ligaments.

Figure 11. The assistant holds the tenacula upward toward the symphysis as the surgeon identifies the uterosacral ligaments on both sides. Downward pressure of the index finger of the left hand on the posterior wall of the vagina helps to expose them. A row of sutures approximates the ligaments, helping to obliterate the enterocele defect and to pull the cervix back into the hollow of the sacrum.

Figure 12. The sutures have been tied and the neck of the enterocele sac is now firmly attached to the posterior wall of the uterus. The opening into the abdominal cavity is automatically closed.

Figure 13. The cervical traction is released by removing the tenacula.

Figure 14. The true neck of the enterocele sac is brought forward by the traction on the cut fringe and a purse-string suture laid in place, snugged down and firmly tied.

Figure 15. The redundant portion of the hernial sac is then excised as the assistants keep the edges on tension with clamps.

Figure 16. Allis clamps are applied to the incised edges of the posterior vaginal wall. This adds to the exposure of the upper portion of the levator ani muscles. Interrupted catgut sutures are then placed in the levator muscles on either side as the operator pushes back the rectum with the left index finger. The sutures are not tied but clamped and left long.

Figure 17. After placing a series of sutures in the levator muscles the surgeon now closes the fascia over the rectum with interrupted sutures.

Figure 18. All sutures are now tied, bringing the levators together high up in the vaginal canal, and the surgeon begins the closure of the vaginal epithelium. Each suture is held on tension after tying to facilitate the placing of the next suture.

Figure 19. Holding the last suture in the vaginal epithelium on tension to improve the exposure, the surgeon now places interrupted sutures in the perineal body. These are designed to build up the perineal body at the introitus.

Figure 20. The vaginal wall is now closed and the operation completed by placing and tying interrupted sutures in the skin below the vaginal closure. An inlying catheter is placed in the bladder.

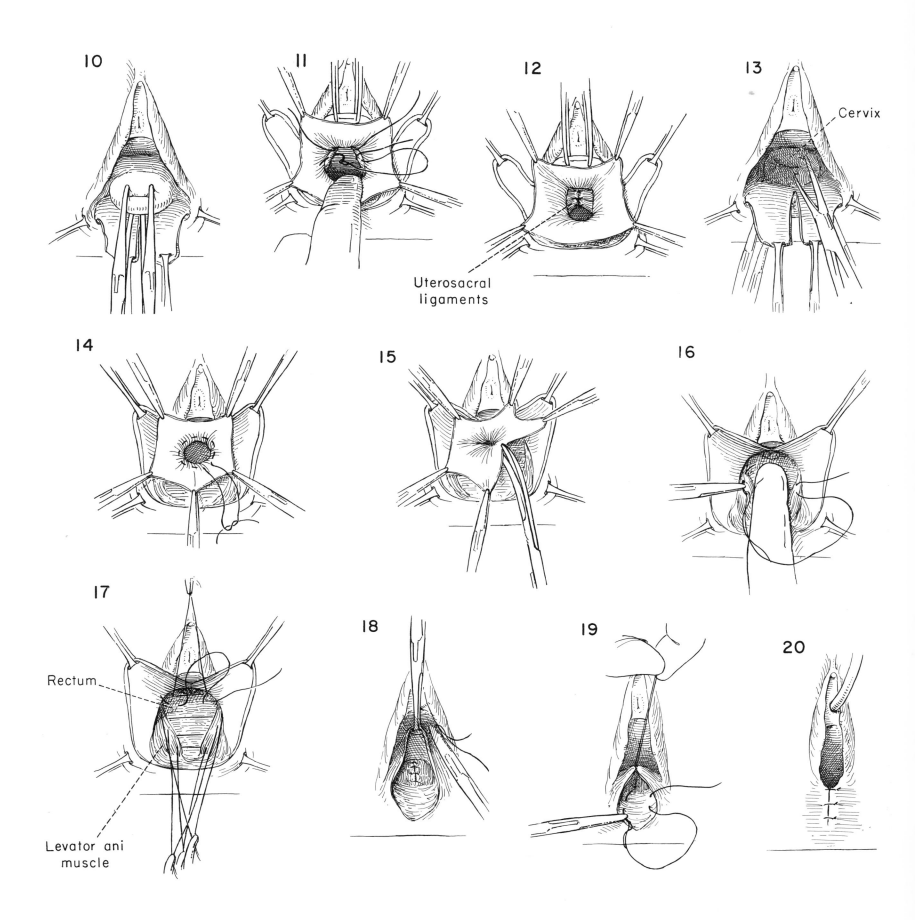

Uterosacral ligaments

Cervix

Rectum

Levator ani muscle

HEMORRHOIDECTOMY

The most satisfactory surgical management of a hemorrhoid involves excision of the dilated and tortuous veins which produce it. The redundancy of the perianal skin folds must be trimmed away, for these loose tags will continue to annoy the patient and create the suspicion that the operation has been unsuccessful.

A minimum of mucosa should be removed with the hemorrhoid to leave as little scar as possible within the anal canal. Precise hemostasis will prevent postoperative hemorrhage. No attempt is made to close any part of the wound, for an abscess is likely to develop beneath such closures.

Figure 1. This shows the area of vulva and anus with the patient in the lithotomy position. All major hemorrhoids will be found in the five, seven or 11 o'clock position. Dilatation of the anal sphincter will simplify exposure. This should be done slowly with graduated dilators, but should be carried to the point at which three fingers can be inserted with ease.

Figure 2. One usually operates first on the most posterior pile, so that blood oozing from small vessels will not obscure the field at any time. The hemorrhoid is picked up with two grasping forceps, one on the main body of the varix and the other on the corresponding skin tag. A V incision is made through the skin. Excellent exposure is offered if a right-angled retractor with a concave blade is held just opposite the hemorrhoid by an assistant.

Figure 3. A small vessel beneath the skin is clamped, the dissection continued further under the varix, and the vessel tied with fine catgut.

Figure 4. The incisions are extended up into the mucosa on either side of the hemorrhoid. These are planned deliberately to remove as little mucous membrane as possible, allowing the edges of the wound to fall together easily and heal with minimum scar.

Figure 5. The hemorrhoid is elevated forcibly and a Kocher clamp secured along its base, flush with the bowel wall.

Figure 6. The hemorrhoid is amputated.

Figure 7. A catgut suture is begun about ¼ inch from the tip of the clamp.

Figure 8. This suture is tied once and is intended to include the major vein at its upper end.

Figure 9. The suture is continued over and over the clamp.

Figure 10. The ends of the suture are held on light tension in the axis of the clamp, which is now opened, disengaged from the tissue and withdrawn through the loops of the suture.

Figure 11. The two ends of catgut are tied securely. This provides excellent hemostasis.

Figure 12. This shows the operation completed, with three hemorrhoids excised.

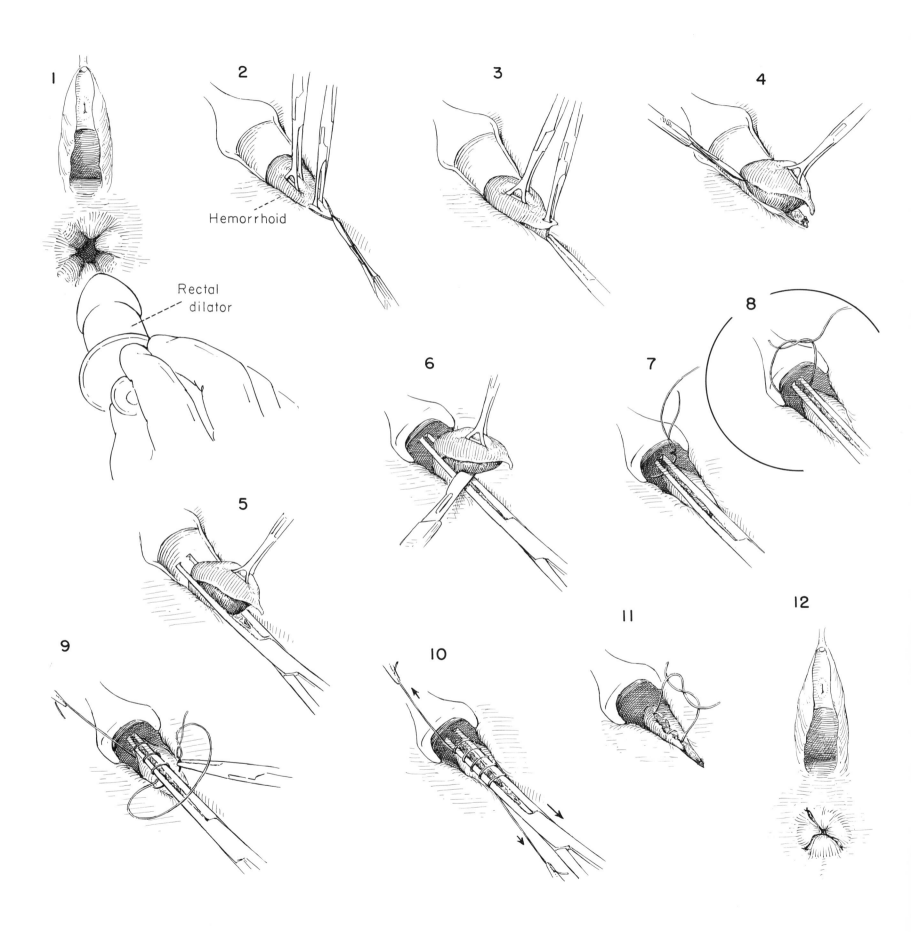

Hemorrhoid

Rectal dilator

CONSTRUCTION OF AN ARTIFICIAL VAGINA

The patient with congenital absence of the vagina usually becomes aware of it when she consults her physician for the first time in her teens because she has not had a menstrual period or later in life when she plans to be married. The absence of the vagina may be total or partial and is usually accompanied by complete absence, or at best incomplete development, of the uterus. In many instances the patient will have normal ovarian function and normal secondary sex characteristics.

It is possible to construct an artificial vagina which will function satisfactorily in the marital relationship even though the patient will never be able to become pregnant or have a menstrual period.

The timing of the reconstruction is of prime importance. Although in the past it has been customary to wait until marriage is imminent, this produces such severe emotional problems that it is now considered wiser to wait only until the patient understands the problem and the importance of her full cooperation. The patient is obliged to wear an obturator constantly following the operation until the time of her marriage to avoid the tendency to stricture.

There are two phases in the construction of the artifical vagina. The first, shown on this plate, concerns itself with developing the free space between the bladder and the rectum. This can be done bloodlessly and with relative ease. Care must be taken not to damage the urethra, bladder or rectum.

INSET A. This anatomic reconstruction shows the congenital absence of the uterus as well as the total lack of any vaginal canal. The amount of dimpling of the skin at the perineal body will vary and is shown in this patient with an arrow pointing to it. The area normally occupied by the vagina is not fused but is made up largely of areolar tissue.

Figure 1. Before attempting to make any incision it is advisable to establish normal landmarks. The labia and clitoris lie free and appear to be normal. The urethra and anal opening are in normal position.

Figure 2. The assistant holds two Allis clamps on tension. They are placed some distance apart on the skin on either side of the dimpled area. The surgeon places a clamp on the skin in the midline below the urethra and keeps it on traction as he prepares to make a transverse incision in the skin at the point of election.

Figure 3. Allis clamps are placed on the upper edge of the incision and held on traction. The nurse assists by pulling downward on the clamps placed on the lower edge. The surgeon then gently separates the areolar tissue from the upper skin flap with scissor dissection.

Figure 4. As the dissection continues deeper into the cavity, the surgeon must keep a close eye on the position of the anterior rectal wall.

Figure 5. The index finger placed in the rectum helps in orienting the surgeon in determining the position of the rectum in relation to the newly created cavity.

Figure 6. With the position of the rectum outlined, the surgeon now gently separates the areolar tissue away from the skin flap with his right index finger. All clamps are held on traction while this is done.

Figure 7. A Kelly clamp is inserted through the urethra and advanced into the bladder. This will aid in determining the position of the bladder wall.

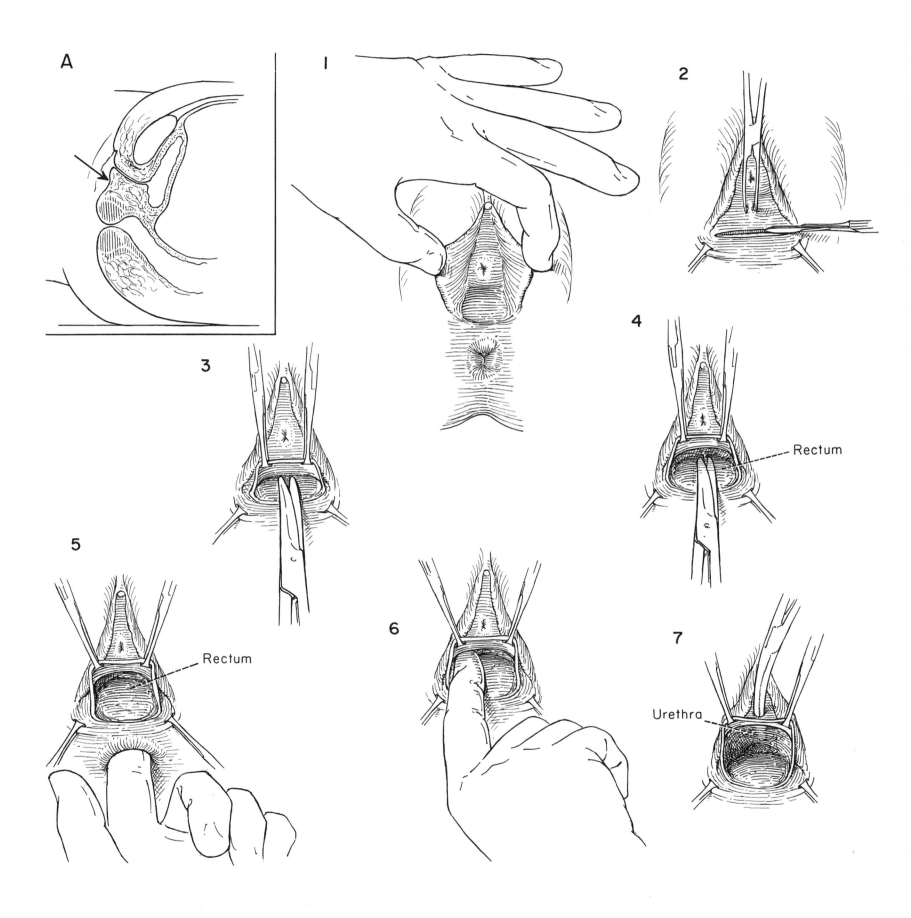

The second phase of the operation is concerned with the problem of obtaining skin to cover the obturator which must be placed in the newly created opening. It may be taken from a nonhairy area on the abdomen or thigh. The best place to take it, however, is from the skin over the buttocks. The skin is of fine texture, contains no hair, heals readily and leaves no visible evidence that the patient is aware of. A piece of skin large enough to cover the plastic obturator is readily obtained with an electric dermatome. The skin graft is sutured around the plastic mold before it is inserted in the opening prepared at the same operation. When it is removed in 10 days for cleansing and inspection, complete epithelialization has usually taken place. The obturator is fixed in place and held there with a male type cotton binder.

Figure 8. The assistants maintain traction on the clamps on the edges of the opening the surgeon has made with the caliber of the plastic obturator on which he will place the skin graft.

Figure 9. If the opening is not large enough to receive the plastic obturator the surgeon has two choices: he may choose to use a smaller size obturator, or he may enlarge the opening by inserting the index finger of his left hand in the opening, pushing away the rectum and making a linear incision of the skin in the midline.

Figure 10. The skin graft has been previously taken from the buttocks with the patient lying prone. The dermatone is usually set at .018 inch. This provides the optimum thickness of skin for use as a split thickness graft. The fat underlying the area from which the graft is taken is not traumatized and healing of the donor site is rapid.

The graft is stretched out on a sheet of rubber and kept moist with saline while the patient is turned and placed in the lithotomy position and the raw vaginal aperture is constructed.

In this illustration the graft is peeled off the rubber and applied to the obturator with the external surface of the skin in apposition to it.

Figure 11. The skin graft is gently teased out to its full length to completely cover the obturator. Patches are inserted to give complete coverage and the edges sutured to each other with fine catgut.

Figure 12. The assistants keep traction on the clamps while the surgeon inserts the skin-covered obturator in the space. The obturator is fashioned with a flat surface on top and so designed that no undue pressure is exerted on the urethra.

Figure 13. The obturator is fixed in position by placing a catgut suture through the skin on either side.

Figure 14. Several turns are made around the end of the obturator and the suture tied. An inlying catheter is inserted in the bladder.

INSET B. This drawing demonstrates the anatomic relationships.

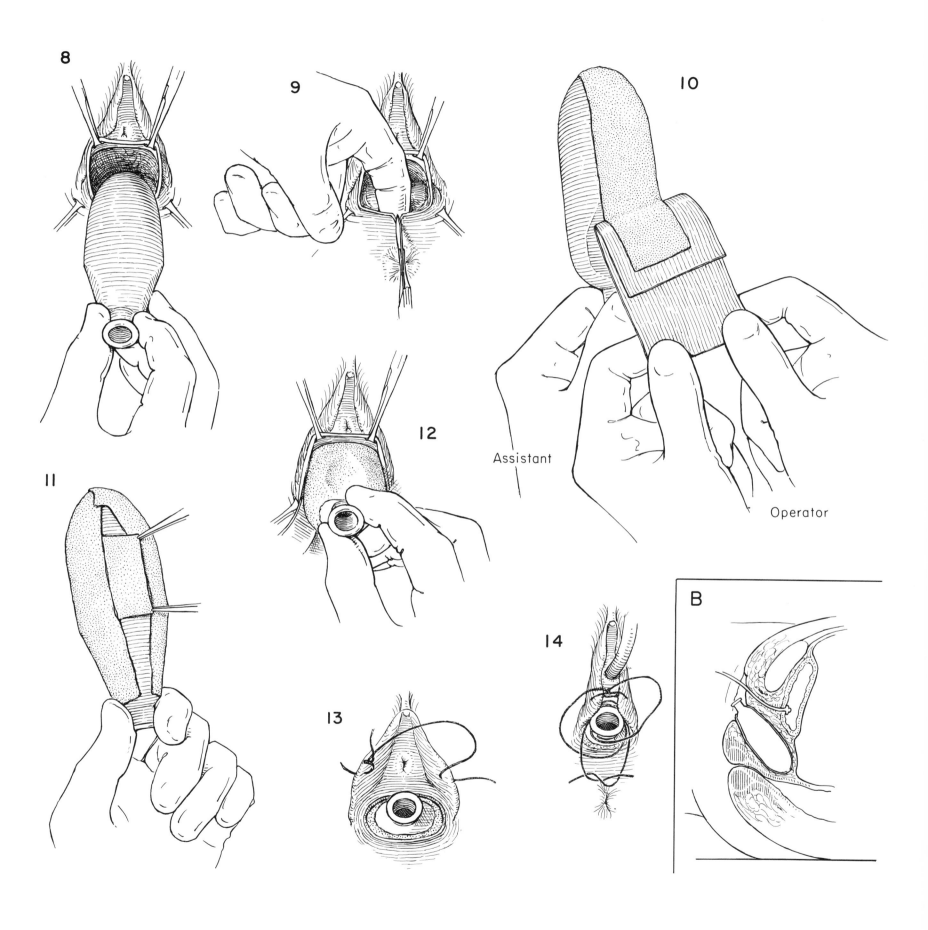

8

9

10

Assistant

Operator

11

12

13

14

B

COMBINED VAGINAL AND ABDOMINAL REPAIR OF AN ENTEROCELE

When the surgeon feels that the repair of an enterocele by the vaginal approach leaves some question as to the permanency of the pelvic floor reconstruction, it may become necessary to add abdominal intervention with obliteration of the posterior cul-de-sac to the repair already accomplished from below. The details of the vaginal portion of the operation have been described in pages 262-265. A brief recapitulation is presented here in Figures 1 to 5.

Figure 1. The posterior vaginal wall is placed on stretch by Allis forceps at the lateral angles while the surgeon incises the bridge between them.

Figure 2. With the vaginal wall flaps developed as in a rectocele, the enterocele sac is separated from the bulging, underlying rectum.

Figure 3. The sac is then entered and the peritoneal cavity exposed. A purse-string suture closes the neck of the sac and the redundancy is excised. The surgeon now decides to strengthen the repair from above. The uterosacral ligaments will not be sutured from the vaginal side, but attacked through the abdomen.

Figure 4. Interrupted sutures are placed in the levator ani muscles and retracted downward while additional interrupted sutures close the fascia in the midline above the levator repair.

Figure 5. All sutures are tied and cut and the edges of the vaginal wall brought together and the perineal body sutured. The skin edges are closed.

Figure 6. The abdomen is then opened through a left paramedian incision.

Figure 7. The uterus is held upward, exposing the purse-string suture of the vaginal repair lying between the uterosacral ligaments. The ligaments will be brought together in the midline to reinforce the repair. An interrupted silk suture is placed in the right uterosacral ligament just below the cervix.

Figure 8. The same suture picks up the region of the neck of the sac and then continues on through the left uterosacral ligament in the same corresponding position on the left side.

Figure 9. Several such sutures are placed, tied and cut. The abdomen is then closed in the usual manner.

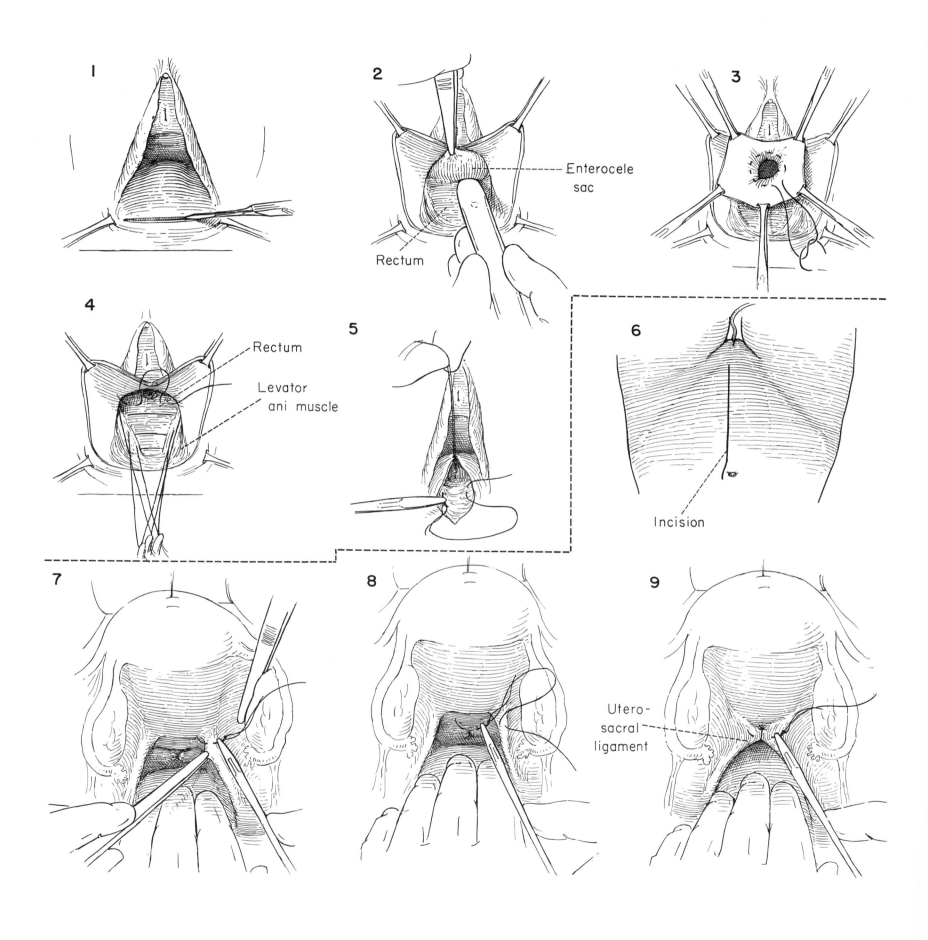

PROLAPSE OF THE VAGINA FOLLOWING TOTAL HYSTERECTOMY

On rare occasions the vaginal vault may prolapse following a total hysterectomy. This is always distressing, but the problems are compounded if the patient is in the active sexual age and patency of the canal must be preserved. In the older patient in whom the sexual factor may be of no consequence, the problem can be satisfactorily handled by obliterating the vagina. The surgeon may wish to try to bring the supporting structures together after again repairing the cystocele and rectocele. If an adequate operation has been done the first time, the chances of success are minimal and there is the possibility that the situation may be made worse. Dyspareunia can be as distressing as the original complaint and is very apt to occur if much reconstructive surgery is attempted in the upper vagina.

A variety of operations have been devised to deal with the problem of vaginal vault prolapse, including various types of sling operations using the patient's own fascia from a number of different anatomic sources. Satisfactory results also appear to follow the use of a Mersilene gauze strip, which is well tolerated by the patient when the vagina is tacked back to the posterior bony wall of the pelvis using the strip as suture material.

Figure 1. The vaginal stump is retracted downward with Allis forceps. The anterior vaginal wall has been separated from the bladder as in the first steps of the advancement of the bladder. The lower edges of the posterior vaginal wall are held downward as the wall is incised in the midline.

Figure 2. The fibrous strands holding the vessels to the vaginal wall are carefully divided and then further reflected off the wall with the knife handle on both sides. To facilitate these moves the vaginal wall is held on tension and the bladder pulled toward the midline.

Figure 3. The bladder is then gently pushed upward off the anterior peritoneum with the thumb.

Figure 4. Interrupted sutures are placed in the bladder wall to either side of the midline as in cystocele repair.

Figure 5. The sutures are tied and cut, infolding the bladder and advancing it upward.

Figure 6. Interrupted sutures approximate the raw edges of the anterior vaginal wall incision in the midline.

Figure 7. The vaginal stump is replaced in the canal and the posterior wall exposed. Allis forceps on the lateral edges provide exposure as a transverse incision is made on the vaginal wall above the fourchette.

Figure 8. An Allis forceps in the midline holds up the posterior vaginal wall as interrupted sutures are laid in the levator muscles.

Figure 9. An Allis forceps holds the vaginal wall upward as the surgeon places the first of the interrupted sutures which will approximate the edges in the midline.

Figure 10. The vaginal portion of the operation has been completed as the cystocele and perineum are repaired.

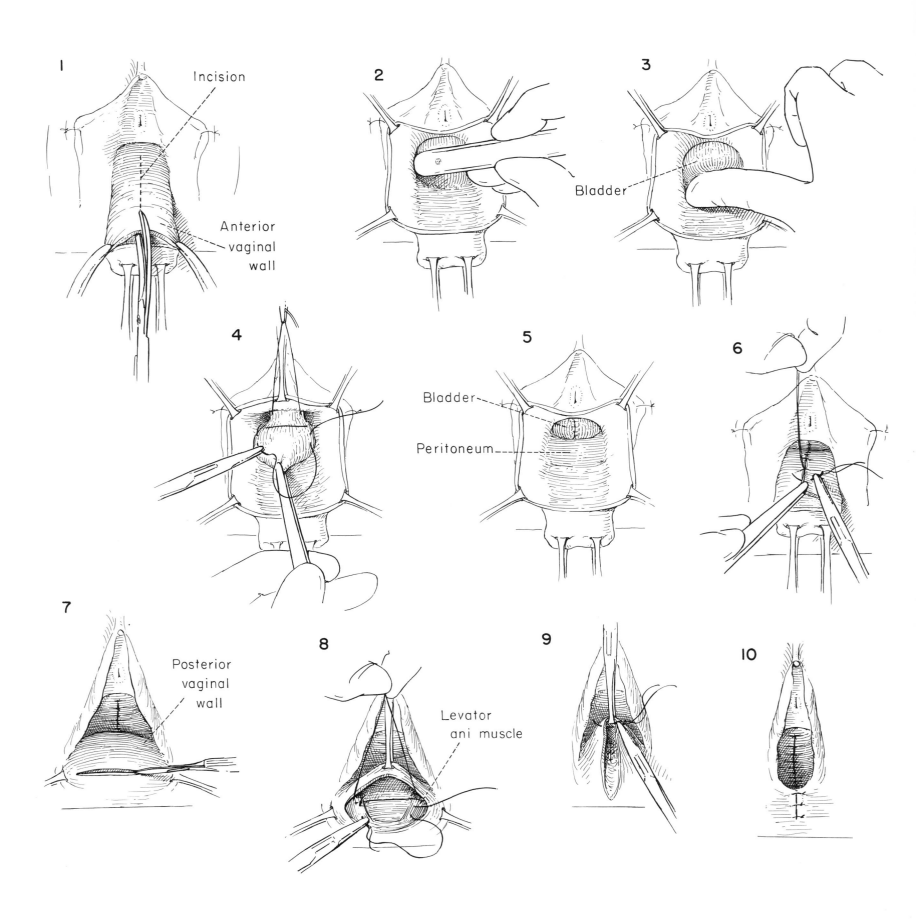

Figure 11. The abdomen is now opened through a paramedian incision.

Figure 12. The skin and fat of the abdominal wall are dissected laterally to expose a wide segment of the anterior rectus fascia on either side of the midline. The fascia is then incised in the midline from just below the umbilicus to the symphysis in the following manner: Two ½-inch transverse incisions are made to either side at the upper end. Parallel incisions are dropped from the outer end of either transverse incision to the symphysis, developing two fascial strips still securely attached at the lower end. The surgeon separates the strip from the rectus muscle beneath as the assistant holds it on tension with clamps. Both flaps are cleaned to their point of attachment at the symphysis. There they hang free. The rectus muscles are separated and the peritoneum identified.

Figure 13. The assistant and the surgeon pick up the peritoneum and open it.

Figure 14. Retractors in the wound expose the depths of the pelvis. The intestine is packed back. The peritoneum just posterior to the bladder is incised and a bladder flap developed. The apex of the vaginal stump is identified. A stitch is placed in it and tied. The long ends are held in a clamp.

Figure 15. The surgeon then grasps the lower edge of the peritoneum on the left side. It is pulled toward the midline as he bluntly separates the peritoneum from the rectus muscle, gradually forming a retroperitoneal tunnel along the path of the round ligament.

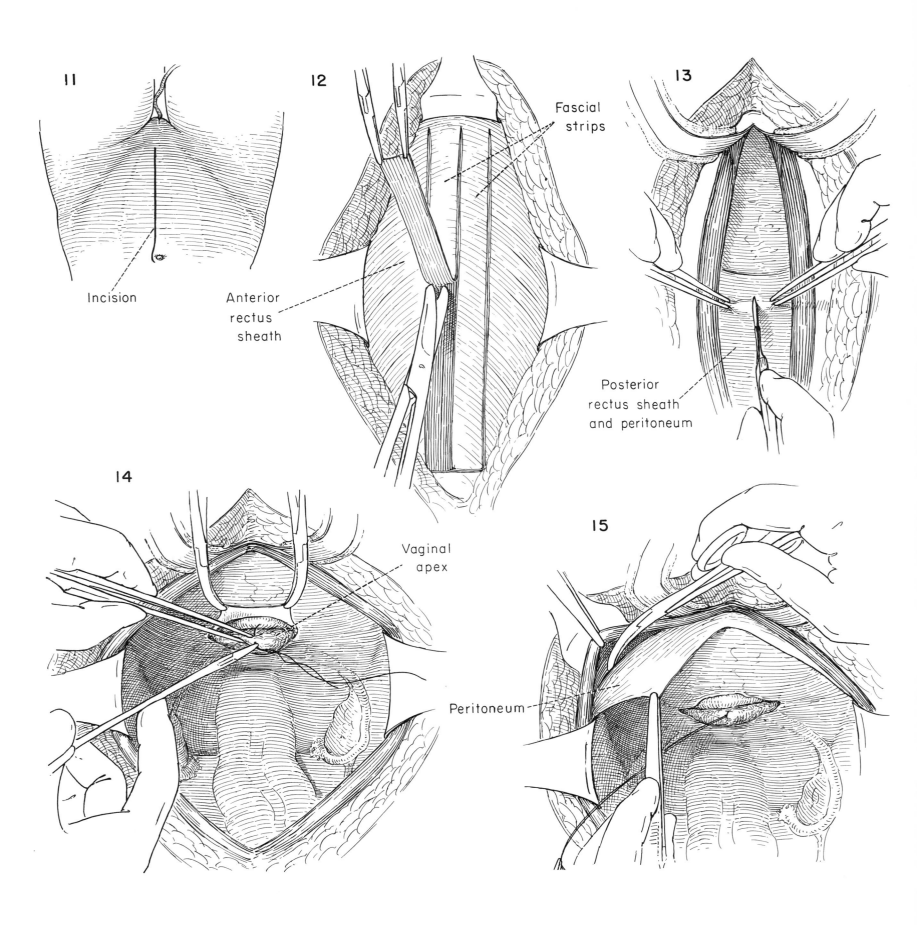

11 Incision

12 Fascial strips
Anterior rectus sheath

13 Posterior rectus sheath and peritoneum

14 Vaginal apex

15 Peritoneum

Figure 16. The Kelly clamp then grasps one strand of the stay suture previously placed on the vaginal apex. This is drawn through the tunnel to emerge on the abdominal wall.

Figure 17. A curved needle is threaded on the single catgut strand and led through the free end of the fascial strip as a mattress suture on the left side and tied, and the needle removed.

Figure 18. The surgeon then gently pulls on the suture and in this manner the fascial strip is drawn through the tunnel, its free end appearing within the abdomen while the other end remains attached at the symphysis. The same maneuver is repeated on the right side.

Figure 19. Each fascial strip is then sutured to the vaginal apex with interrupted silk sutures while the bladder flap is elevated.

Figure 20. Additional stitches secure the fascial strips to each other.

Figure 21. The opening in the peritoneum is closed with the bladder under direct vision. The wound is repaired in layers in the usual fashion.

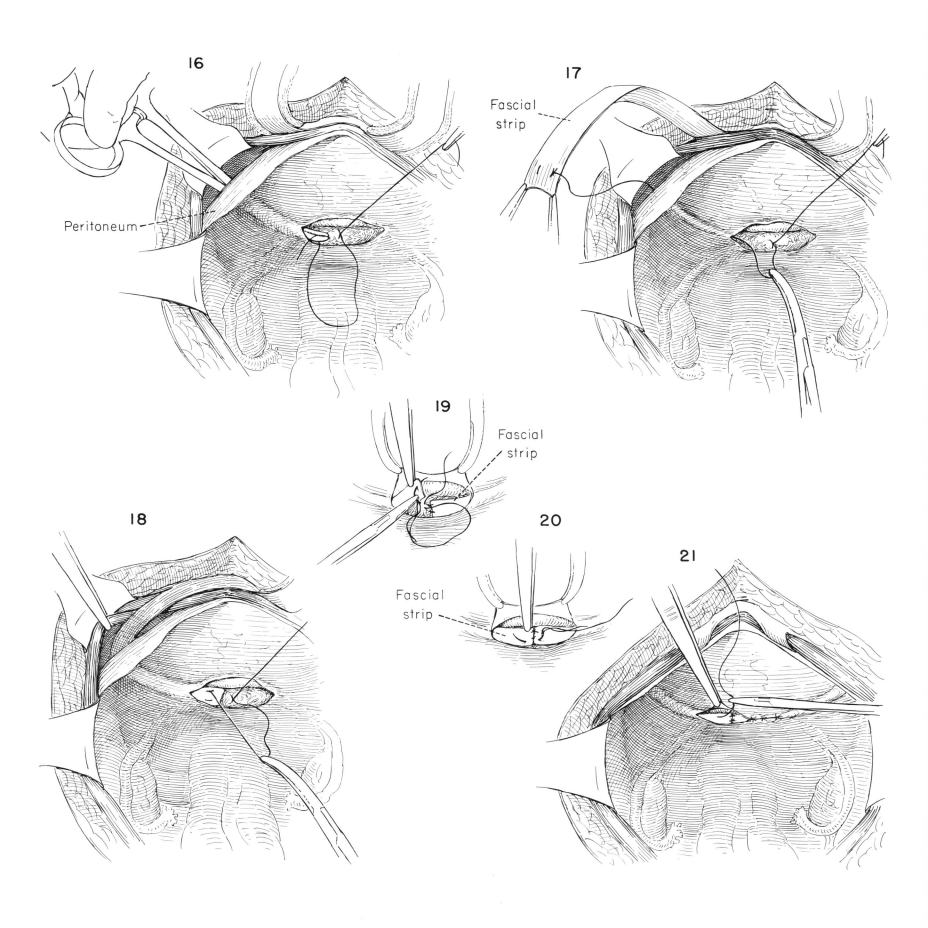

16

Peritoneum

17

Fascial
strip

19

Fascial
strip

18

20

Fascial
strip

21

Alternative Method Using Mersilene Strip for Suspension

Figure 1. After completion of the vaginal procedure, the abdomen is prepared, draped and opened.

Figure 2. The first step after packing of the small intestine and sigmoid out of the pelvis is to dissect the bladder away from the apex of the vagina. An incision has been made in the peritoneum overlying the bladder wall. The anterior wall of the bladder has been freed from the anterior peritoneal flap which is now being elevated by Kelly clamps placed on its edge. The posterior wall of the bladder has been cleaned from the anterior wall of the vagina enough to identify the vagina as a separate structure. The surgeon now grasps the anterior vaginal wall with long forceps and places the first interrupted catgut suture. This is held long and not tied.

INSET A. In order to identify the vaginal apex, avoid sewing through its full thickness. First and foremost, to extend the apex as close as possible to the sacrum, the assistant introduces his index finger into it. The thrust up and backward is maintained until the Mersilene strip is securely tacked down.

Figure 3. The surgeon now retracts the sigmoid to the left side with a Deaver retractor, exposing the posterior peritoneum overlying the hollow of the sacrum and its promontory. A longitudinal incision is then made as the assistant and the surgeon pick up the peritoneum with long forceps.

Figure 4. The assistant holds up the lateral edge of the posterior peritoneal incision while the surgeon frees the undersurface of an areolar attachment, clearing a space for the introduction of the stitch ligatures which will anchor the Mersilene gauze strip.

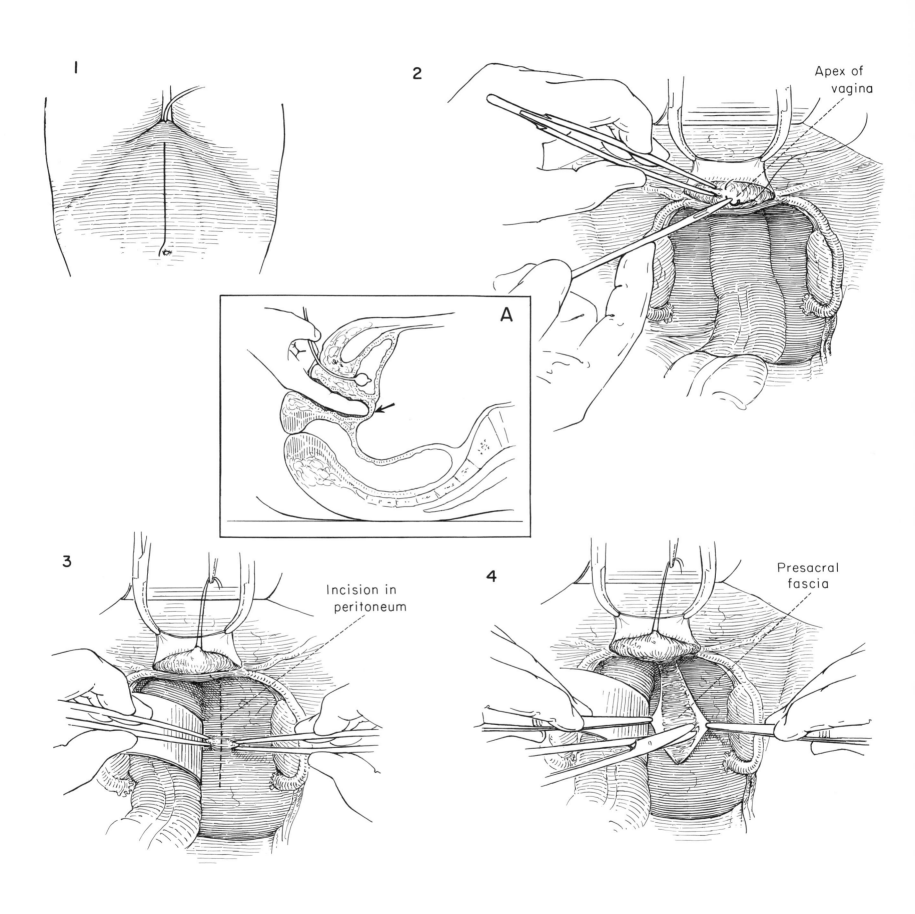

1

2

Apex of vagina

A

3

Incision in peritoneum

4

Presacral fascia

Figure 5. The peritoneal edges are placed on traction to provide exposure to the operative field. The stay suture on the vagina is held on tension as the surgeon places the first interrupted catgut suture through the Mersilene gauze strip and the vaginal wall. This is done at two points to ensure firm fixation.

Figure 6. This illustration indicates that the two sutures through the tape and the vaginal wall have been tied. To reinforce the fixation a third stitch passes through both strands of the folded tape and into the posterior vaginal wall. The tape is now firmly anchored to the vagina at the lower end.

Figure 7. The surgeon must now fix the two ends of the tape to the posterior wall of the bony pelvis. The assistant holds the peritoneal edge back with forceps to expose the operative field. A Deaver retractor pulls the sigmoid to the left. The first suture has been placed through the tape on the right leading edge and into the periosteum of the bony sacrum as the surgeon maintains traction on the strip to keep it taut.

Figure 8. Both ends of the tape are stitched to the periosteum of the sacrum. Sutures are placed on each edge. The redundant portion of both strands of tape are then cut off. The free ends are similarly tacked down to bone.

Figure 9. This view shows the two arms of the Mersilene tape in place fixed to the apex of the vagina at the lower end and to the sacrum in a V formation at the proximal end.

Figure 10. The entire area is now being peritonealized. All sutures and foreign body material lie behind the peritoneal cover.

INSET B. The diagram demonstrates the points of attachment and the direction the tape takes in suspending the vagina. Note that the pull is not only upward but backward as well. In this position it most closely simulates the normal ligamentous support to the upper part of the vagina. Observe that the apex is well suspended and that the vaginal canal is patent.

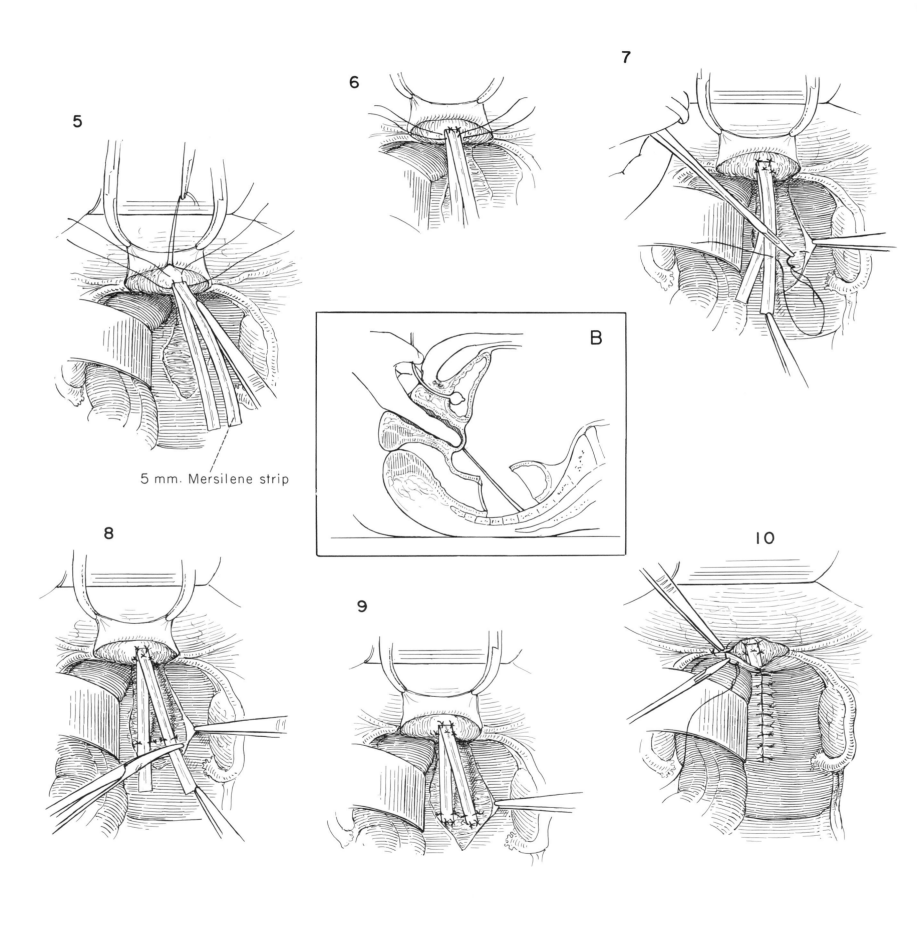

5

6

7

5 mm. Mersilene strip

B

8

9

10

THE SLING OPERATION FOR STRESS INCONTINENCE

The majority of patients with symptoms of stress incontinence can obtain relief when the surgeon corrects the sagging neck of the bladder and plicates the internal sphincter. This is true when the clinical findings, supplemented by cystogram studies taken during drainage, indicate that there has been loss of the vesicourethral angle. The operations performed through the vagina occasionally fail and more surgery is needed. The reasons for the failure are not often immediately apparent. They could be due to poorly executed surgical procedures, more intensive disruption of the sphincter musculature than was obvious at the time the original repair was done or perhaps the failure to recognize that a posterior rotational defect was present in the urethra. The latter would show up only when chain cystogram studies were done and the lateral view examined.

When previous operations have failed to correct the stress incontinence, the surgeon may wish to employ a combined vaginal and abdominal surgical approach to the problem. The bladder neck is exposed through the vagina. An abdominal incision is made and the superior surface of the rectus fascia exposed. A long longitudinal strap of fascia is developed. It is freed from the underlying muscle and is detached at the upper end. The lower end is left intact at the point of its insertion in the symphysis. The long strap of fascia is then passed beneath the urethra and bladder neck and brought up through the muscle on the opposite side and sutured to the upper surface of the rectus.

The secret of the operation is to maintain a bloodless field and to apply the proper amount of tension to the fascial strip so that the sling supports the urethra without cutting into it. This is more readily accomplished when the combined approach is used, for everything then can be seen and felt.

Figure 1. The bladder has been advanced off the cervix and the sulcus between lateral vaginal wall, urethra and bladder thoroughly developed. This sulcus may be extended upward beneath the symphysis without bleeding when the steps outlined in page 210 are followed closely.

Figure 2. One end of a strip of rubber (empty Miller wick) is placed in the left sulcus lateral to the urethral wall and advanced upward with smooth forceps as the bladder is held down.

Figure 3. The same maneuver is repeated on the right with the other end of the same strip of rubber. This illustration shows the sling of rubber beneath the neck of the bladder. Both ends have disappeared behind the symphysis alongside the urethra.

Figure 4. An inlying catheter is placed in the bladder and the vaginal wall closed. Note that no attempt is made to repair the neck of the bladder or urethrocele from below.

Figure 5. The patient is then placed in Trendelenburg position and a midline incision made.

Figure 6. The skin and fat are dissected back, widely exposing the anterior rectus sheath. This is incised in such a way that a strip of fascia is outlined, beginning at the umbilicus and attached to the pubis. The free end is grasped with clamps and the strip freed from the underlying muscle.

Figure 7. The rectus muscles are now developed through the length of the incision and the peritoneum freed from the undersurface until the prevesical space is entered.

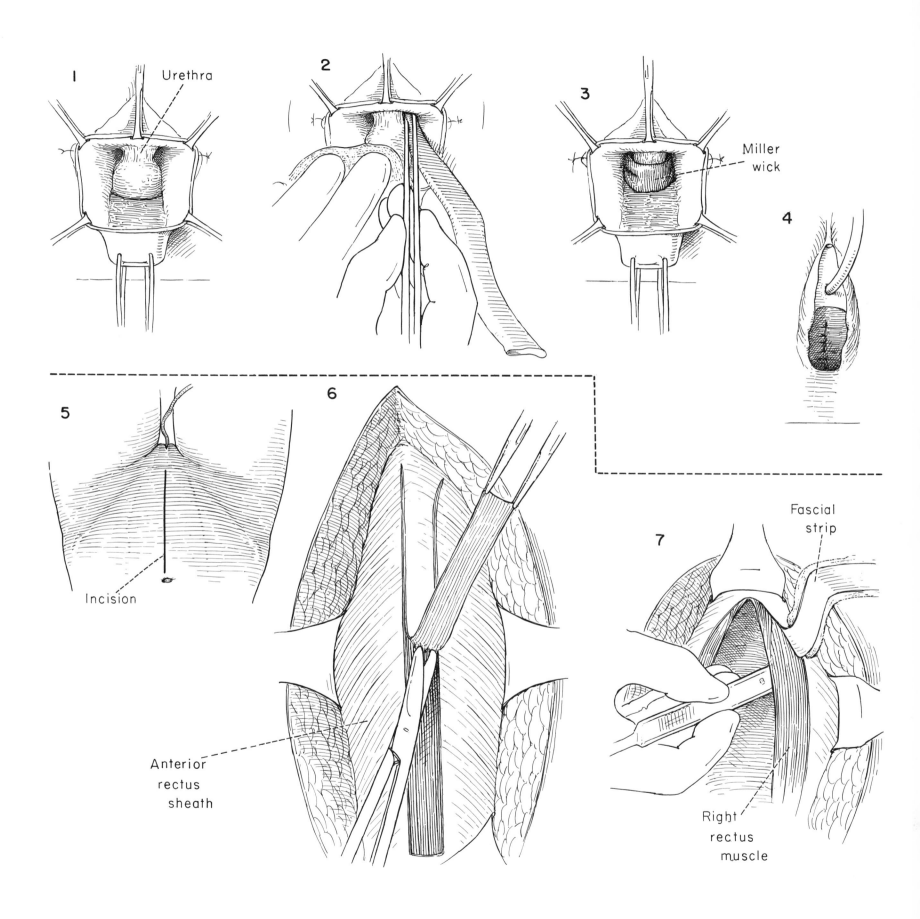

1 Urethra

2

3 Miller wick

4

5 Incision

6 Anterior rectus sheath

7 Fascial strip

Right rectus muscle

Figure 8. Retractors are placed to either side of the wound and in the midline over the symphysis. Laying the flat of the hand on the anterior bladder wall, the surgeon pulls the bladder away from the undersurface of the symphysis with a raking motion of the fingers.

Figure 9. The bladder is pulled to the left to expose the right side of the urethra. The free end of the rubber strip presents, and the surgeon grabs it with a clamp and pulls it gently upward. This should not be done too forcefully, for the other end is not attached to anything. The same move is made on the left side and both ends of the rubber strip are pulled upward, thus forming a sling beneath the urethra.

Figure 10. The free end of the fascial strip is led through the body of the right rectus muscle about 1 inch from the medial border.

Figure 11. The free end of the fascial strip is then sutured to the right arm of the rubber stirrup.

Figure 12. The surgeon holds the bladder out of the way as he gently leads the fascial strip through the tunnel underneath the bladder neck by pulling on the left free end of the rubber guide. If it does not slide freely, the fascia should be withdrawn slightly and gentle traction again applied until it appears.

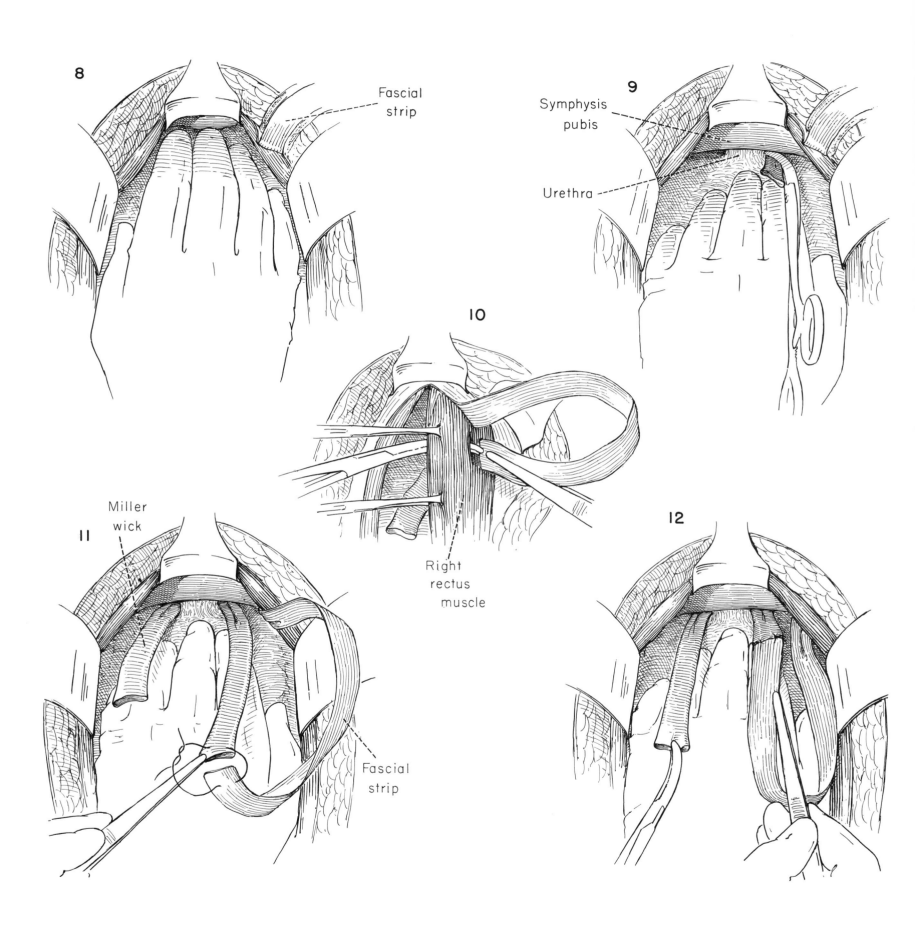

8

Fascial strip

9

Symphysis pubis

Urethra

10

Right rectus muscle

Miller wick

11

Fascial strip

12

Figure 13. The surgeon holds the bladder back and brings the free end of the fascial strip through on the left side. The rubber strip is then detached.

Figure 14. The abdominal wall is retracted to the left while the assistant retracts the edge of the left rectus muscle toward the midline. With Allis forceps holding the muscle and Kelly clamps on the fascia, the surgeon then tunnels through the lower end of the rectus muscle 1 inch from the medial border and close to the symphysis.

Figure 15. The anterior rectus sheath is then held medially and incised just over the opening in the muscle tunnel as the skin is held back with a retractor.

Figure 16. With the abdominal wall retracted, the surgeon introduces the tips of a Kelly clamp through the opening in the fascia and muscle and grasps the free end of the fascial strip.

Figure 17. As the muscle and fascia are held taut the fascial strip is led through them out onto the superior surface of the left rectus fascia. The amount of tension on the strip is of utmost importance. It should be snug enough to support the neck of the urethra without necrosing it through too much pressure. This is a matter of the surgeon's judgment. The excess is then cut off.

Figure 18. The end is sutured to the anterior rectus fascia.

Figure 19. To close the defect left in the anterior rectus sheath when the flap was fashioned it will be necessary to mobilize the lateral margin. The wound is closed in layers, first approximating the muscle borders in the midline.

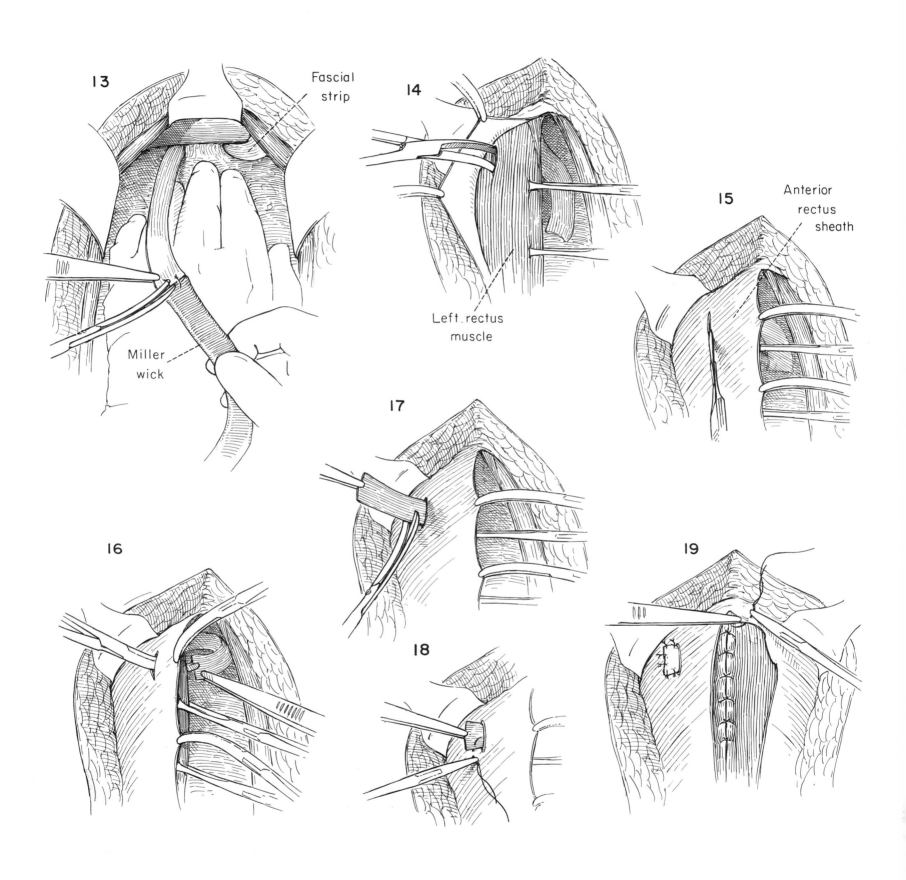

13

Fascial strip

Miller wick

14

Left rectus muscle

15

Anterior rectus sheath

16

17

18

19

VAGINAL REPAIR OF VESICOVAGINAL FISTULA

The majority of vesicovaginal fistulas encountered today result from surgical trauma. Usually they are small and appear at the vaginal apex on the anterior vaginal wall just above the transverse scar left by a previous hysterectomy. The repair is complicated by the inaccessibility of the fistula. This problem is minimized when the patient is placed in the prone rather than the lithotomy position.

There are certain principles to follow to obtain a successful repair: (1) The surgery should not be attempted too soon after the fistula is noted. An adequate blood supply is essential for tissue regeneration; too hasty attempts at reconstruction can result in failure because of poor tissue response. (2) Proper exposure must be established during the operation. All sutures must be identified and seen at all times. (3) A successful repair depends more on adequate mobilization of the bladder wall and fistulous opening than it does on the type of suture material used. The tissues must approximate without tension. (4) Adequate postoperative drainage must be maintained by catheter during the healing phase.

These illustrations show the steps of a vaginal repair of a small fistula occurring after a hysterectomy. Note that the prone position is used.

Figure 1. The patient is placed on the table with her face down. The thighs are abducted and the table is broken at the level of the pelvis, flexing the thighs. The knees rest on the lower portion of the table. This allows the surgeon easy access to the vagina and has the distinct advantage of allowing him to operate on top of the fistula rather than working from below upward.

Figure 2. Retractors are placed in the vagina, exposing the bladder with its fistulous opening. To make the fistulous tract more accessible a Foley catheter is inserted in the fistula. This is preferable to the use of stay sutures, which tend to pull out.

Figure 3. The balloon in the catheter is inflated. The assistant maintains traction on the catheter, bringing it up into view so the surgeon can dissect the vaginal epithelium away from the entire circumference of the opening.

Figure 4. The separation is carried out widely on all sides of the fistula, exposing the bladder wall with the fistula in the middle.

Figure 5. The surgeon and the assistant pick up the edges of the vaginal epithelium as the operator enlarges the opening by incising the vaginal wall in a lateral direction.

Figure 6. With the fistulous tract dissected completely free, the Foley catheter is removed and stay sutures placed on the edges of the opening. The surgeon now excises the fistulous tract.

Figure 7. The surgeon now picks up the bladder wall on either side of the fistula with a fine atraumatic catgut suture and places the first of a series of interrupted sutures.

Figure 8. Each suture is held up as the next one is placed. Note that the stitch is placed in the musculature and does not enter the interior of the bladder.

Figure 9. A second row of interrupted sutures is placed, reinforcing the original line.

Figure 10. The defect in the vaginal epithelium is converted into a transverse ellipse and closed with a series of interrupted sutures at right angles to those in the bladder wall.

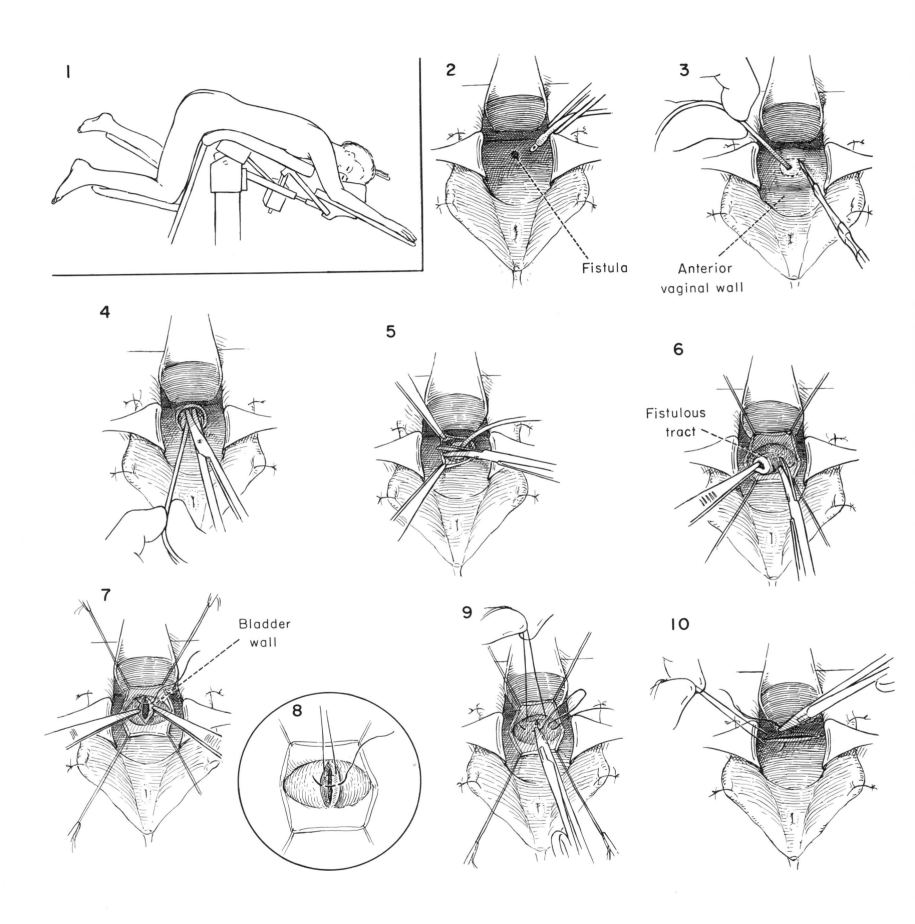

1

2 Fistula

3 Anterior vaginal wall

4

5

6 Fistulous tract

7 Bladder wall

8

9

10

TRANSVESICAL REPAIR OF VESICOVAGINAL FISTULA

When preoperative cystoscopy and preliminary investigation place the fistula in close proximity to the ureteral outlet in the bladder, vaginal repair may prove to be too blind a procedure. Direct attack on the fistula through the bladder has the advantage that it may be carried out under direct vision.

INSET A. This diagram demonstrates the position of the fistula in relation to the bladder neck and urethra. The vagina is packed with gauze to elevate the floor of the bladder and aid in exposure.

Figure 1. A short midline incision is made in the abdominal wall.

Figure 2. The peritoneum in the lower wound is separated from the rectus muscle bundles with the knife handle.

Figure 3. A retractor provides exposure as the peritoneal reflection is identified in relation to the bladder wall. It is retracted upward with gentle traction of the fingers.

Figure 4. With the peritoneum held upward with the Deaver retractor laid over gauze, the surgeon and assistant grasp the anterior bladder wall and incise between Allis clamps.

Figure 5. A self-retaining retractor is placed in the bladder opening. Further exposure is provided by retractors at opposite ends of the incision. The trigone of the bladder is identified, and a catheter is placed in the ureteral opening close to the fistula to demonstrate the course of the ureter in the bladder wall.

Figure 6. Surgery is begun by outlining a narrow rim of bladder wall around the fistulous opening.

INSET B. Although the gauze pack in the vagina does help to elevate the bladder floor, additional measures make the fistulous tract even more accessible. This is done by inserting a Foley type catheter into the opening in the bladder. When the balloon is distended and the catheter is held on traction, it is much easier for the surgeon to get at and dissect out the tract. The surgeon is seen circumcising the fistulous opening.

VESICOVAGINAL FISTULA
TRANSVESICAL REPAIR

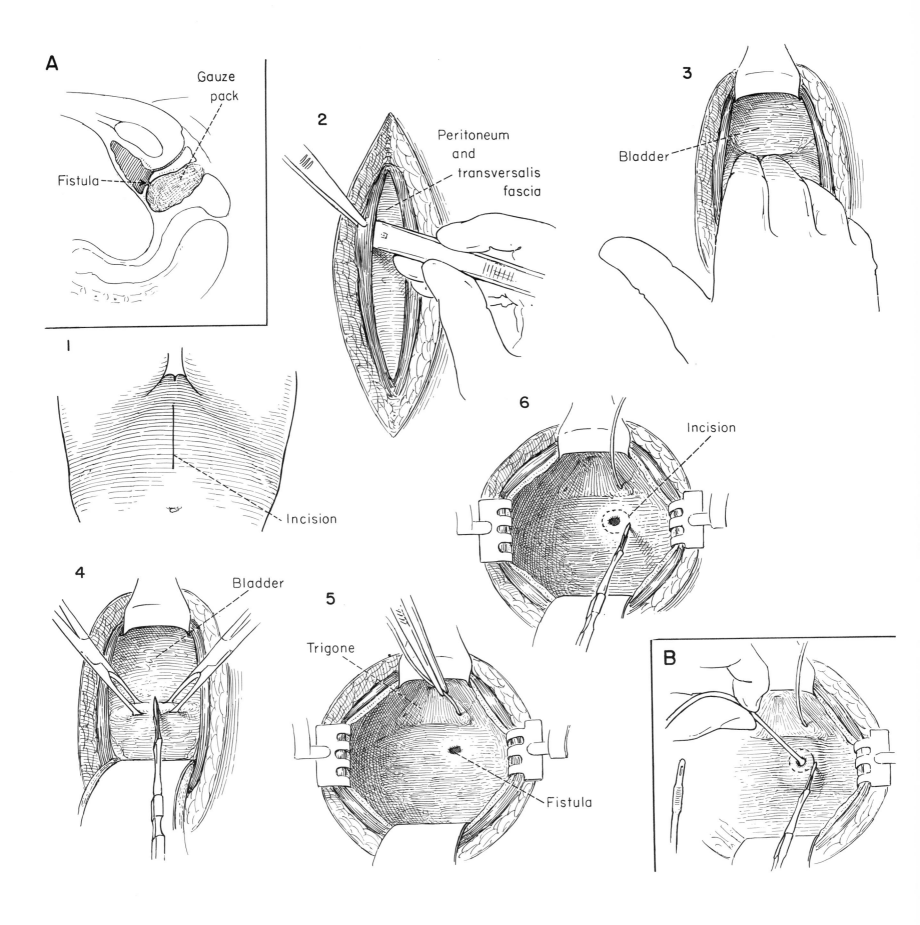

A Gauze pack

Fistula

1 Incision

2 Peritoneum and transversalis fascia

3 Bladder

4 Bladder

5 Trigone

Fistula

6 Incision

B

Figure 7. Since the dissection around the fistulous tract must extend laterally, the ureteral catheter in the right ureter is a great help in locating the intravesical portion of the lower ureter. The dissection should be carried out in all directions sufficiently widely to produce identification of bladder and vagina and to provide enough mobility so that the structures can be brought together without tension.

Figure 8. When the vaginal wall has been exposed widely enough and the fistulous tract sufficiently mobilized, the Foley catheter may be removed. The assistants hold back the bladder epithelium while the surgeon holds the tract on tension with forceps and excises it.

Figure 9. The vaginal wall opening is closed vertically with a series of interrupted catgut sutures. When all are placed, they are tied and cut.

Figure 10. A second layer of interrupted catgut sutures is placed in the vaginal wall.

Figure 11. The bladder musculature is closed transversely with a series of interrupted catgut sutures.

Figure 12. A running row of fine atraumatic catgut approximates the mucosa.

Figure 13. The bladder wall incision is then closed with a series of interrupted catgut sutures starting at the lower end. Each is tied and held as the next suture is placed.

Figure 14. An opening is left at the dome of the bladder for a Foley catheter, which is held in place with an interrupted catgut suture placed in the bladder wall and through the catheter where it is tied. When the balloon is filled, the catheter should fit snugly against the dome of the bladder.

The wound is then closed and a Penrose drain placed in the prevesical space at the lower end of the wound.

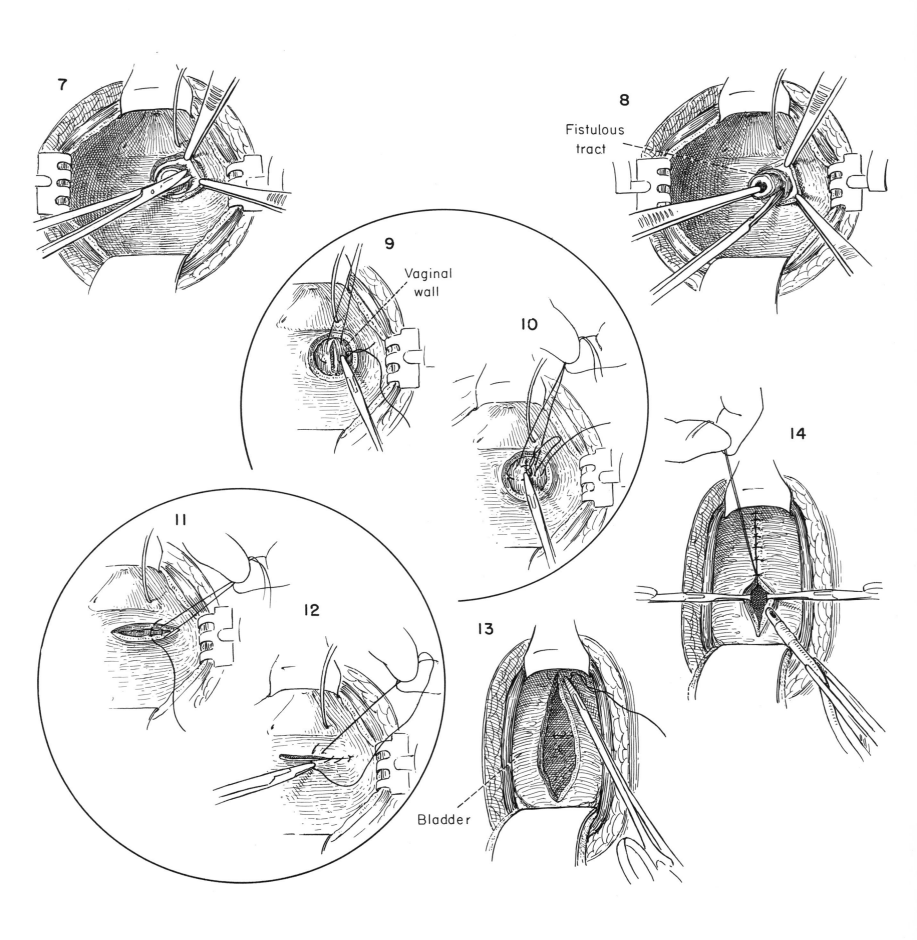

7

8

Fistulous
tract

9

Vaginal
wall

10

11

12

13

Bladder

14

REPAIR OF VESICOVAGINAL FISTULA THROUGH THE ABDOMINAL CAVITY

In certain instances the fistula between bladder and vagina may appear in an area remote from the ureteral opening into the bladder. Inaccessible from below, it is so situated that the approach through the bladder may be less direct than an approach through the abdominal cavity.

INSET A. This shows the anatomic position of the fistula in relation to the vaginal canal, which is packed with gauze to provide a firm surface for dissection.

Figure 1. The abdomen may be opened through a paramedian incision. A transverse or Pfannenstiel incision may be used, depending on the preference of the operator.

Figure 2. The patient is in the Trendelenburg position. The abdominal wall is held back by the self-retaining retractor after packing the intestine out of the lower pelvis. A Deaver retractor is placed in the midline below to aid in the exposure. The vaginal apex with its peritoneal cover is identified in relation to the bladder wall. The surgeon and assistant pick up the peritoneum with forceps as the former incises it.

Figure 3. Kelly clamps are placed on the peritoneal edge as the surgeon separates it from the bladder lying beneath.

Figure 4. With the anterior wall of the bladder denuded of peritoneum, the surgeon retracts the posterior wall of the bladder and begins to dissect it free from its attachments to the vaginal stump. Continuation in this plane of dissection will demonstrate the fistulous tract, which is then transected.

Figure 5. The assistant continues to elevate the bladder by traction on the anterior peritoneal bladder flap as the surgeon elevates the bladder wall, revealing the fistulous opening into the bladder, as distinct from that entering the vaginal canal.

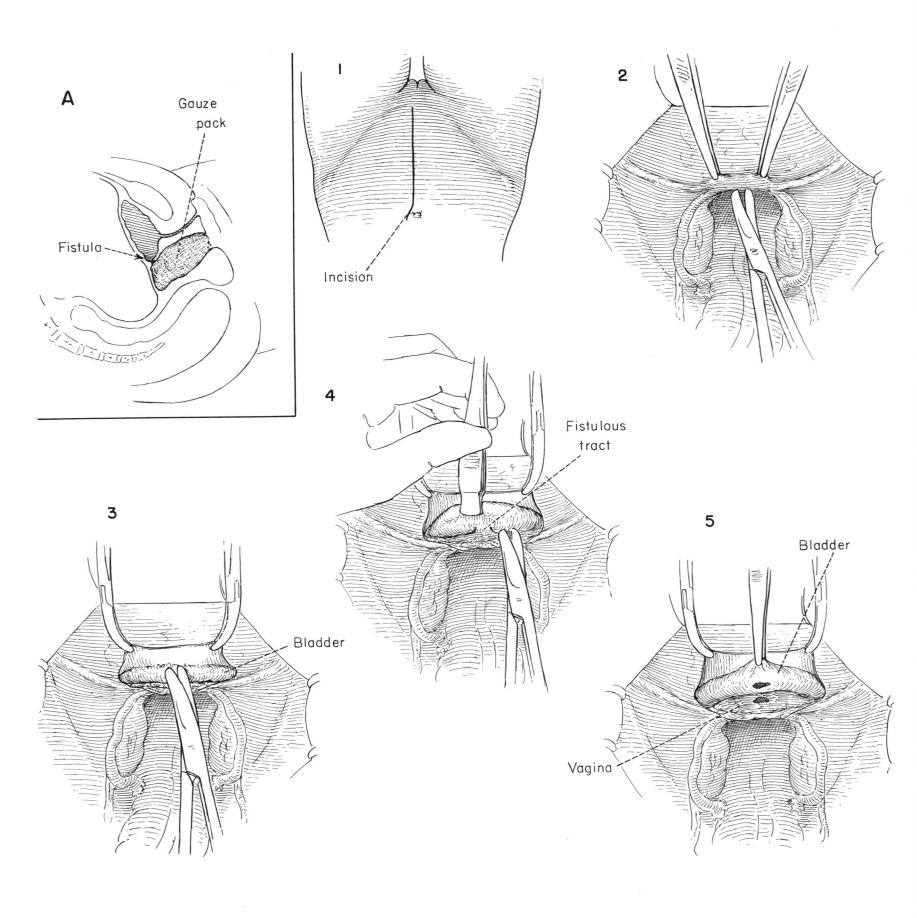

A

Gauze
pack

Fistula

1

Incision

2

4

Fistulous
tract

3

Bladder

5

Bladder

Vagina

Figure 6. With enough bladder wall freed so that the sutures may be approximated without tension, the surgeon picks up the bladder wall on either side of the fistulous opening and introduces an atraumatic catgut suture in the bladder wall, taking care not to enter the bladder mucosa. Each stitch is held as the next one is placed.

Figure 7. The initial row of sutures is tied and cut. A second layer is similarly laid into the bladder wall. When all are in place, they are tied and cut, thereby burying the first line of sutures.

Figure 8. The bladder closure is now complete. The bladder is then retracted with the forceps handle as the fistula opening in the vagina is exposed. A series of interrupted catgut sutures is placed in the vaginal wall on one side of the opening into the vagina and then on the other. These sutures are placed transversely or at a right angle to the initial reparative sutures in the bladder wall. When all are in position, they are tied and cut.

Figure 9. With the bladder still retracted, a second reinforcing layer of interrupted sutures is laid in place in the vaginal wall, tied and cut, thereby burying the primary vaginal suture line.

Figure 10. The opening in the peritoneum at the vaginal apex is now closed with a running stitch to cover all raw surfaces.

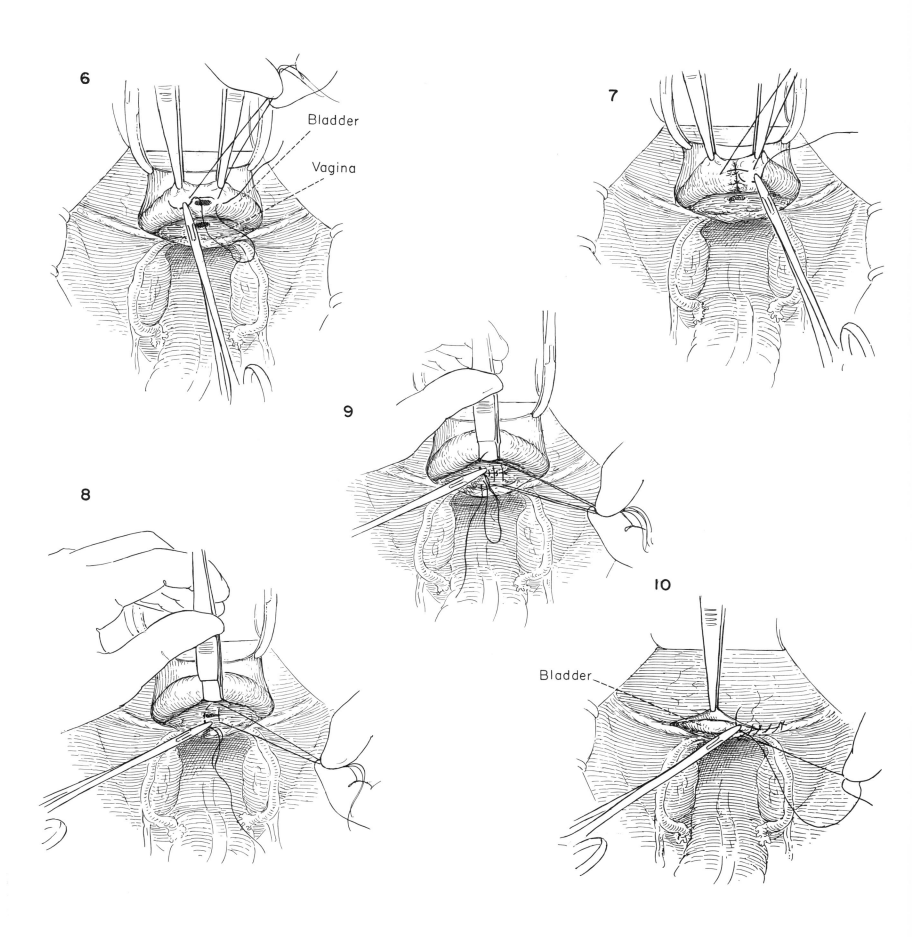

6

Bladder

Vagina

7

9

8

10

Bladder

Figure 11. To divert the urinary stream during the period of healing, a suprapubic cystotomy should be done. Kelly clamps on the lower edges of parietal peritoneum are placed on tension, and the peritoneum is stripped from the underlying muscles, laterally exposing the bladder.

Figure 12. With the palm of the right hand the surgeon strips the peritoneum off the dome of the bladder.

Figure 13. The anterior wall of the bladder has now been laid bare. It is grasped near the dome below the level of the peritoneal reflection. The interior of the bladder is entered by incising the wall between Allis forceps.

Figure 14. The edges of the bladder opening are steadied with forceps as a Foley catheter is introduced into the bladder.

Figure 15. The balloon is filled and the catheter pulled snugly up against the dome of the bladder. The opening in the wall around the catheter is closed with interrupted sutures, one of which fixes the catheter in place.

Figure 16. A catgut suture is then started through the right rectus fascia and muscle to pick up the bladder on either side of the catheter; it emerges at the same relative position on the left after passing through rectus muscle and fascia.

When the wound is closed, with a drain in the prevesical space, tying of this suture will hold the bladder up to the abdominal wall and at the same time prevent the tube from lying against the symphysis, thus avoiding a possible osteomyelitis.

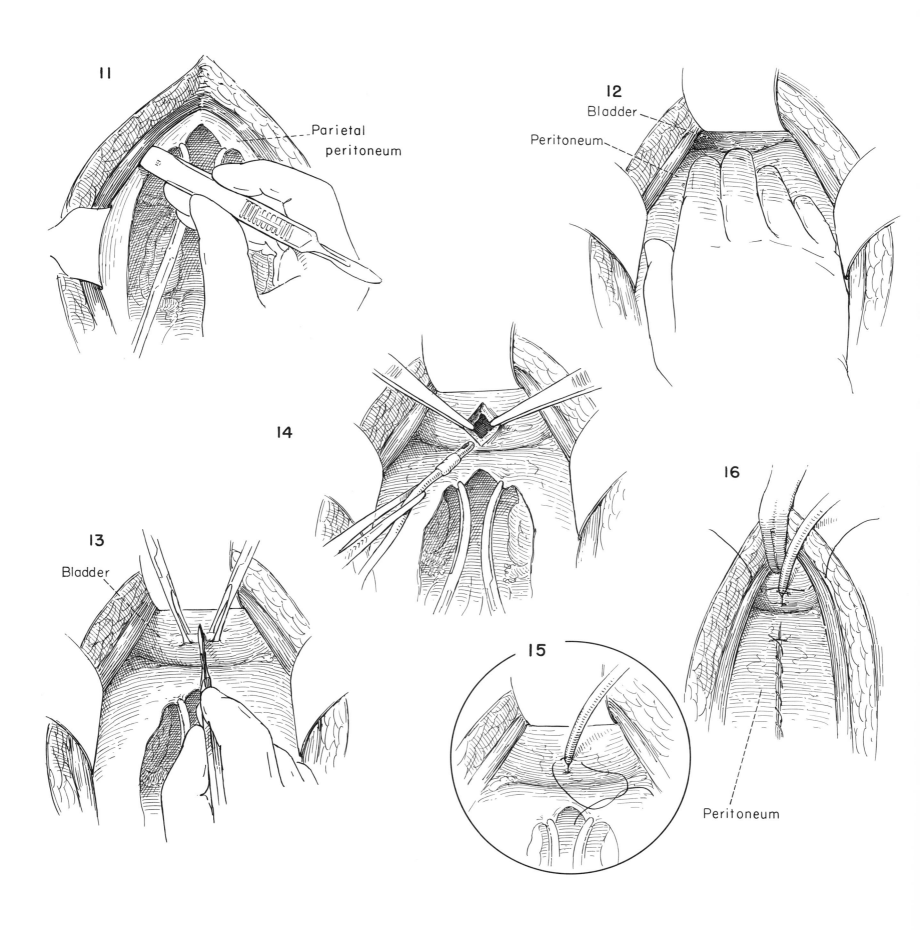

RECTOVAGINAL FISTULA

The same principles that applied in the obliteration of a urinary fistula are of equal importance when the patient has a rectovaginal fistula. The rectovaginal fistula is much more accessible, which is an advantage, but the surgeon faces an additional problem because the continual passage of fecal material over the reconstructed fistulous opening interferes with the normal processes of tissue healing. It is of the utmost importance that no distention should be allowed to occur. These problems are peculiar to the rectovaginal type of fistula. Careful dilatation of the anal sphincter at the conclusion of the operation will help to prevent this.

Many of the rectovaginal fistulas are small and can be readily mobilized and repaired with a simple purse-string closure.

Figure 1. The posterior vaginal wall is held up by Allis forceps at four equally spaced points to provide a fixed surface for the surgeon to circumscribe the fistulous tract by making an incision through the vaginal epithelium with a knife.

Figure 2. The incised vaginal edge is picked up around all sides of the tract and separated from the anterior wall of the rectum for a short distance.

Figure 3. The edges of the vaginal wall are pulled downward with clamps as the surgeon advances the tips of the scissors upward in the midline, staying close to the undersurface of the posterior vaginal wall.

Figure 4. The vaginal wall is then incised in the midline, thus exposing a wide area of anterior rectal wall.

Figure 5. The surgeon picks up the margin of the fistula and excises it with the scissors.

Figure 6. A purse-string suture of catgut on an atraumatic needle is laid in the rectal wall around the fistulous opening. The stitch should be in rectal wall musculature and should not penetrate the rectal mucosa.

Figure 7. This purse-string suture is then tied and cut. A second layer of interrupted sutures is placed first on one side of the closed fistula and then the other. Several such sutures are placed. When a sufficient number are in place, they are tied and cut, thereby burying the purse-string closure.

Figure 8. The levator muscles are brought together in the midline with interrupted catgut sutures, tied and cut.

Figure 9. Redundant vaginal wall is trimmed down, and the edges of the vaginal wall are then closed.

Figure 10. This shows the completed closure with the fistula repaired.

RECTOVAGINAL FISTULA

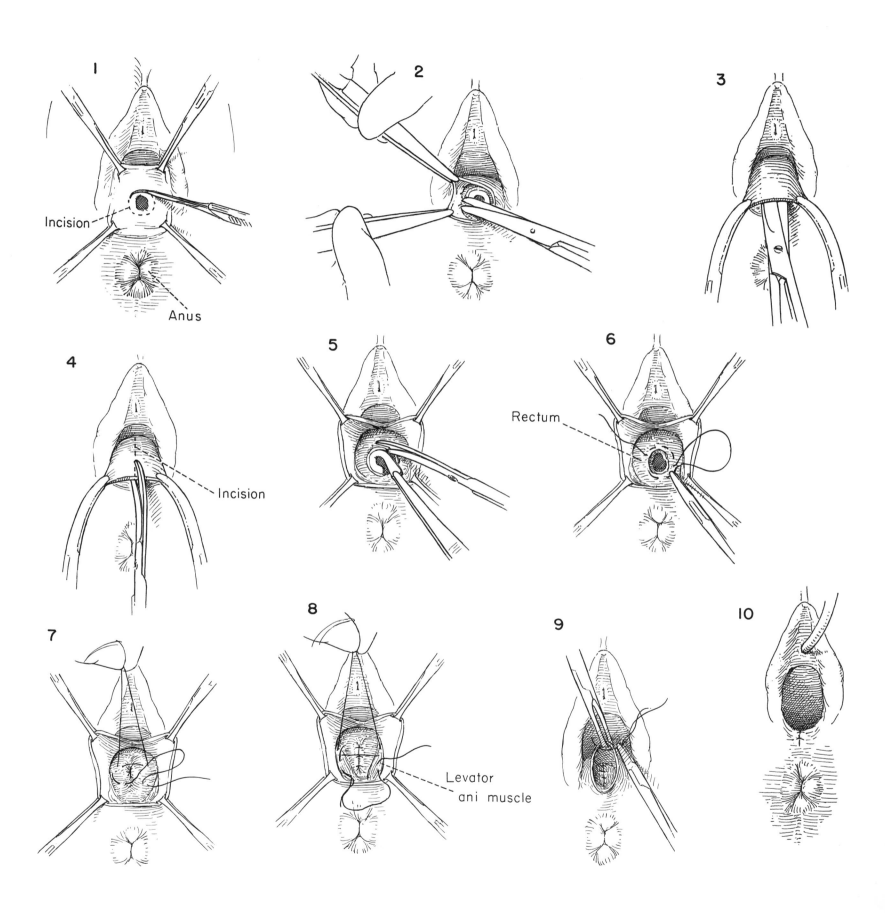

1 Incision Anus

2

3

4 Incision

5

6 Rectum

7

8 Levator ani muscle

9

10

RECTOVAGINAL FISTULA NEAR ANAL SPHINCTER

When there is extensive loss of tissue near the anal sphincter, it is impossible to mobilize enough rectal wall to use a purse-string suture. In this situation it is better to convert the fistula into a third degree tear. The rectal wall must be mobilized sufficiently widely to permit the mucosal edges to come together without tension.

Figure 1. The large midline defect is seen in fairly close proximity to the anal opening. An incision is made through the full thickness of the vaginal wall around the fistula.

Figure 2. When it is obvious that insufficient bowel wall can be developed to permit closure without tension, the opening is converted into a third degree tear by cutting through the narrow bridge in the midline.

Figure 3. Allis clamps are placed on either side of the vaginal outlet. The plane between vagina and rectum is developed as tension is maintained. This dissection is carried well above the fistula.

Figure 4. Kelly clamps will be necessary to maintain adequate traction as the posterior vaginal wall is freed. The flap is then split in the midline.

Figure 5. The edges are held up, exposing a wide surface of anterior rectal wall and the levator ani muscles on either side. The scarred edges of the fistulous opening are excised.

Figure 6. The surgeon picks up the rectal wall and places an interrupted suture first on one side of the rectal wall and then the other, without entering the mucosa. The entire defect is closed in this manner as the sutures are tied and cut.

Figure 7. A second reinforcing layer is similarly introduced, tied and cut.

Figure 8. Nerve hooks pick up the divided ends of the sphincter muscle on either side. These are held on tension as the surgeon approximates the ends with interrupted catgut sutures.

Figure 9. The levators are brought together by a series of interrupted catgut sutures. These are held long as the redundant bowel above is reduced with a few shallow stitches in the fascia overlying it.

Figure 10. After the sutures have been tied and cut, the posterior vaginal wall defect is closed with interrupted catgut sutures.

Figure 11. These sutures are tied and cut and the operation is complete.

RECTOVAGINAL FISTULA NEAR ANAL SPHINCTER

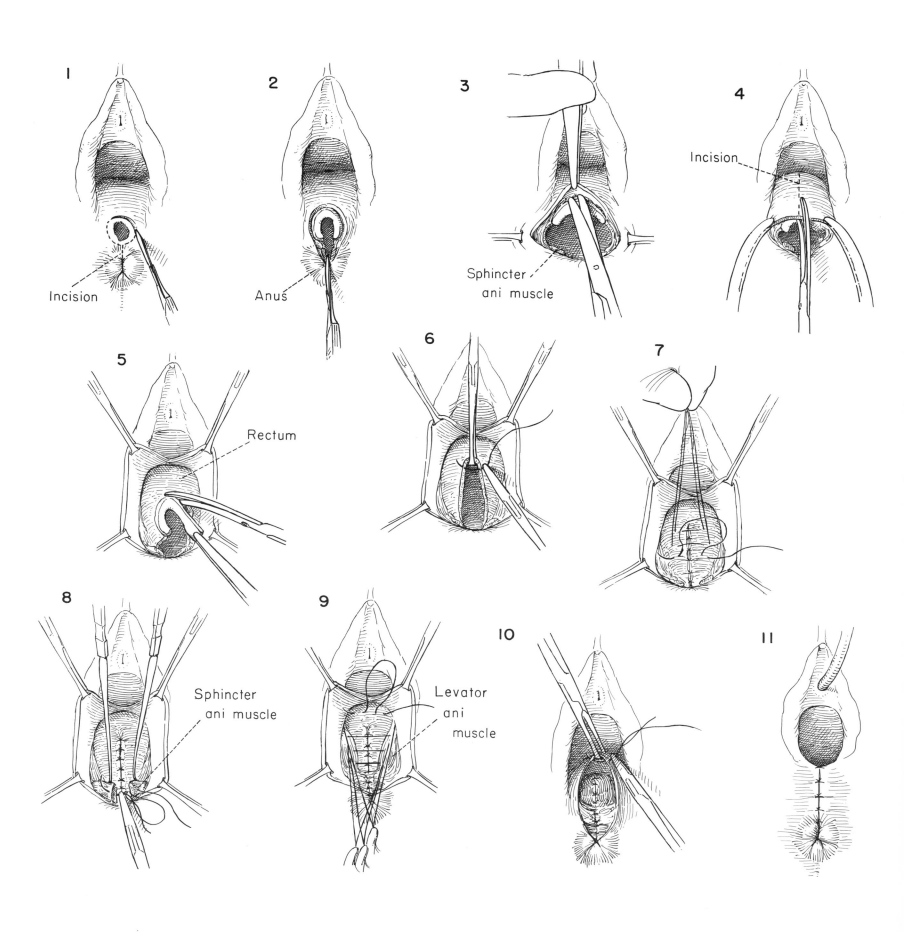

BIOPSY OF THE CERVIX

When there is a visible erosion or an area of cervical epithelium that fails to stain dark brown with aqueous iodine (Schiller's solution), a sample of this tissue must be obtained. This specimen should contain a piece of the adjacent normal tissue as well as that under suspicion. This will give the pathologist a basis for comparison. Many types of punch biopsy forceps are available, but the best instrument of all is the scalpel.

When no suspicious areas can be seen but symptoms or cytologic studies suggest the need for investigation, it is vital that tissue be removed from all areas that might harbor malignant changes in the epithelium. The first step would be fractional curettage. This means the removal of tissue separately from the endocervical cavity and from the fundus of the uterus. The material obtained from each area should be set aside and specifically labeled.

When the portio of the cervix is under suspicion, particularly if an erosion is present, the entire squamocolumnar junction should be excised in the form of a cone. This must be done with a knife and not an electric cautery in order to avoid damage to the tissue that must be examined. If oozing follows the removal, the affected area may be sutured or cauterized.

This method provides a higher degree of accuracy than the method commonly used of taking biopsies from each of the four quadrants of the cervix.

Endocervical Biopsy

Figure 1. With the patient in lithotomy position the anterior vaginal wall is elevated and the cervix exposed. It is then held on traction with two tenacula placed on the anterior lip.

Figure 2. The endocervical canal is first scraped with a curette which collects the tissue as it comes free. The material obtained is set aside and labeled. The surgeon then proceeds with the evaluation of the rest of the endometrial cavity in both upper and lower portions.

Figure 3. The canal of the cervix is gently dilated.

Wedge Biopsy of Exocervix

Figure 4. Any suspicious area should be excised. The specimen must contain the full epithelial layer and enough stroma for comparison.

Figure 5. The small specimen obtained is marked and saved for special pathologic scrutiny.

Cone Biopsy of Squamocolumnar Junction

Figure 6. When there is an erosion present, the entire squamocolumnar junction should be excised. A circular incision is drawn around the external os with a narrow pointed blade.

Figure 7. The knife is then thrust obliquely through the muscle beneath the circle until the tip enters the endocervical canal. With short sawing strokes which follow the circle, a cone of tissue is excised completely surrounding the external os.

Figure 8. This specimen is carefully lifted out and sent to the pathologist for study. Frequently the irregular contour of the cervix will make it necessary to accomplish this in two or more fragments. All should be examined microscopically.

Figure 9. If there is significant oozing from the raw surfaces light cauterization will usually control it.

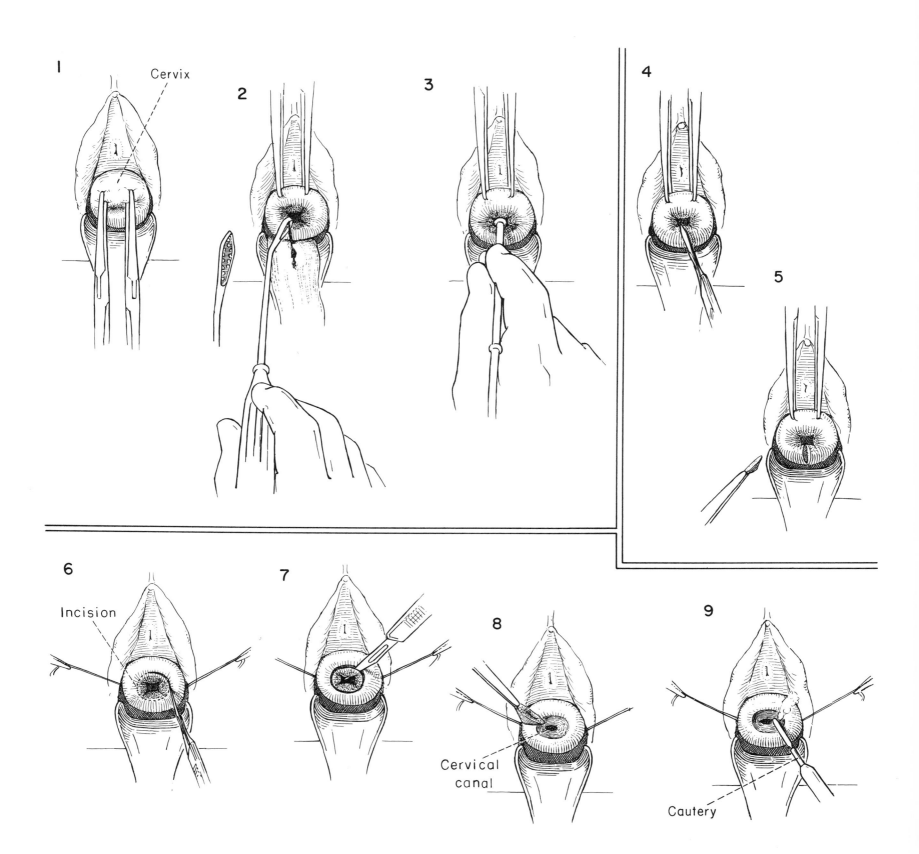

CAUTERIZATION OF THE CERVIX

In the face of marked erosion or ectropion of the endocervical mucosa or deeply seated chronic infection within the tortuous racemose glands of the cervix, all of which give rise to persistent, tenacious and distressing leukorrhea, radial cauterization of the cervix has much to recommend it. Depending on the depth of cauterization desired, this procedure may be used in either the office or the operating room. The more superficial lesions can readily be treated as an office maneuver.

Figure 1. The cervix is exposed and tenacula applied. Moist gauze protects the vulva. Linear streaks are made with a cautery radially from the external os as the central point and carried as deeply into the musculature as desired. The tip of the cautery blade should not carry a white hot heat.

Figure 2. Successive linear striations are made from the central focal point, leaving segments of tissue between the cauterized streaks.

THERAPEUTIC CONIZATION OF THE CERVIX

Figure 3. When the surgeon would like to remove the extensive erosion and he is not concerned about pathologic interpretation of the specimen, he may elect to use a Hyam's type of cautery which removes a core of tissue.

This is a very simple procedure but can be made even more so if the surgeon will place a figure-of-eight suture through the vaginal epithelium and into the muscle of the cervix at about the level of the internal os. This is done on both sides. The sutures are then clamped and left long to provide traction on the cervix. The absence of tenacula makes it much easier for the surgeon to get a good cone of tissue.

The tip of the Hyam's conization instrument is inserted into the canal to the full extent of the cutting wire.

INSET A. This diagram shows the type of the coning point. The width of the erosion or ectropion will determine the size of the conization tip to be used.

Figure 4. The instrument is made moderately hot and gradually turned.

Figure 5. The procedure is continued through a full circle.

Figure 6. The cone of tissue is removed en bloc. Any bleeding points should be touched with a coagulating current.

INSET B. A sagittal section of the uterus shows the area of excision. Dilatation of the cervical canal at frequent intervals during the period of healing will help to prevent any stenosis.

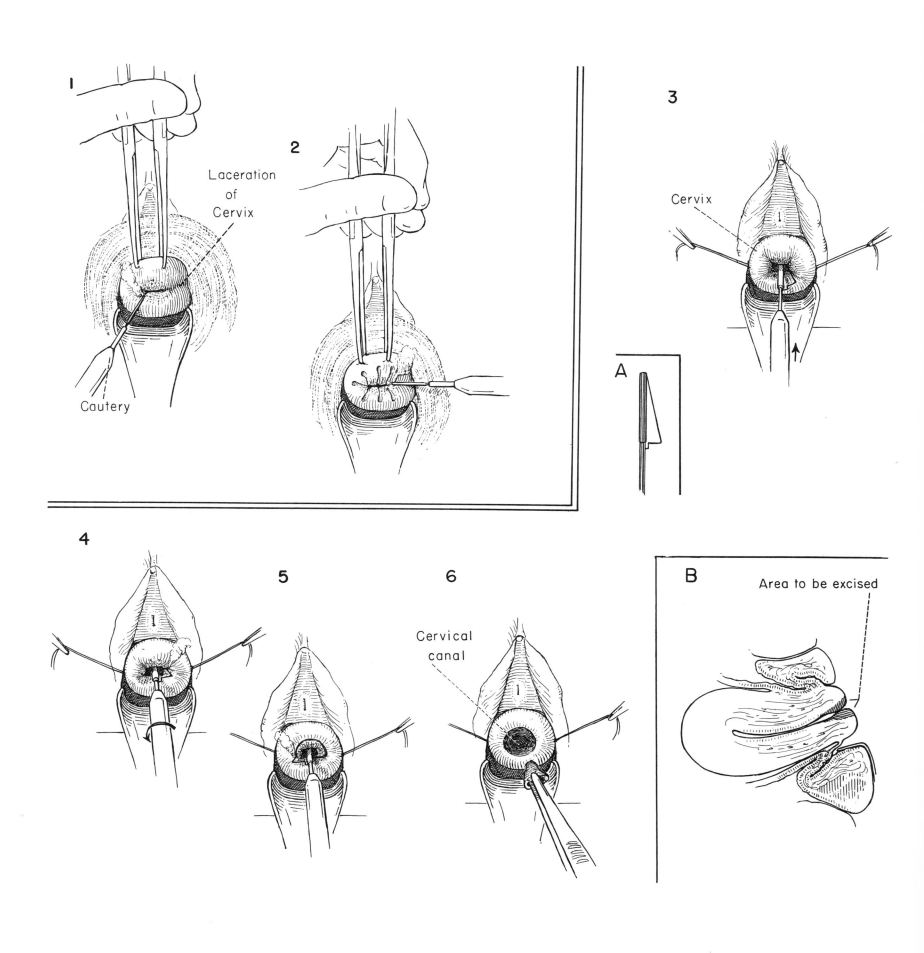

LOW AMPUTATION OF THE CERVIX

This operation is offered when scarring and deformity of the cervix are extensive. It may be done as a definitive procedure for a lacerated or infected cervix with exposure of the endocervix, or as a part of other operations such as the Manchester.

The vaginal portion of the cervix is transected at the level of the fornices and the stump is covered with full thickness flaps of epithelium from the anterior and posterior vaginal walls.

Preliminary dilatation of the canal is important. It is also essential that the canal be checked for patency at the conclusion of the operation and after several menstrual periods in the convalescent phase.

In these illustrations the operation is being done for a badly lacerated cervix with exposure of the endocervix.

Figure 1. Tenacula are applied to the cervix, which is then held upward to permit the introduction of a probe. Thorough dilatation and curettage are performed.

Figure 2. The labia are stitched to the surrounding skin with interrupted catgut sutures. The cervix is held down and the vaginal wall incised transversely just above the cervix. The incision carries through the full thickness of the wall.

Figure 3. The tenacula turn the cervix upward, and the posterior vaginal wall is similarly incised, thus encircling the cervix.

Figure 4. Allis forceps are placed on the edges of the incision on the anterior vaginal wall. Countertraction is applied to the tenacula on the cervix as the vaginal wall is stripped upward.

Figure 5. The posterior cervix is freed from the vagina in similar fashion.

Figure 6. By elevating the detached vaginal wall on the left side with Allis forceps, the lower attachments of the cardinal ligament to the cervix are exposed; they are clamped just above the site chosen for amputation. The same maneuver is carried out on the right side.

Figure 7. The cardinal ligaments are cut and secured with suture ligatures.

Figure 8. Amputation of the cervix is carried out at the point of election, using circumferential sweeps of the knife and bevelling slightly toward the fundus. New tenacula are applied to the lateral corners of the cervix to maintain traction as the distal fragment is cut free.

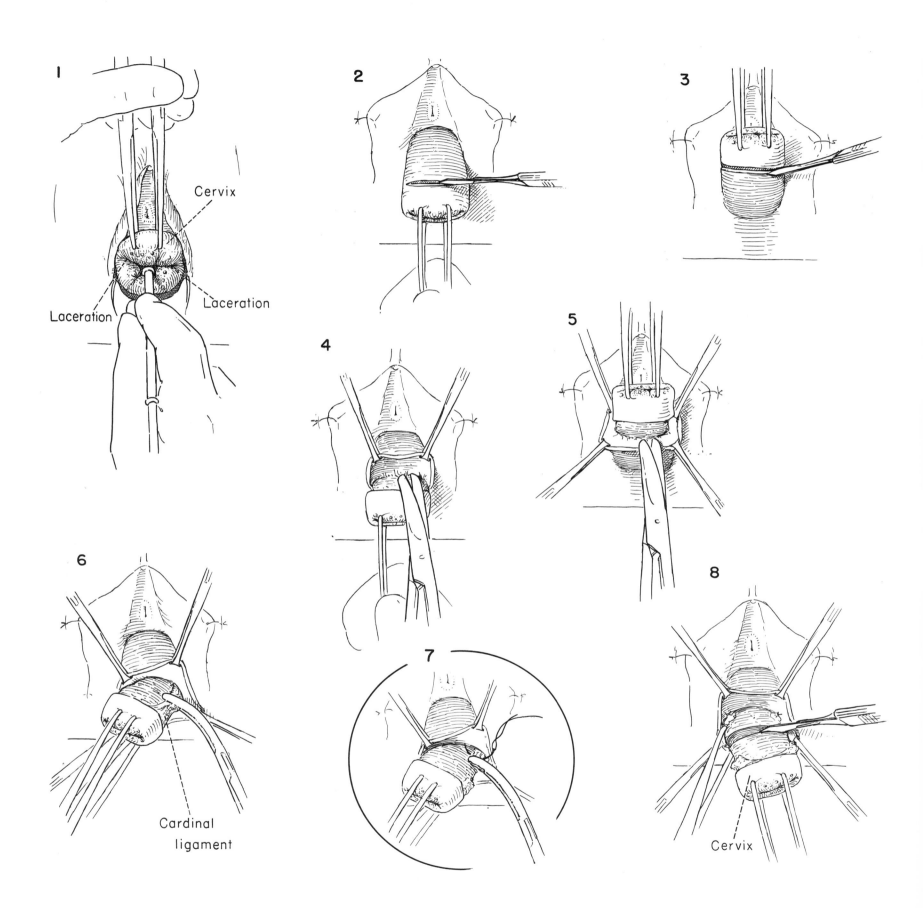

Figure 9. Note that the vaginal epithelium has been stripped back from the entire circumference of the cervix for a considerable distance. In this manner a free flap is provided which will be used to cover the raw cervical stump. It should lie easily in this position without tension.

A curved needle with a cutting point is used to pass one end of a catgut suture through the posterior vaginal wall at its midpoint. There it is tied. A second needle is threaded on the other free end of the suture.

Figure 10. The surgeon passes one of the cutting point needles through the cervical wall from the canal out through the muscle to emerge on the vaginal side about ¾ inch below the original tie.

Figure 11. This step is repeated with the cutting needle on the other free end of the suture. This stitch emerges through the vaginal wall about ¼ inch lateral to the first one.

Figure 12. As this suture is tied the flap of the vaginal wall is drawn up into the cervical canal covering it on the posterior wall.

Figure 13. The anterior vaginal edge is to be brought over the cervix in identical fashion. Here the stitch is placed in the center of the flap.

Figure 14. The second suture is being placed through the substance of the cervix.

Figure 15. The epithelium is drawn neatly into place as the stitch is tied.

Figure 16. The flap hangs loosely at either lateral corner. The surgeon then begins a stitch at one anterior lateral corner, passing through the vaginal wall and into the substance of the cervix to obliterate dead space and to help to control any bleeding from the cervical branch of the uterine artery. A similar suture is placed on the opposite side. These sutures are held long until all raw edges are approximated. They are then tied.

Figure 17. The patency of the cervical canal is checked by introducing a medium-sized dilator.

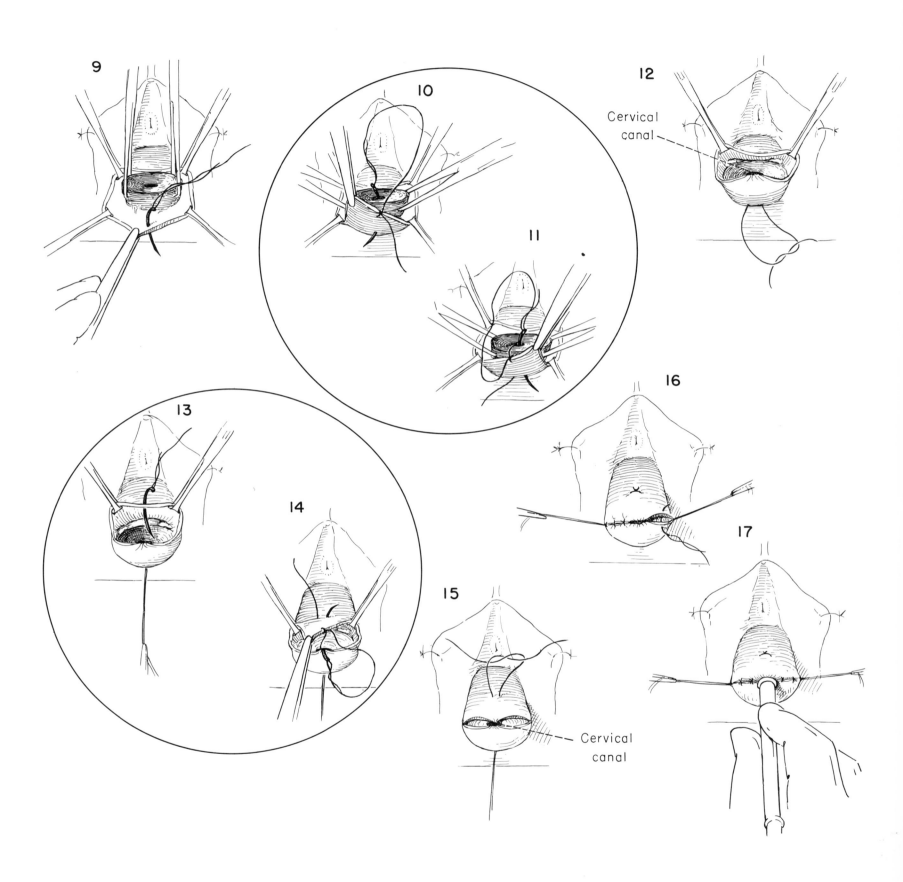

TRACHELORRHAPHY

In the past, trachelorrhaphy was commonly done for repair of a lacerated cervix with exposure of the endocervix as a prophylaxis against subsequent development of carcinoma. Today it is less frequently used than conization, yet it has a definite place in surgical therapy.

Figure 1. The anteriop lip of the cervix is grasped with a tenaculum on the side away from the laceration. A second tenaculum is placed on the corresponding position on the posterior lip.

Figure 2. Beginning on the lower edge, so that blood running down does not obscure the field, the surgeon outlines the scarred laceration.

Figure 3. The incision continues around the area outlined, bevelling medially as one gets deeper.

Figure 4. A heart-shaped piece of tissue is removed. Troublesome bleeding from the cervical branch of the uterine artery will be encountered if the excision extends too far laterally on the cervix.

Figure 5. The most lateral of the stitches should therefore be placed deep into the muscle, carrying through both edges of the incision. The surgeon should use fine wire rather than catgut sutures to minimize sepsis and adverse tissue reaction.

Figure 6. The sutures are drawn to the right and the most lateral suture tied first. Each suture is held long until the next is tied. It is then cut. The wire sutures are removed in the convalescent period when healing is complete.

Bilateral Trachelorrhaphy

If the laceration is bilateral, both areas are excised before beginning the repair.

Figure 7. A typical bilateral laceration of the cervix with exposed endocervix is shown. Tenacula are applied for traction.

Figure 8. The epithelial surfaces on either side are outlined for excision. Since the space between will form one half the circumference of the endocervical canal, care must be taken to leave enough epithelium.

Figure 9. The flaps are excised.

Figure 10. Fine wire sutures are laid in place, and the ends of each suture are held in a snap.

Figure 11. The sutures are drawn together, bringing the raw surfaces of the anterior and posterior cervix in contact. They are tied and cut after testing of the canal for patency. Removal in the office will be necessary after two weeks.

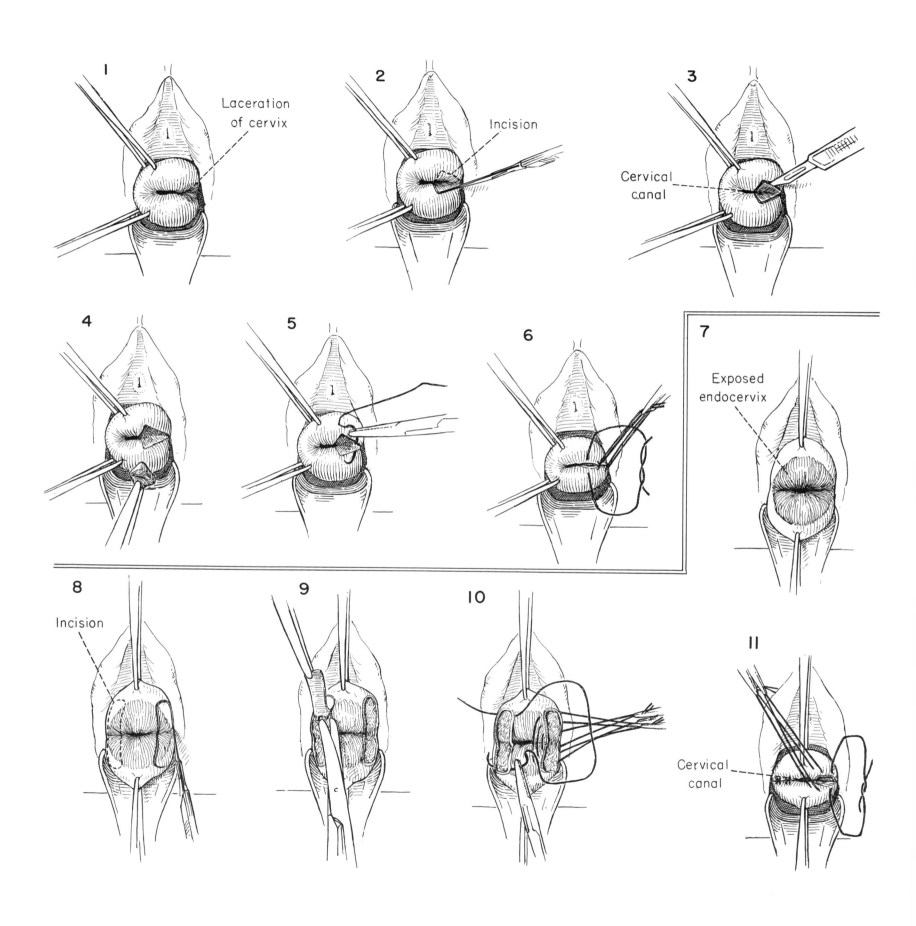

EXCISION OF CYST OF BARTHOLIN'S GLAND

Cystic enlargement of Bartholin's gland is a fairly frequent and well recognized gynecologic entity. Although the enlargement may regress to the point where only a firm hard kernel can be felt on one side or other of the vulva, its natural history is that of repeated though intermittent recrudescence. It also has a marked tendency to become infected. A definite effort should be made to remove the gland in its entirety without rupture.

Treatment of the acutely infected cyst is often best accomplished by simple incision and marsupialization.

Figure 1. The labia are tacked to the skin with interrupted catgut sutures. An incision is made laterally following the natural curve of the introitus through the skin at its junction with the vaginal epithelium.

Figure 2. Allis forceps are applied to the edge of this incision. The incised edge on the vaginal side is elevated as the surgeon separates the connective tissue bands holding the vagina to the underlying cyst wall.

Figure 3. As the dissection progresses in this plane more clamps are placed on the edge of the vaginal wall to provide countertraction to that offered by the surgeon as he gently retracts the cyst wall with the tips of his fingers laid over gauze. In this manner the dissection proceeds around the circumference of the cyst on its medial side.

Figure 4. This may be a bloody operation. By staying in the plane close to the cyst wall in the dissection and by isolating and clamping each vessel as it is encountered, the amount of blood loss may be considerably reduced. The cyst is completely enucleated from its bed. A final attachment will always be found at the upper pole. This is clamped and cut.

Figure 5. The individual vessels are tied.

Figure 6. To obliterate dead space and to cut down a persistent venous ooze, a series of interrupted catgut sutures are placed in the depths of the cavity. When all are placed, they are tied and cut.

Figure 7. A second layer further obliterates the dead space by burying the first line of sutures.

Figure 8. The skin edges are loosely closed with interrupted catgut sutures. A slip of rubber wick is left in the cavity to prevent hematoma.

EXCISION OF CYST OF BARTHOLIN'S GLAND

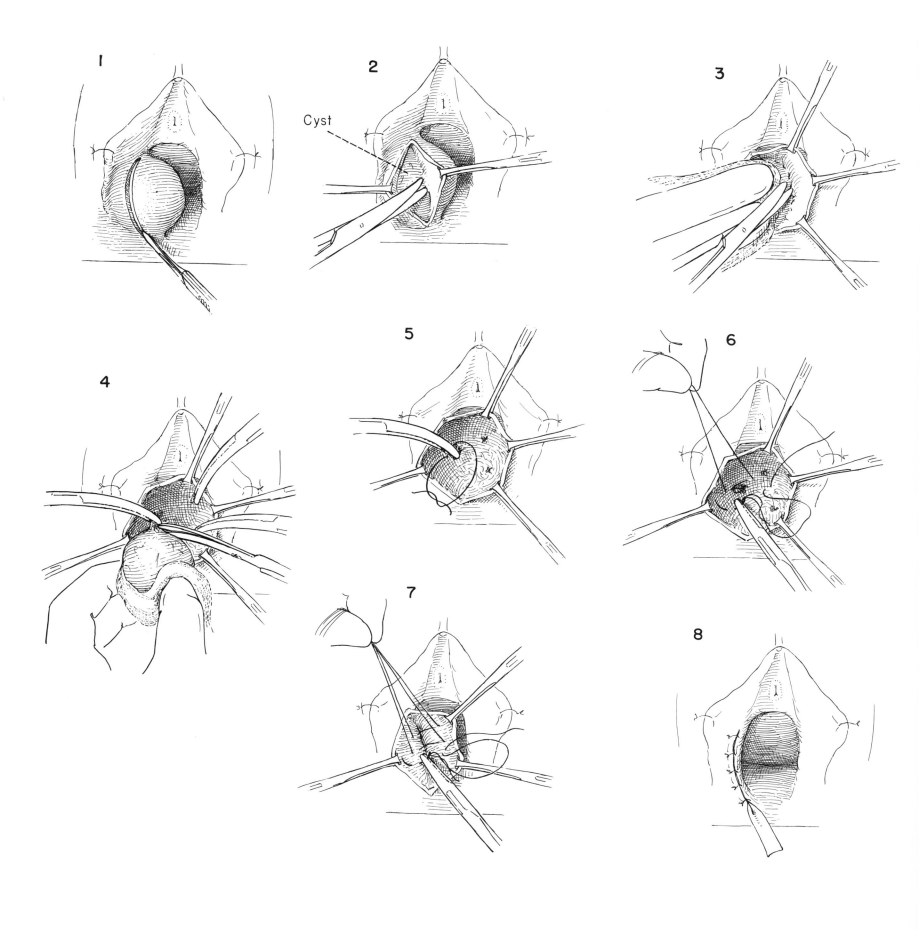

Cyst

SIMPLE VULVECTOMY

This procedure involves the removal of all the vulva, including the labia and the clitoris. The inner border of excision is the junction between keratinized and squamous epithelium surrounding the urogenital vestibule. The operation is designed only to remove diseased or abnormal skin and just enough fat to permit easy closure without tension. It is inadequate for treatment for malignant disease in this area but can be employed as a prophylactic measure in the prevention of subsequent malignant disease.

The closure is usually a simple matter. To avoid the later development of a rectocele it is always wise to perform a perineorrhaphy in conjunction with the simple vulvectomy.

Figure 1. This outlines the incisions to be made. The amount of skin to be removed depends on the amount of disease present. The inner incision encircles the vagina and urethra.

Figure 2. The labia are held upward with Allis forceps on either side as the surgeon pulls down on the anterior vaginal wall and incises the epithelium above the urethral opening.

Figure 3. The incision continues on both sides and across the midline posteriorly.

Figure 4. The surgeon then turns his attention to the outer margin of excision. Beginning in the midline on the mons veneris above the clitoris, the incision extends around the vulva on both sides, removing as much skin as necessary. Individual vessels are clamped, tied and cut as they appear.

Figure 5. The incision is deepened around the entire circumference of the vulva as the skin edges are held back with rake retractors. The upper edge of the skin to be removed is pulled downward to expose the suspensory ligament of the clitoris, which is then clamped and divided.

Figure 6. The lower edge of the incision is then grasped with Allis clamps and the posterior vaginal wall dissected free of the perineal body and rectum.

Figure 7. The lower skin edge is then turned down and held on traction as the surgeon breaks through into the inner incision from below.

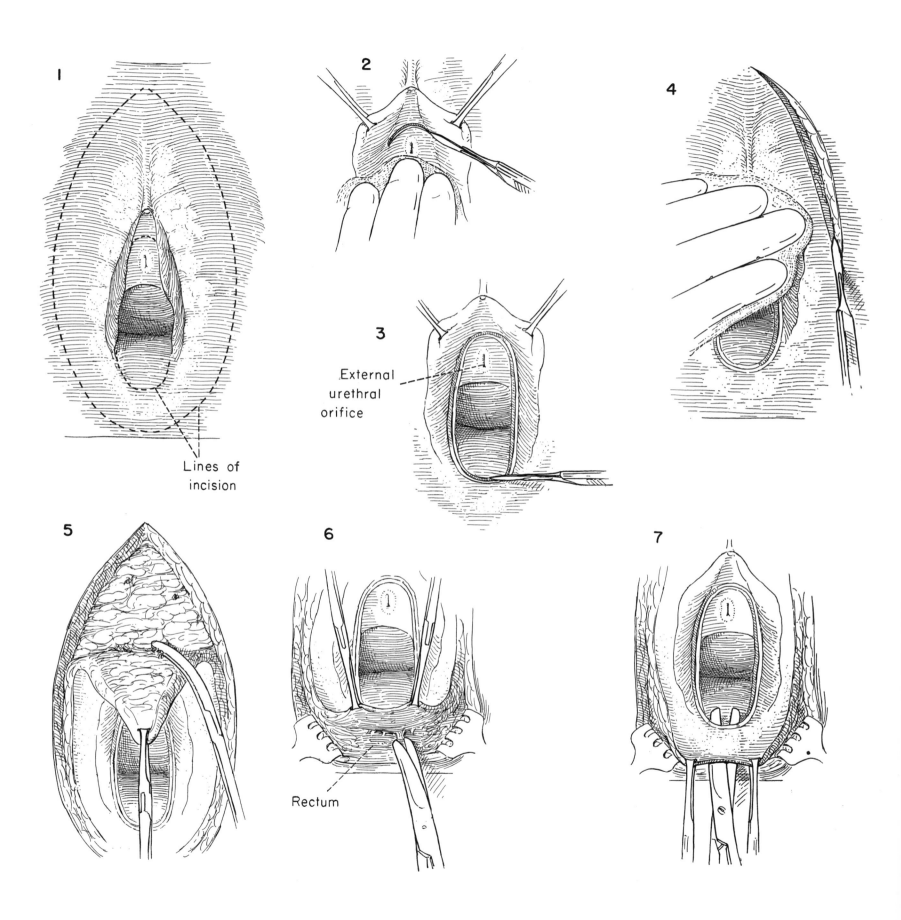

1

Lines of incision

2

3

External urethral orifice

4

5

6

Rectum

7

Figure 8. Traction is provided on the left lateral margin of skin to be removed, pulling it toward the midline as the surgeon undermines the skin, bevelling the knife toward the vaginal canal. The lateral skin edges are held back with rake retractors.

Figure 9. The dissection then continues in this plane until the incision in the vaginal wall is met. In this manner the entire vulva is removed. It is not necessary to remove large amounts of fat or expose the fascia of the deeper muscles.

Figure 10. The entire specimen has been removed, and any bleeding vessels secured. Traction is applied in a downward direction to the corners of the posterior vaginal wall. The tips of the scissors hug the undersurface of the vaginal wall as they are forced upward in the midline. A flap of posterior vaginal wall is created.

Figure 11. The posterior vaginal wall flap is then turned upward, exposing the levator muscles. The surgeon places the first of a series of interrupted catgut sutures parallel to each other in each muscle bundle.

Figure 12. All these sutures are then tied and cut. Additional stitches reconstruct the perineal body.

Figure 13. The skin edges above the vaginal outlet are approximated with interrupted silk. The surgeon then places a series of interrupted silk sutures around the entire circumference of the vagina to bring the skin edges together with the vaginal epithelium.

Figure 14. The closure is complete. Drains are unnecessary. The bladder is placed on constant drainage.

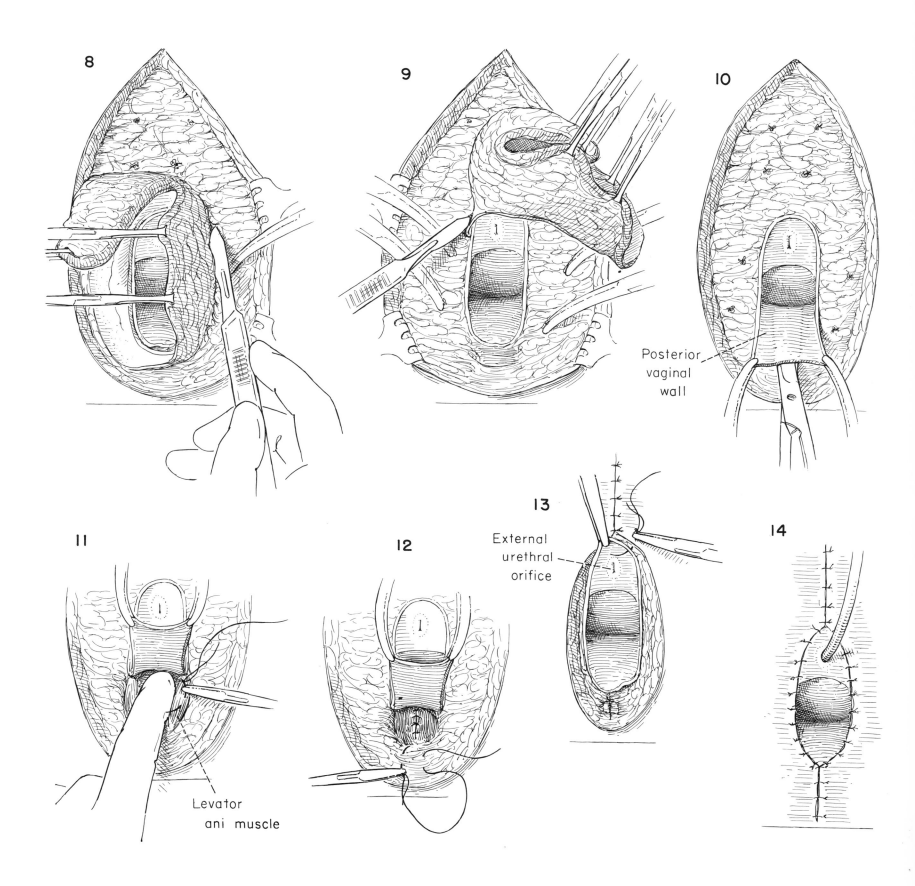

8

9

10

Posterior
vaginal
wall

11

12

13

External
urethral
orifice

14

Levator
ani muscle

Section III

Operations for Malignant Disease

WERTHEIM HYSTERECTOMY WITH PELVIC LYMPHADENECTOMY

This operation was designed for the treatment of cancer of the cervix. It is peculiarly appropriate to this because the life history of cervical cancer tends to keep it confined to the primary site, to the tissues immediately adjacent to the cervix and to the regional nodes in the iliac and obturator areas. Also, it fulfills the basic concept for the treatment of malignant disease anywhere; namely, that the operation remove en bloc the organ of primary involvement, its adjacent structures and the pathways of lymphatic spread. This is in contrast to the operations performed for benign lesions which are extended laterally only occasionally to permit total local excision of the growth.

The Wertheim operation removes the contents of the pelvis from one obturator fossa to the other. The regional nodes that are located along the common iliac, hypogastric and external iliac vessels and in the area immediately beneath the external iliac vein and above the obturator nerve are also excised. In order to encompass the lymphatic tissue that extends from the side wall of the pelvis to the paracervical and paravaginal area adjacent to the primary tumor in the cervix, the bladder and ureters must be completely freed from the vagina.

The important part of this operation is the meticulous en bloc resection of the lymphatic channels in the paracervical and paravaginal area. The magnitude of this dissection creates a definite risk of damage to the bladder floor and ureter. To remove less tissue in order to reduce the chance of creating a ureterovaginal or vesicovaginal fistula is to increase the likelihood of leaving cancer behind.

INSET A. The best way of preventing fistulas and performing an adequate excision of potential cancer-bearing tissue is to have a thorough knowledge of the anatomy of the area and to operate in a dry surgical field. The surgeon should be able to anticipate where each structure will normally be encountered. It is a cardinal principle that each step be carried out under direct vision in a field unobscured by blood and unencumbered by clamps.

This anatomic drawing shows the major blood supply in the area to be dissected in relation to the structures to be preserved, namely, the bladder and rectum.

Figure 1. After examination and preparation of the vagina, the bladder is placed on constant drainage and the abdomen prepared and draped. The abdomen is opened through a midline incision; after exploration of the upper abdomen, the intestine is packed off. The uterus is held on traction by a tenaculum on the fundus. The assistant and the surgeon pick up the peritoneum of the avascular area of the broad ligament as the surgeon incises it.

Figure 2. With the uterus on traction the surgeon introduces his index finger into the subperitoneal space and gently teases away the areolar tissue, pushing the bladder medially. This is done on both sides.

Figure 3. Kelly clamps are placed on the leading edge of the incised peritoneum and held upward on traction. The surgeon then incises the peritoneum intervening between the two openings. Care must be taken not to damage the underlying bladder wall.

Figure 4. The anterior wall of the bladder is then dissected from the undersurface of the peritoneum for a short distance as the assistant holds the clamps on tension.

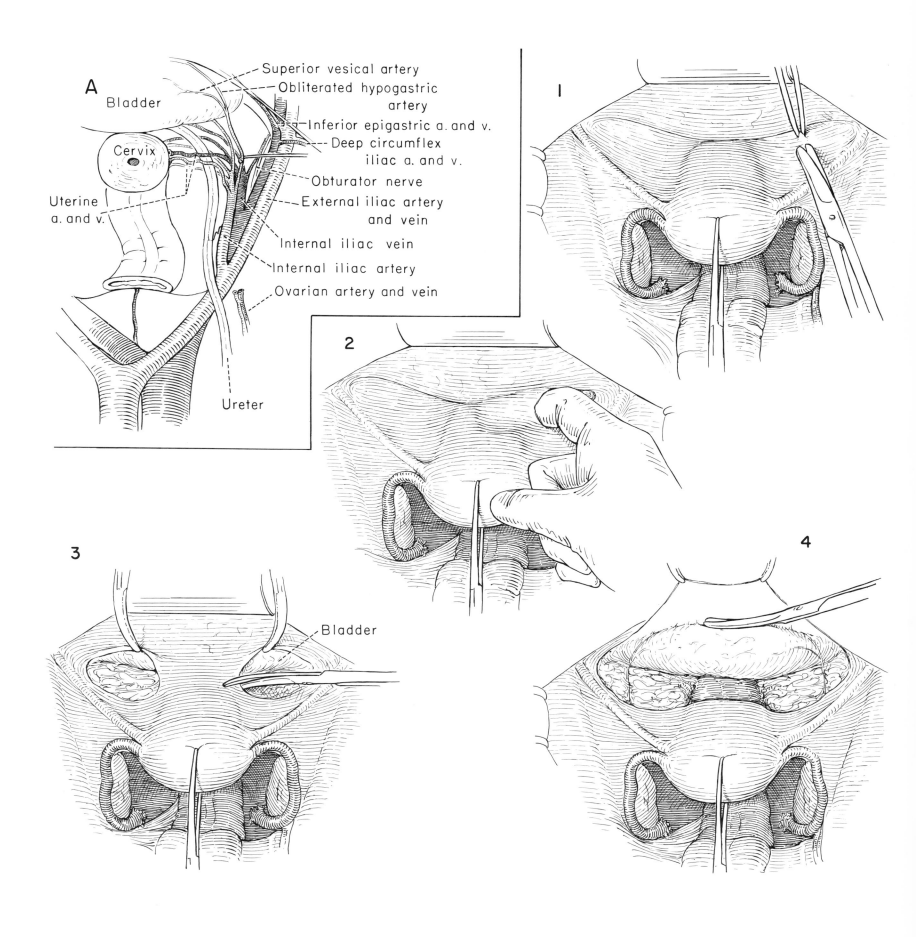

A

Bladder

Cervix

Uterine a. and v.

Superior vesical artery

Obliterated hypogastric artery

Inferior epigastric a. and v.

Deep circumflex iliac a. and v.

Obturator nerve

External iliac artery and vein

Internal iliac vein

Internal iliac artery

Ovarian artery and vein

Ureter

1

2

3

Bladder

4

Figure 5. The uterus is drawn sharply toward the symphysis. The surgeon picks up the right tube and ovary to expose the sigmoid and the posterior peritoneum. The course of the ureter beneath the peritoneum can be traced, beginning at the point at which it crosses the common iliac vessels and descends into the pelvis along the lateral wall.

Figure 6. With the uterus held on tension and the ovarian vessels retracted to permit better view of the course of the ureter, the peritoneum is incised in a longitudinal direction just lateral to the course of the ureter. The ovarian vessels are then identified and isolated from the underlying ureter. The surgeon elevates the vessels and draws a ligature through and ties it. Kelly clamps are applied and the vessels divided.

Figure 7. The pedicle is then secured with a stitch ligature.

Figure 8. The uterus is drawn medially and the peritoneum incised along the path shown by the dotted line. Stitch ligatures are placed in and around the round ligament. They are held long while the ligament is divided. This will expose the areolar tissue overlying the structures of the pelvic wall.

Figure 9. While the surgeon and assistant maintain traction on the uterus and the severed pedicles, the surgeon with gentle finger dissection separates the central mass from the lateral wall. This is the paravesical space, lying between the external iliac and hypogastric vessels, and is easily opened.

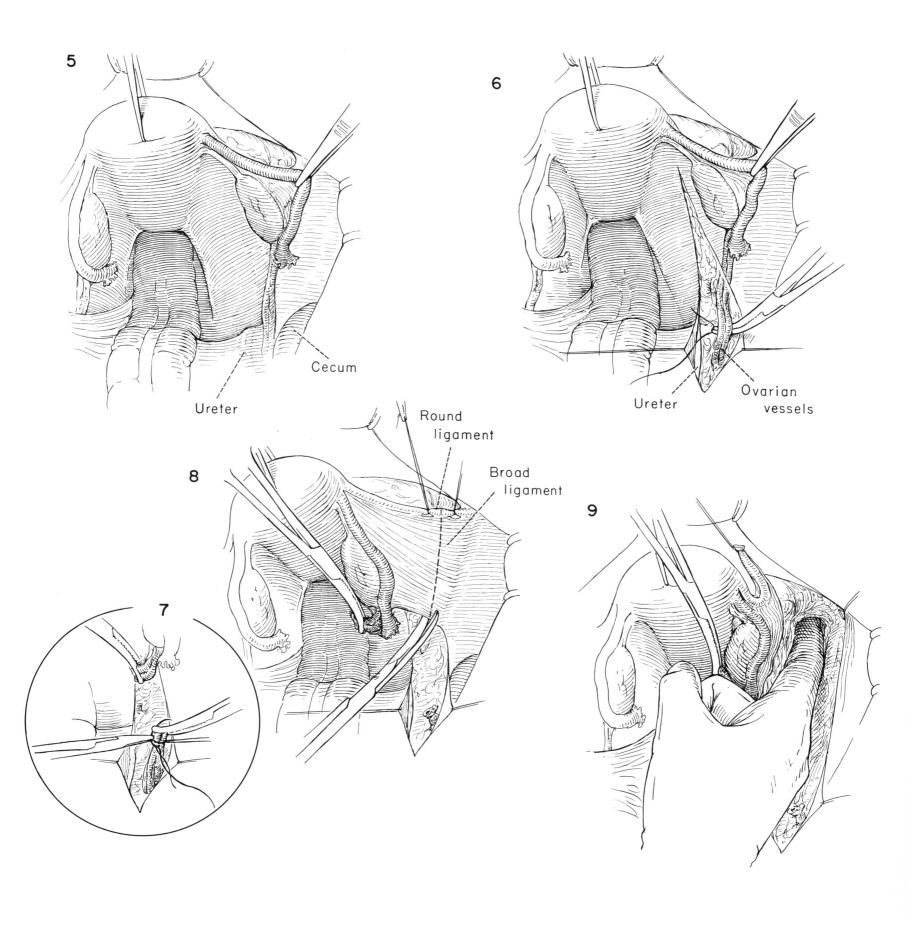

5

Cecum

Ureter

6

Ureter

Ovarian vessels

7

8

Round ligament

Broad ligament

9

Figure 10. The uterus is pulled upward by the assistant who also places the round ligament on tension by drawing it toward him with forceps. The surgeon then replaces the clamp on the divided end of the ovarian vessels with a tie of the ligature on the round ligament.

Figure 11. The uterus continues to be drawn upward in the midline by traction. The sutured ends of the ovarian and round ligaments are then tied around the tenaculum. This maneuver keeps them up out of the operative field and gives the surgeon greater freedom of movement as well as better visualization.

Figure 12. The uterus is drawn to the opposite side by applying traction to the tenaculum to which the adnexa are attached. Stay sutures are then placed on the medial edge of the incised peritoneal edge. These are held on traction as the surgeon exposes the internal iliac artery by dissecting the areolar tissue away from its superior surface. A small but constant branch to the ureter arises about 1.5 cm. below the bifurcation.

Figure 13. With traction on the uterus and stay sutures maintained, the surgeon identifies the uterine artery at the point of its origin on the internal iliac. He must isolate the superior vesical artery from the uterine artery before he places a clamp on the latter vessel.

Figure 14. With the superior vesical artery out of the way the surgeon places a second clamp on the uterine artery medial to the clamp previously applied. Firm traction on the uterus and stay suture maintains tissue planes and facilitates the separation of the vesical artery and permits the proper application of the clamps for the simple reason that it can be seen.

Figure 15. The uterine artery is then divided between clamps and both ends ligated. In the interest of better exposure and greater freedom of movement in a field unencumbered by clamps, it is always a good idea to tie the lateral end and remove first the clamp closest to the assistant.

Figure 16. This shows a very important step. Traction is again maintained on the uterus and stay sutures. The surgeon notes the course of the ureter lying on the medial flap of peritoneum. The anatomic position of the internal iliac artery is identified. The surgeon's index finger can then be gently inserted into a completely bloodless area along the side of the rectum. Care should be taken to insert the finger gently, staying on the medial side toward the rectum to avoid damaging the internal iliac vein which lies just below and deep to the artery.

In this manner the posterior attachments of the uterosacral ligament to the posterior wall of the bony pelvis are isolated. The "web" containing the uterine vein and vaginal wall vessels as well as all the paravaginal lymphatic channels are thus developed and identified as the septum between the paravesical and pararectal spaces.

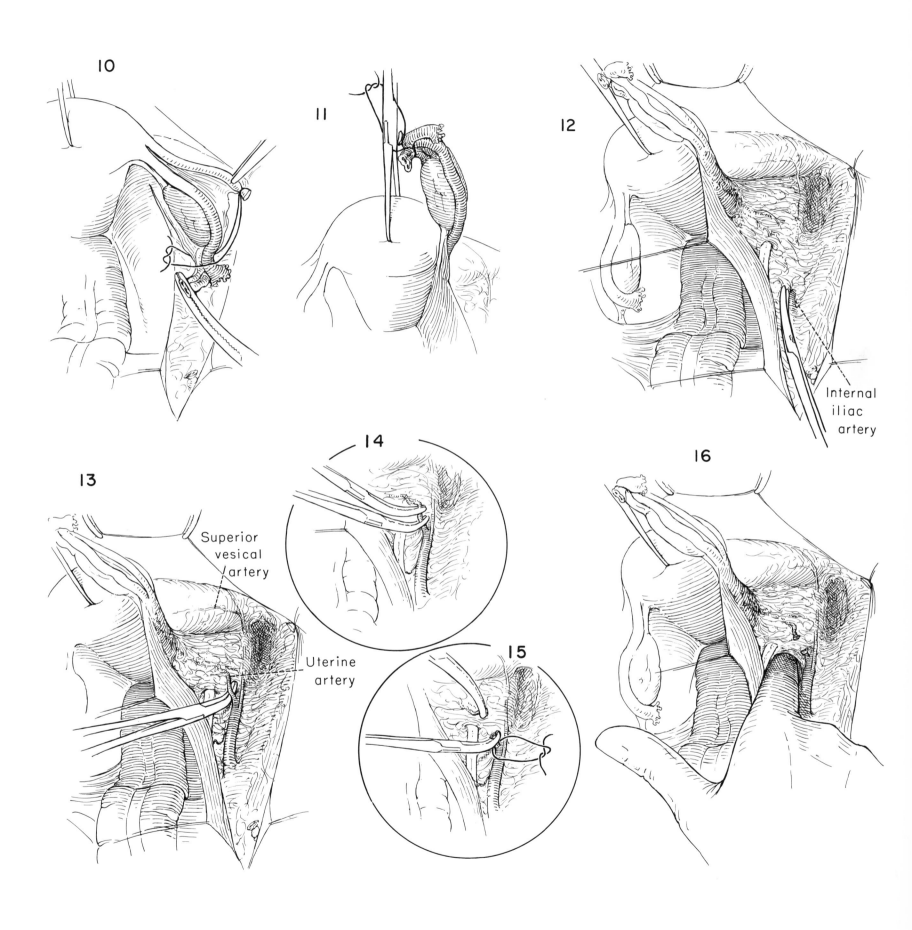

Figure 17. This important part of the dissection concentrates on the paracervical and paravaginal tissues. The ureter as well as the blood supply to bladder and vagina lie in this area. A meticulous dissection is needed to prevent blood loss and to keep the field dry so that all structures can be identified and damage to them avoided.

The uterus and adnexa are drawn to the side opposite the area to be dissected. The ureter is located medially and the hypogastric artery is seen in its upper portion. It is essential that the superior vesical artery be spared to preserve the blood supply to the bladder.

The hypogastric and superior vesical arteries are in close proximity and follow the same course. The surgeon picks up the vessels and holds them on tension as he dissects the tissue from beneath them as they pass onto the bladder wall.

Figure 18. The dissection now turns to the other side as the assistant draws the uterus to the right to expose the operative field. Steps 6 through 17 are repeated on the patient's left side. The surgeon may find the exposure better and the dissection easier if he will take his position on the right side of the patient.

Figure 19. One of the most dangerous parts of the dissection arises when the surgeon traces the ureter down into the bladder and dissects it free from the tissue containing the lymphatics lying within it. This can be accomplished much more easily and with much less danger if the uterus can be brought up out of the depths of the operative field. The next four illustrations are of great importance.

The uterus is drawn upward in the midline. The peritoneum adjoining the two operative fields is to be incised on either side of the rectosigmoid in the manner indicated by the dotted line. Essentially all of the cul de sac is removed.

Figure 20. The assistant continues traction on the uterus in an upward direction, inclining it slightly to the left. A small vein retractor is placed medial to the ureter. The ureter is teased away from the overlying peritoneum, usually at a level just below the small artery which enters it from the internal iliac. The surgeon picks up the sigmoid, pulling it to the left.

Figure 21. With the uterus pulled to the left, the ureter retracted and the posterior peritoneum on tension it is now possible to incise as planned and to leave the cul de sac on the specimen side of the subsequent dissection.

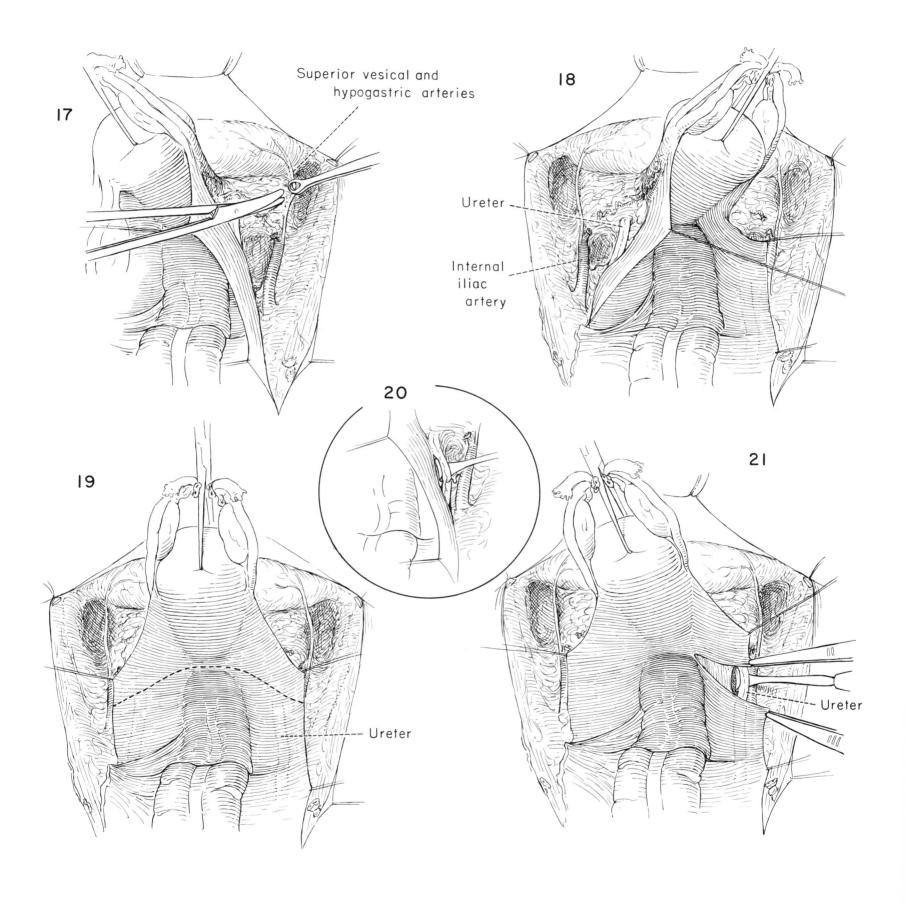

17

Superior vesical and
hypogastric arteries

18

Ureter

Internal
iliac
artery

19

20

21

Ureter

Ureter

Figure 22. Clamps are placed on the peritoneum. These clamps and the uterus are drawn upward to expose the pararectal space with the ureter lying free within it. The dissections shown in Figures 19, 20 and 21 are now repeated on the opposite side of the patient.

Figure 23. The assistant applies upward traction toward the symphysis on the tenaculum on the fundus and the two Kelly clamps placed on the peritoneal edge. The surgeon draws the rectosigmoid upward and backward with the outstretched fingers of the left gloved hand as he dissects the rectum away from the posterior wall of the vagina.

Figure 24. The dissection continues downward along both sides of the rectum, separating the bowel from the deep uterosacral ligaments. Any bleeding vessels encountered are immediately individually clamped and secured with stitch ligatures. The operative field is kept entirely free of clamps. This is extremely important because the surgeon must have an unrestricted view of the area to be dissected. Furthermore, if bleeding is encountered he must be able to identify the source so that he may move freely and easily and not have to fight his way through a group of clamps. When one reaches the level at which the vagina is later to be transected, the posterior dissection is finished.

Figure 25. The surgeon now turns his attention toward the bladder and begins to dissect it free from the lower end of the cervix and the anterior vaginal wall. The importance of freeing the posterior attachments of the uterus now becomes apparent. Instead of having to do deep in the pelvis the meticulous dissection required to free up the ureter and bladder, the uterus now moves up into the wound where the dissection can be carried out much more easily and with less risk.

To facilitate this dissection the assistant draws the uterus upward and backward toward the patient's head while the surgeon picks up the bladder wall with long smooth forceps and begins to separate the bladder from the anterior vaginal wall in the obvious plane of cleavage.

22

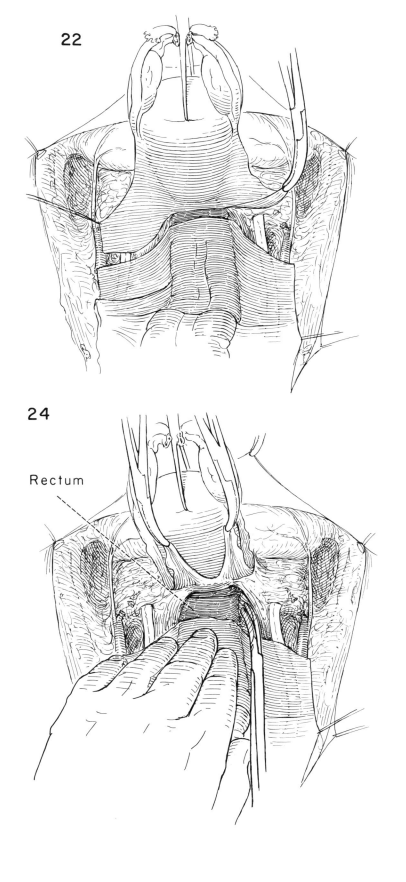

23

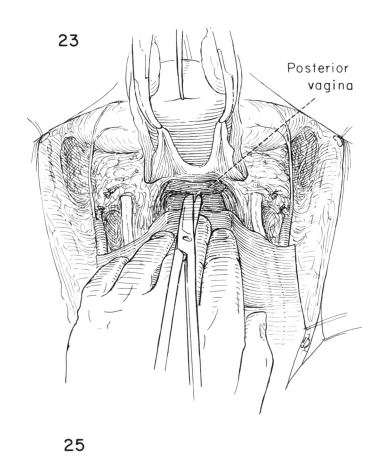

Posterior vagina

24

Rectum

25

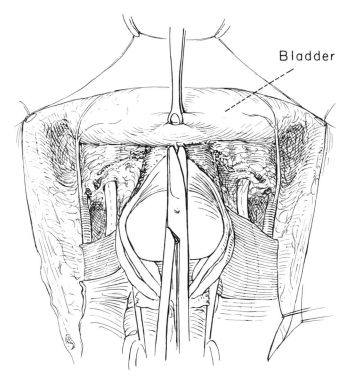

Bladder

Figure 26. This portion of the dissection must be carried out with the greatest of care. Primarily the operation is designed to deal with cervical cancer. In its growth pattern cancer of the cervix often spreads in an antero-posterior direction as well as laterally. The surgeon must assure himself that in separating the bladder from the anterior wall of the vagina he is not dissecting through an area of potential extension of cervical cancer. The dissection must be made close to the bladder wall to avoid the possibility of leaving disease upon it. There is always the danger that in so doing the surgeon may enter the bladder or seriously jeopardize its blood supply.

To minimize the danger inherent in both problems traction is essential. The assistant keeps the uterus on tension by pulling it backward and upward. The bladder is picked up with nontraumatizing tissue forceps and in this fasion the cleavage plane between the bladder and vagina becomes more definite. With long, blunt-end scissors the separation is made and the dissection carried well down on the anterior vaginal wall.

Figure 27. With the bladder well advanced off the anterior vaginal wall the surgeon now turns his attention toward the ureter. The basic aim is to dissect the ureter free from (a) the tissues that lie above the ureter and form the superior surface of a tunnel (within this tissue lies the uterine artery), and (b) the tissue lying beneath the ureter which contains lymphatic channels and a bundle of small veins, including the uterine vein. The mobilization of the uterus previously accomplished posteriorly makes this dissection easier because it is more accessible.

The assistant draws the uterus to the opposite side while the nurse or second assistant applies gentle traction to a small vein retractor and draws the ureter laterally, keeping it on light traction. The surgeon then begins to dissect the ureter away from the tissues which surround it.

Figure 28. To expose the course of the ureter as it passes beneath the tunnel of tissue which contains the uterine vessels and its terminal branches, the assistant now pulls the uterus upward and backward while the nurse or second assistant keeps the ureter under light traction.

With all tissues on tension the surgeon picks up the bladder wall and gently inserts a small Moynihan clamp within the tunnel and above the presenting surface of the ureter.

Figure 29. This tissue is then clamped and a second clamp is applied; the tissue between them is divided.

This illustration shows the uterus, ureter and bladder on tension. The tissue held within the clamps is then secured with a stitch ligature.

Figure 30. With all structures held on tension and the clamps removed it is now possible for the surgeon to identify the ureter as it emerges from below the tunnel and runs along the side of the vaginal wall before it enters the bladder base.

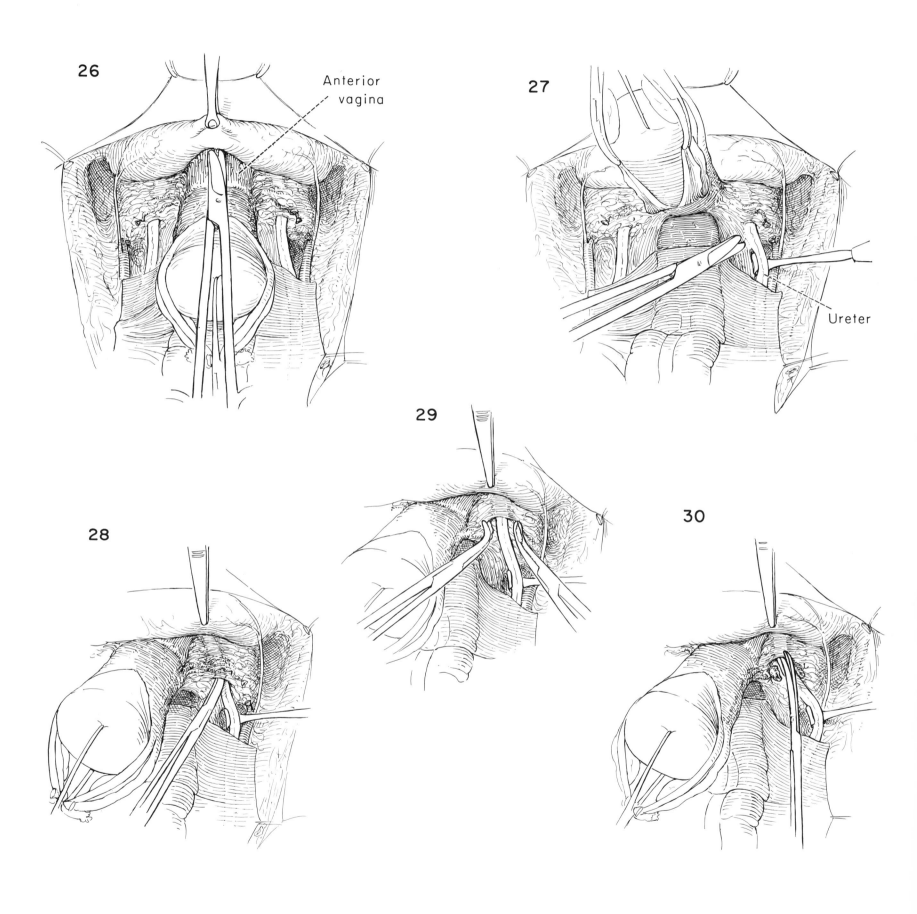

26

Anterior
vagina

27

Ureter

29

28

30

Figure 31. The tissue lying over and above the superior surface of the ureter has been divided. The ureter must be lifted out and away from the posterior wall of the tunnel. This must be done with great care to avoid trauma to the ureter itself and to prevent excessive blood loss, for this can be a very bloody area because of the extensive venous blood supply.

The small retractor is moved downward toward the bladder and is held on gentle tension. The surgeon elevates the bladder at the point at which the ureter enters it and gently dissects the tissues from its underside.

Figure 32. When the ureter is free of all attachments down to the point at which it enters the bladder, the surgeon directs his attention to the most lateral portion of the bladder itself. This aspect is now dissected free of the underlying tissue which contains the paravaginal lymphatic channels. Gentle elevation of the bladder demonstrates the correct plane.

Figure 33. The same steps are repeated on the opposite side. Again to make the dissection easier the surgeon would do well to change his position at the operating table and move to the side opposite the area he wishes to work on.

In this view the uterus and ureters are on traction while the surgeon holds back the bladder with forceps and begins to insert the clamp into the tunnel.

Figure 34. The uterus and its supports are now drawn sharply toward the symphysis and, with all structures on tension, the surgeon completes the posterior dissection of the specimen away from the side wall of the rectum.

Figure 35. This dissection is completed on both sides. The lateral extensions of the deep uterosacral ligament now are prominently displayed.

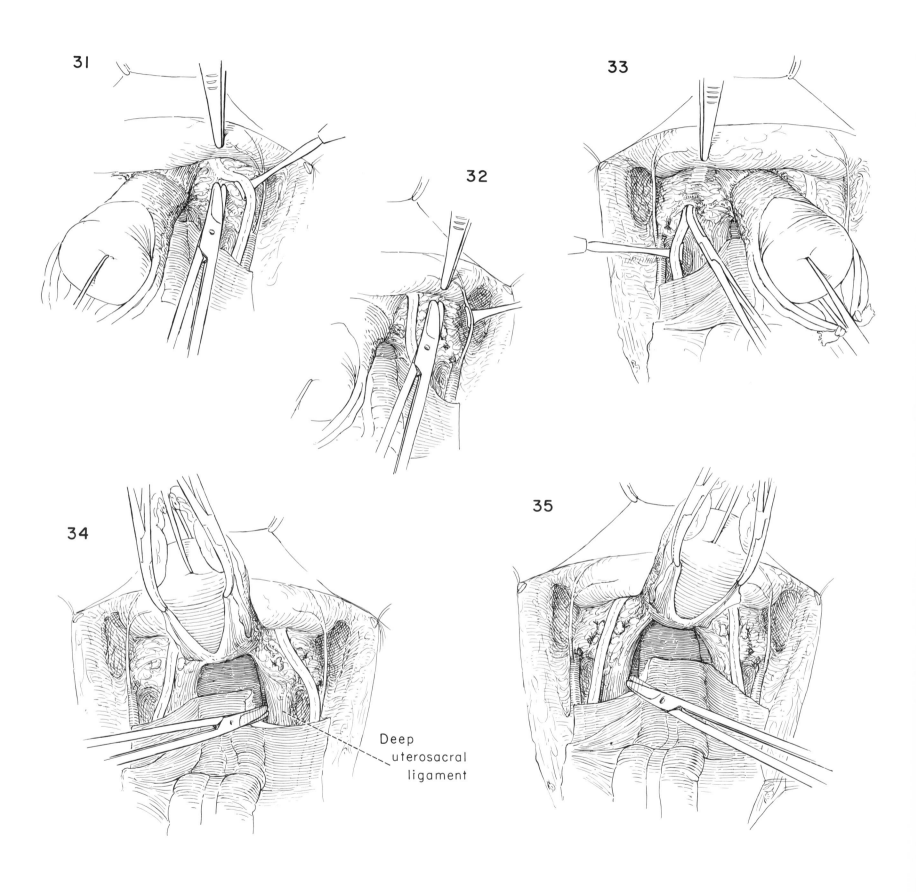

Deep
uterosacral
ligament

Figure 36. All the dissection up to this point has had as its main purpose the exposure of the lymphatic tissue lateral to the vagina and bladder as well as around the ureter and rectum. This block of tissue must be removed for it is within this area that cancer of the cervix extends after it has left its primary point of origin within the cervix. The addition of a pelvic lymphadenectomy to the operation cannot improve the five-year survival figures unless the dissection of the paravaginal and paracervical tissue is adequate.

To facilitate the exposure of this important area the assistant draws the uterus to the opposite side and holds it on traction. With the ureter and superior vesical and hypogastric artery held out of the way the surgeon applies a large Moynihan clamp close to the posterior pelvic wall at the base of the deep uterosacral ligament. Care must be taken in applying the clamp not to damage the internal iliac vein, which is in close proximity. The tissue is cut and the clamp replaced with a stitch ligature.

Figure 37. This illustration demonstrates the so-called web which is made up of the paravaginal and paracervical lymphatic channels as well as the terminal branches of the hypogastric artery which supply the vagina.

When the tissues have been freed from the side wall of the rectum a free cleavage plane is created. The landmarks are the ureter lying medially and the hypogastric artery laterally. This cleavage plane is entirely bloodless. With the uterus held on traction to the opposite side the surgeon can safely insert the index finger into this bloodless space lying posterior to the web. With the finger so placed the surgeon now grasps the web between index and middle fingers. The web contains much of the blood supply to the lower pelvis, except for the superior vesical and hypogastric arteries, and the lateral terminal branches of the hypogastric such as the gluteal, the pudendal and the obturator arteries.

Figure 38. The uterus is drawn firmly to the opposite side and the vein retractor beneath the ureter lifts it up out of the way as the surgeon applies two large Moynihan clamps as far out laterally as he can without compromising the hypogastric artery and veins.

Figure 39. The tissue between the clamps is then divided and secured with a stitch ligature. It is always wise to suture the tissue in the medial clamp first. The major source of the blood supply takes origin from the lateral side. With the medial clamp removed after suturing, the surgeon has easy access to the remaining clamp. All tissues are under direct vision.

Figure 40. The entire tissue within the web covers too wide an area to be included in one clamp; several bites will be required. In this illustration the uterus is again pulled to the opposite side and the ureter lifted free of the web lying beneath and lateral to it. Another clamp is then placed on the remaining pedicle. Again the tissues will be divided and secured with the web lying beneath and lateral to it. Another clamp is then placed on the remaining pedicle. Again the tissues will be divided and secured with stitch ligatures, beginning on the medial side. The clamps are then removed.

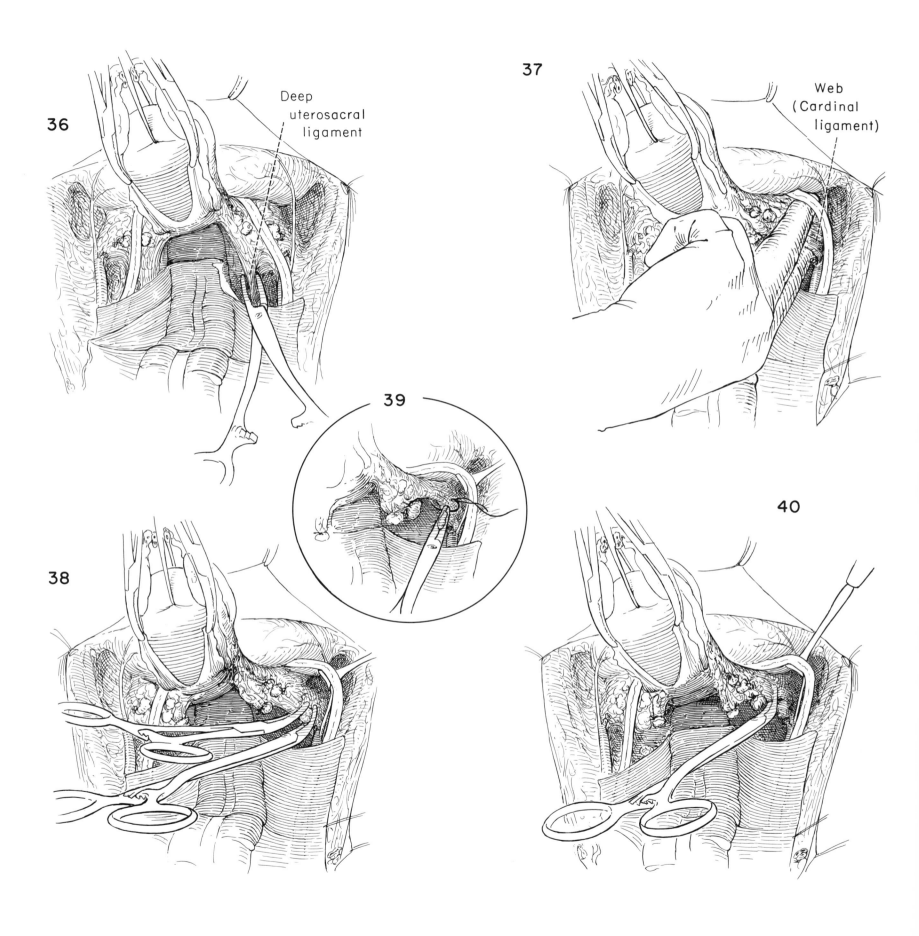

36

Deep uterosacral ligament

37

Web (Cardinal ligament)

39

38

40

Figure 41. The last of the clamps is being applied to the tissue in the most distal portions of the web, which is then divided and stitch ligatures applied. The clamps are now removed and the uterus and adjacent lymphatic-bearing material is entirely free of both the side and posterior walls of the pelvis.

Figure 42. With the lateral dissection completed, the focus of attention is on the vaginal wall and the relation of the base of the bladder to it. Fully half of the vagina should be removed. This is more easily accomplished on the anterior and posterior wall than it is laterally.

The assistant draws the uterus upward and backward toward the patient's head and holds the ureter upward and laterally out of the operative field. The surgeon retracts the bladder wall away from the anterior vaginal wall with the handle of the forceps as he completes the anterior dissection.

Figure 43. The uterus is held on firm traction as the surgeon applies a Wertheim clamp across the entire proximal vagina to prevent spillage when the canal is transected. The surgeon should carefully check the position of the ureter, bladder and rectum before placing the clamp.

The surgeon then holds the bladder wall away from the vaginal wall as he applies Heaney clamps on both sides distal to the Wertheim clamp. The vaginal canal is entered by dividing the tissue in the clamp at both angles. It is then secured with a stitch ligature, the ends of which are left long.

Figure 44. This illustration shows the anatomic relation of the different structures in the pelvis after the specimen has been removed. The open vagina can be seen with the two long sutures at the angles. The ureters can be traced into the base of the bladder. The vagina is free of the bladder wall anteriorly and the rectum posteriorly. The side walls of the pelvis are free of all tissue intervening between them and the remaining vaginal wall.

Figure 45. The vaginal canal used to be left open and drains inserted through it directed into the extensive "dead space" deep in the pelvis. The vagina is still left open for drainage, but without wicks. An over-and-over, locking, hemostatic suture secures the cut end.

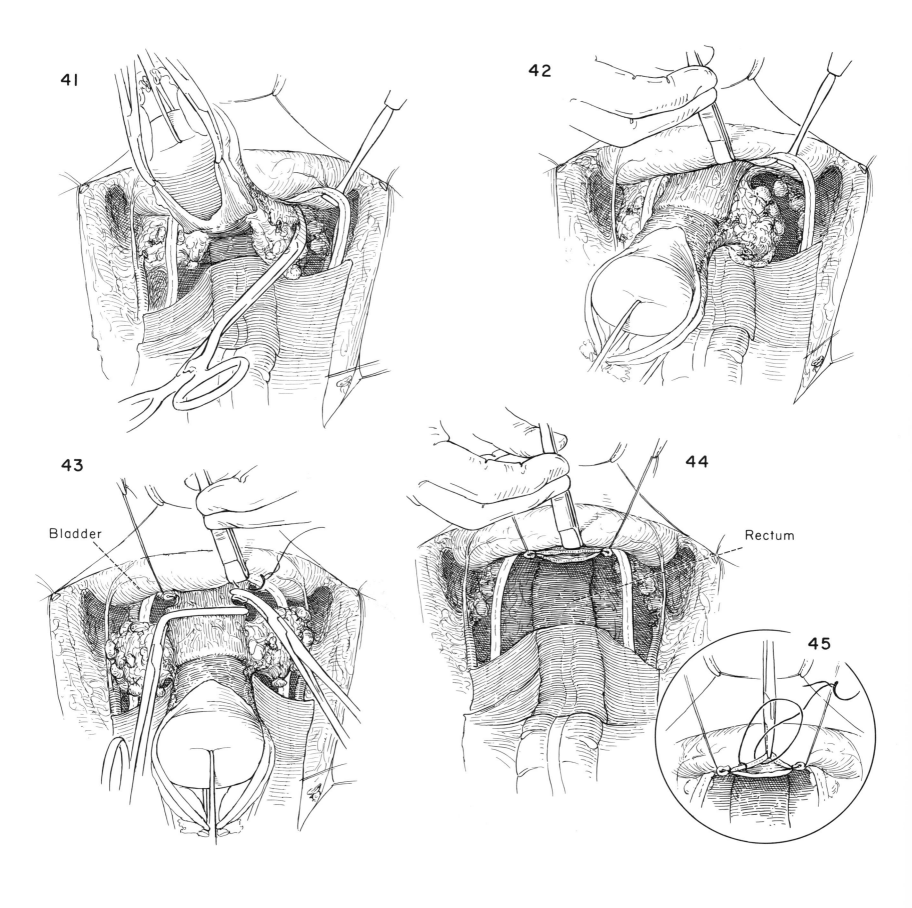

41

42

43

Bladder

44

Rectum

45

With the uterus removed and the pelvic dissection completed, attention now turns to excision of the regional nodes to which cancer of the cervix may reasonably be expected to extend. The first line of defense is the regional nodal chain that lies along the side of and deep to the external iliac artery and vein and between the artery and the vein. A common place to find metastatic nodes is in the so-called obturator space which has the external iliac vein as its upper boundary, the obturator nerve on its lower border and the side wall of the pelvis as its most lateral limit.

If metastasis to nodes is to occur this will be the first place to find them. The second line of defense is the nodal chain that lies in the sacral area and along the side of the common iliac artery. Rarely is it possible to cure a patient who has metastases to the nodes along the side of the aorta. Our dissection, then, is not carried above the bifurcation of the aorta. It is a misconception to measure the character of the Wertheim operation on the extent of the lymphadenectomy alone. The pelvic adenectomy should be meticulous and complete, but the important factor in the Wertheim operation is the extent of resection of the paravaginal and paracervical tissue, not the node dissection. A beautifully performed node dissection cannot produce a cure if the local excision is inadequate.

Figure 46. The dissection begins lateral to the external iliac vessels along the medial border of the psoas muscle. Exposure is provided by a Deaver type retractor placed laterally on the abdominal wall. By use of blunt-end scissors the tissue bundle is stripped away from the medial surface of the psoas.

Figure 47. The dissection continues deep along the medial side of the psoas muscle. Deaver retractors aid in the exposure. There are no arterial vessels encountered in this dissection below the bifurcation of the common iliac artery.

Figure 48. The surgeon now places a small retractor over the external iliac vessels and draws them medially. This permits exposure of the obturator space which lies below the level of the external iliac vein. All tissue is thus freed from the clean pelvic wall down to the obturator nerve.

Figure 49. The mass of connective tissue containing the lymph channels and nodes is then drawn upward and to the right as the surgeon separates it from the superior surface of the common iliac artery and the side wall of the vena cava lying beneath it.

Figure 50. As the surgeon holds up the mass of connective tissue which has been cleaned from the underlying vessels, the internal iliac artery with the stump of the uterine vessel can easily be seen. The bifurcation of the common iliac artery is apparent. At this point there is usually a small nutrient artery which runs laterally to supply the muscle. In the interest of a dry operative field this small vessel should be identified and secured with a fine tie.

Figure 51. To facilitate the removal of the nodes in the common iliac area a Deaver retractor is placed in the upper portion of the wound. A clamp is placed across the tissue at the level of the bifurcation of the common iliac artery and the tissue bundle transected.

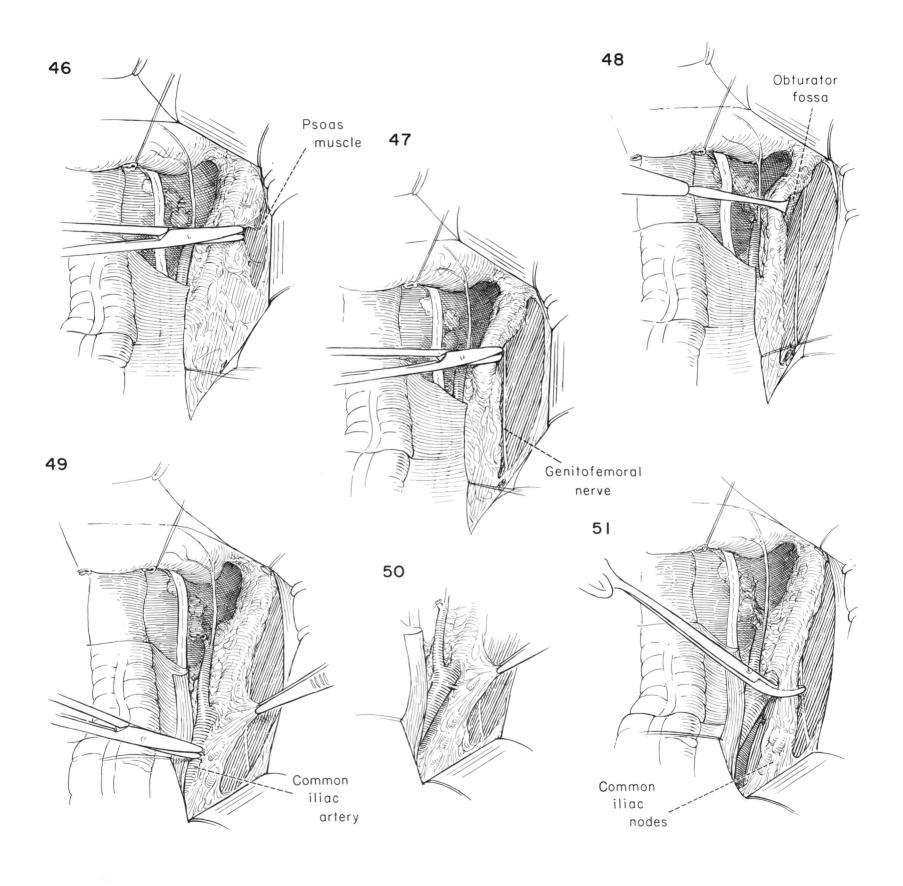

46

Psoas muscle

47

48 Obturator fossa

Genitofemoral nerve

49

50

51

Common iliac artery

Common iliac nodes

Figure 52. The clamp on the upper end is then elevated to be certain that there is no attachment of tissue to the underlying vessels. With the ureter identified and out of the way, another Moynihan clamp is placed high up on the nodal chain. The tissues are then divided and the upper portion of the nodal chain is removed and labeled "common iliac nodes" for later identification.

Figure 53. The tissues within the uppermost clamp are secured with a ligature. This may help to prevent lymphocele.

Figure 54. The dissection of the node-bearing tissue continues. The tissue bundle is incised along the external iliac artery.

Figure 55. Again with the tissue held on tension toward the midline the surgeon gently dissects the areolar tissue away from around the surface of the artery. To make this easier a vein retractor is placed beneath the artery. The cleavage plane is more readily identified when this is retracted and held upward.

Figure 56. The dissection then continues by incising the tissue bundle along the external iliac vein. If the tissues being dissected are held on light traction the excision can be done expeditiously and without danger.

Figure 57. The surrounding fat and lymphatics are easily freed laterally and medially from the vein and allowed to drop into the obturator fossa. The lower limit of dissection is customarily the level at which the deep circumflex iliac vein crosses the major vessels.

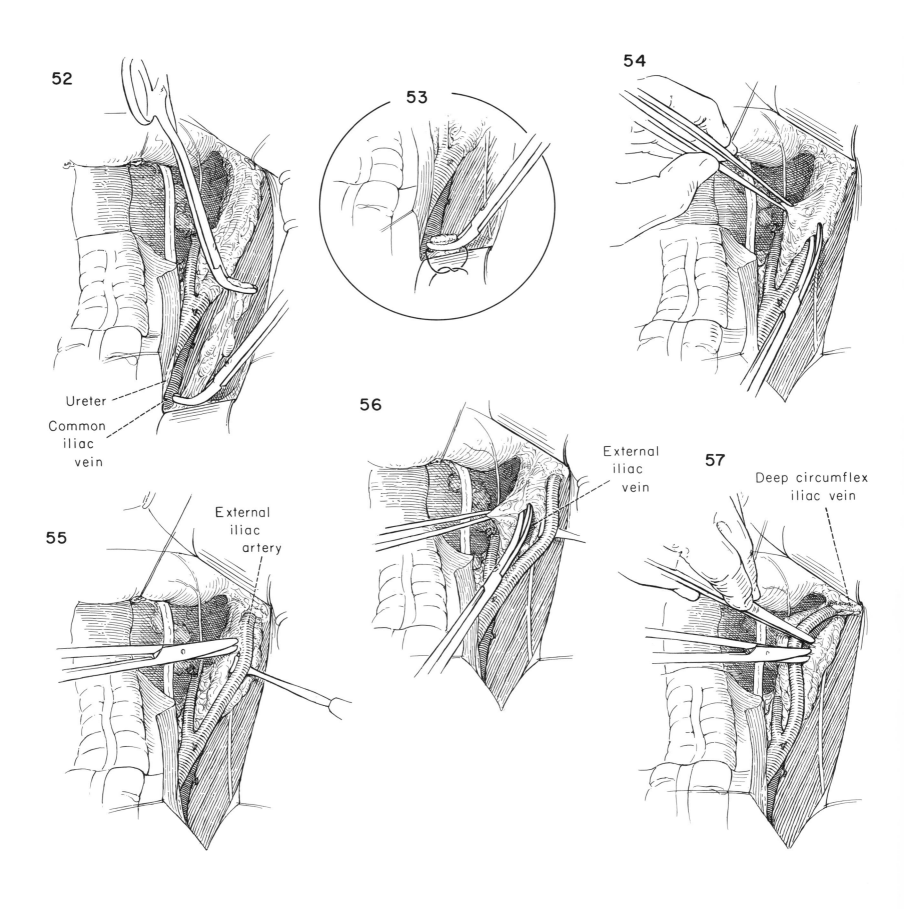

52

53

54

Ureter

Common
iliac
vein

56

External
iliac
vein

External
iliac
artery

55

57

Deep circumflex
iliac vein

Figure 58. One of the most common areas to which cancer of the uterus metastasizes is the group of nodes which lie in the obturator space. The anatomic boundaries are the inferior surface of the external iliac veins, the side wall of the pelvis and, on its deeper portion, the obturator nerve. The external iliac artery and vein are elevated in the retractor and all lymphatic-bearing fat freed from the vessels and the psoas muscle and pushed and pulled medially until they can be delivered into the field of dissection.

Figure 59. The surgeon pulls the block of connective tissue while the assistant retracts the external iliac artery and vein. The dissection is then carried along the inferior surface of the vein, freeing it from all attachments down to Poupart's ligament. Cloquet's node lies medial to the external iliac vein at the most distal point of the dissection.

Figure 60. The surgeon now cleans the tissue from its attachment to the lateral side of the internal iliac artery. This must be done carefully under direct vision for the vein is in close proximity. Frequently a small vessel is encountered on the lateral aspect close to the point of bifurcation of the vessels. This should be clamped and secured.

Figure 61. With the area of the bifurcation cleared and the tissue mobilized, the assistant draws the block of tissue medially as the surgeon continues to separate it from the obturator fossa.

Figure 62. Any small venous branches to the external iliac vein should be identified, clamped, cut and tied as the dissection progresses.

Figure 63. The node-bearing tissue has a tendency to surround the obturator nerve and to hide it from view. It must be identified and the tissue cleaned from it medially. Better exposure can be obtained if the assistant will retract the artery and vein with a vein retractor while the surgeon pulls the contents of the obturator space medially. When freed from the nerve the tissue is removed; the obturator space has been cleared.

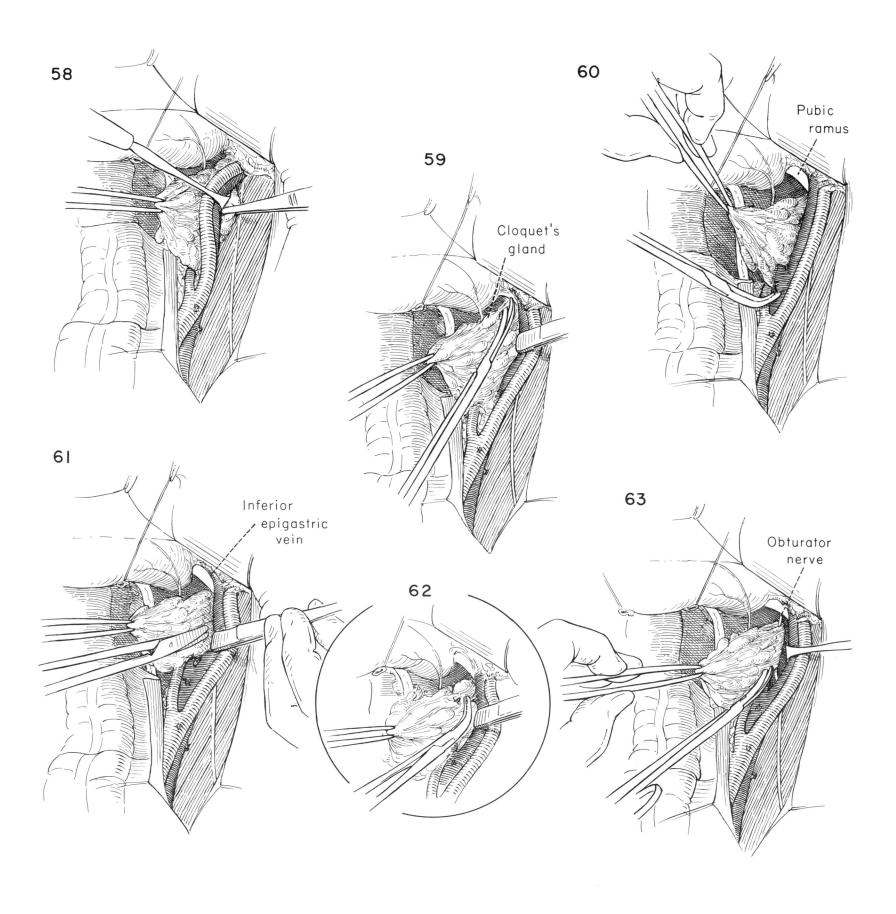

58

59
Cloquet's gland

60
Pubic ramus

61
Inferior epigastric vein

62

63
Obturator nerve

Figure 64. The entire dissection including bilateral pelvic lymphadenectomy has now been completed. This illustration depicts the final appearance of the pelvis.

The important factors to note are:
1. The ureters lying on the inferior surface of the upper edge of the incised peritoneum.
2. The lower portion of the ureter, free of all attachments as it enters the bladder.
3. The transected vagina still held up at the corners.
4. The sutured lateral stumps of the "web."
5. The anatomic position of the vessels following the pelvic lymphadenectomy.
6. The pararectal and obturator space completely free of tissue.

The final steps are concerned with peritonealization and drainage of the dead space that remains after the peritoneum has been sutured.

Figure 65. The surgeon begins the closure of the peritoneum at the lateral angle beneath the cecum. Great care should be taken at this point to so place the sutures that danger of angulating the ureter is avoided. The surgeon retracts and elevates the medial edge of the peritoneum to get a good look at the position of the ureter as he takes the first bite of what is to be a long running peritoneal suture.

Figure 66. The peritoneal closure is being completed. Separate closure of the lateral extensions will reduce the tension on this suture line.

INSET A. It is often considered desirable today to drain the subperitoneal space with suction catheters. When this is to be done, the surgeon must place the drainage tubing deep into the extensive dead space which has been created by the dissection before closing the peritoneum in the midline.

The sharp-pointed steel introducer with its tubing attached is grasped by the surgeon as he elevates the lower abdominal wall on the patient's right side. It passes beneath peritoneum, and through external oblique muscle and fascia, as well as the fat and overlying skin, to emerge at a point on the abdominal wall approximately 2 inches above Poupart's ligament. Great care must be taken to identify the position of the deep epigastric vessels when the surgeon chooses the site of puncture to avoid damaging them.

INSET B. This illustration shows the perforated drainage tube as it rests in position in relation to the other structures left in the pelvis. It should extend deep into the lower reaches of the pelvic cavity medial to the external iliac vessels and lateral to the bladder wall and the obliterated hypogastric and superior vesical arteries. Inasmuch as it is somewhat rigid it should not lie in contact with the vessels.

The catheters are then fixed to the skin with individual silk sutures to prevent them from being dislodged accidentally by traction on them. The peritoneum is closed in the usual fashion.

Note that in this case the vaginal canal itself has been closed to minimize air leak. This method of draining the pelvis is a marked improvement over rubber drains placed through an open vagina.

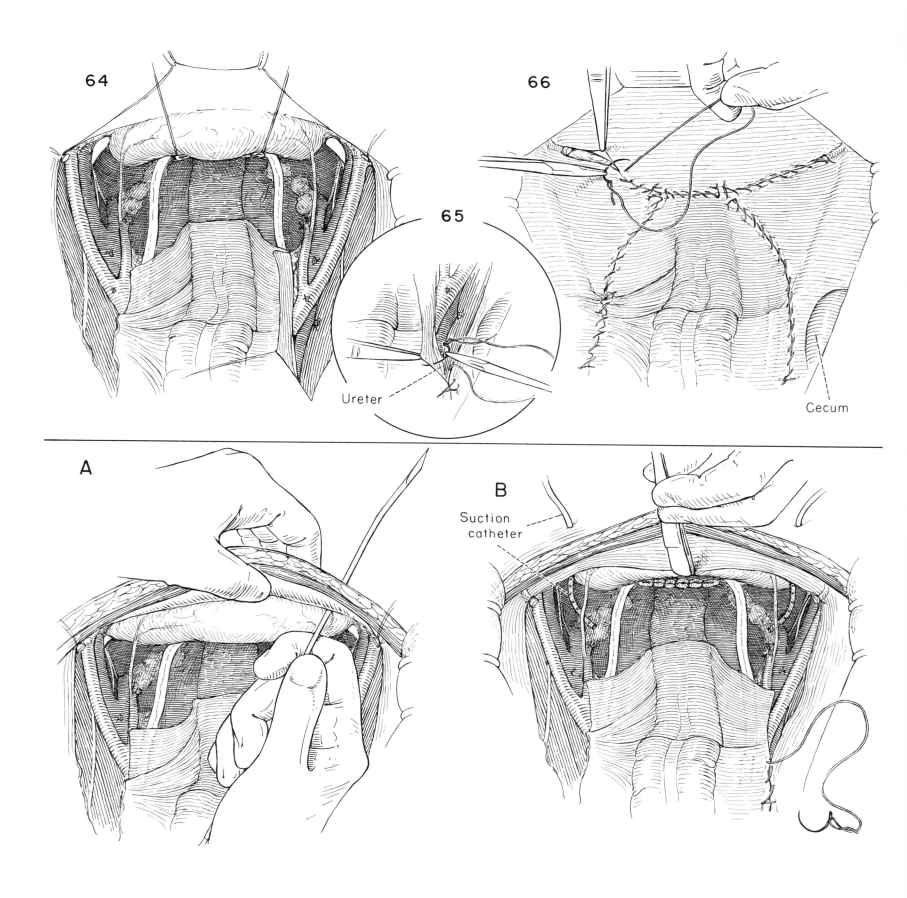

64

65

Ureter

66

Cecum

A

B

Suction
catheter

RADICAL VULVECTOMY WITH BILATERAL
SUPERFICIAL AND DEEP GROIN DISSECTION

This operation exemplifies perfectly the cardinal principles of radical surgery for malignant disease. It is unfortunate that the term radical suggests to many people that the surgeon is carrying out an operative procedure which exposes the patient to excessive risk. A better term might be total, rather than radical, for any operation designed to produce a cure for a malignant process must be extensive enough to encompass the primary tumor and the regional nodal chain to which the cancer can be reasonably expected to extend. The emphasis is on cure, not palliation. To do less than adequate surgery under the mistaken impression that it is conservative management is a tragic error.

The operation described here is performed primarily for malignant disease of the vulva. Since these patients are older and the primary lesion tends to arise on one side of the vulva only, there is a tendency to minimize the amount of surgery deemed to be necessary. Such a point of view completely ignores the life history of these tumors, which metastasize early in their course not only to the nodes on the affected side but to the opposite side as well. A bilateral groin dissection must be an integral part of the operation. Since all the vulvar tissue in a patient with carcinoma is defective, there is no place for local excision or hemivulvectomy. Total removal of the vulva is a basic requirement.

Adequate surgery calls for resection of the nodes in the inguinal, femoral and iliac areas, together with the intervening lymphatic channels, and a radical excision of the entire vulva.

Figure 1. The skin incision we employ for excision of the superficial inguinal and femoral nodes begins at the right anterior superior spine on the abdominal wall, curving down in the crease of the groin. It then crosses in the mons veneris and extends in similar fashion to the anterior superior spine on the left side.

There are other types of incision in common usage. So much undermining of the wound and excision of fat and lymph-bearing tissue is required in the dissection that the wounds collect serum and frequently break down in the healing process. This usually occurs over the femoral vessels. The granulating base required before grafts can be applied takes a considerable amount of time to develop, which increases the length of hospitalization. Low-grade sepsis creates lymphatic blockage and patients are prone to develop edematous legs.

These complications are less likely to occur with the curved incision. If necrosis of the wound edges occurs it usually does so near the midline rather than over vessels. If necessary grafts can be applied earlier on a firm base rather than delayed until a protecting layer of granulations develops over the vessels.

Figure 2. After completing the skin incision the surgeon grasps the upper skin flap and undermines the skin by beveling through the fat in a plane just above the superficial fascia, well up onto the abdominal wall. The assistant clamps individual bleeding vessels as they are encountered.

Figure 3. Attention now turns to the lower skin flap. The assistant elevates the flap as the surgeon dissects through the fat in the same plane used above. The dotted lines in Figure 2 indicate additional incisions at the place where vulvectomy will be done. These facilitate extensive undermining in the femoral area.

Figure 4. Similar dissection is done on the other side. At this point the specimen in both groins has been separated from the overlying skin but left in continuity with the vulva itself.

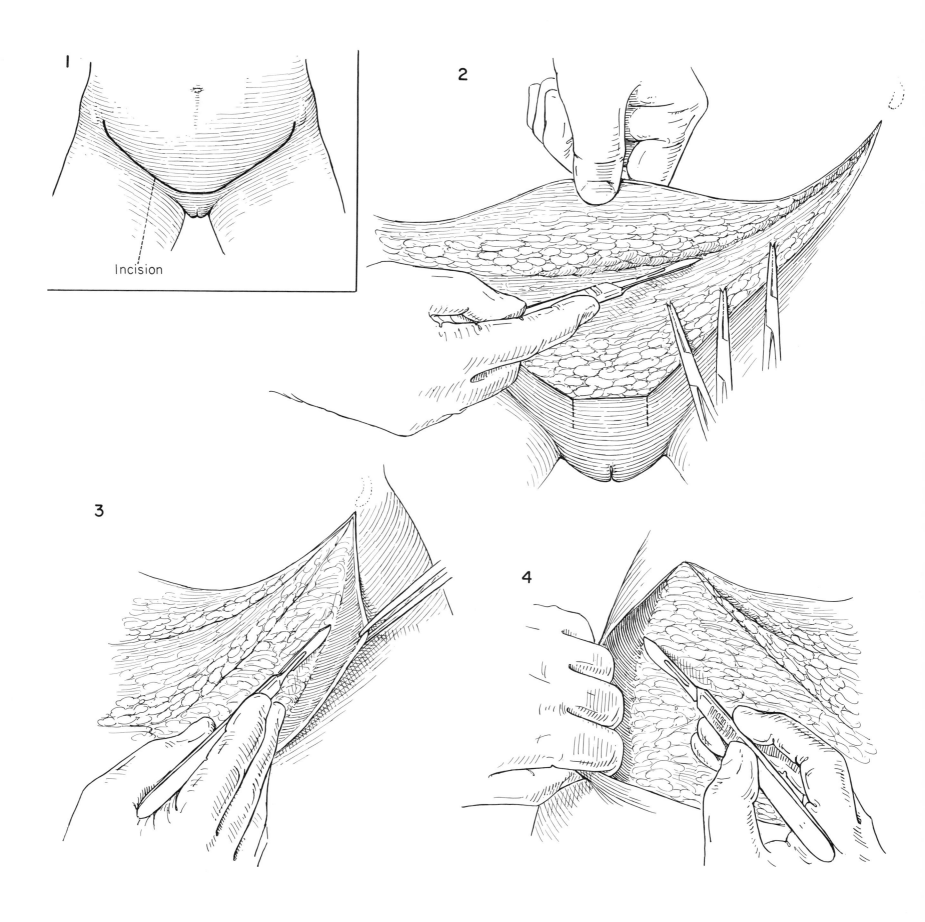

Incision

Figure 5. After completing the dissection in the superficial fatty layer, taking care to leave adequate blood supply to the skin flaps, the surgeon now covers the upper flap with a layer of moist gauze. The deep layer of fat is then dissected from the underlying fascia which covers the external oblique muscle. A knife blade with a rounded sharp end can be most useful in extensive dissections parallel to the surface.

Figure 6. It is important that the operative field be kept dry both during and after the operation. Individual vessels must be secured and tied as they are encountered. The dissection continues across the midline and on downward, separating the specimen from the aponeurosis of the external oblique and rectus muscles.

Figure 7. In this illustration the deeper fatty layer is shown completely dissected free from the fascial layers lying beneath it down as far as the inguinal ligament and rolled down over the lower margin of the incision. The individual vessels appearing through the fascial layer have been clamped and ligated. The clamps on the surface of the specimen will be dealt with in similar fashion.

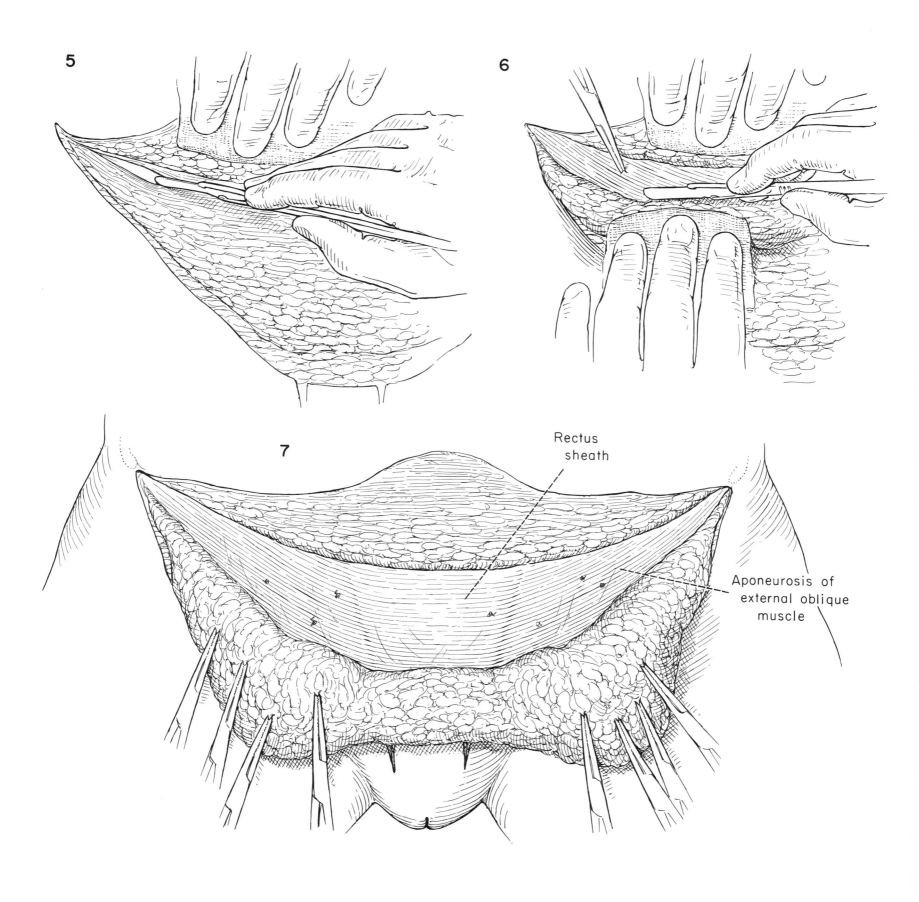

5

6

7

Rectus
sheath

Aponeurosis of
external oblique
muscle

Figure 8. With the deep fatty layer mobilized from the fascia beneath the upper skin flap down to the level of Poupart's ligament, the surgeon now turns his attention to the lower aspect.

The deep fatty layer must be dissected well out laterally on the upper thigh. To accomplish this the assistant elevates the skin with a retractor while the surgeon dissects the fat from the fascia lata.

Figure 9. The tissues are mobilized medially and down, beginning at the inguinal ligament and continuing down the thigh as far as the top of the adductor canal.

The assistant adds to the exposure by retracting the skin flap. The surgeon maintains traction on the mass of fat and nodes, drawing it to the midline as he dissects it free from the fascia lata beneath. The dissection continues medially until the femoral vessels are encountered. When this stage of the excision is completed, the full sweep of the fascia lata is exposed; only a narrow attachment of fatty and lymphatic tissue remains at the level of the inguinal ligament.

Figure 10. At this point the surgeon must establish his anatomic landmarks. He is particularly concerned with the location of the femoral vessels. In this illustration the surgeon can be seen identifying the vessels by palpation at a point just below Poupart's ligament at about its midportion.

Figure 11. With the full knowledge of the position of the femoral vessels the surgeon now continues to dissect the mass of fat and nodes from the inguinal ligament, beginning at the obvious point of attachment laterally.

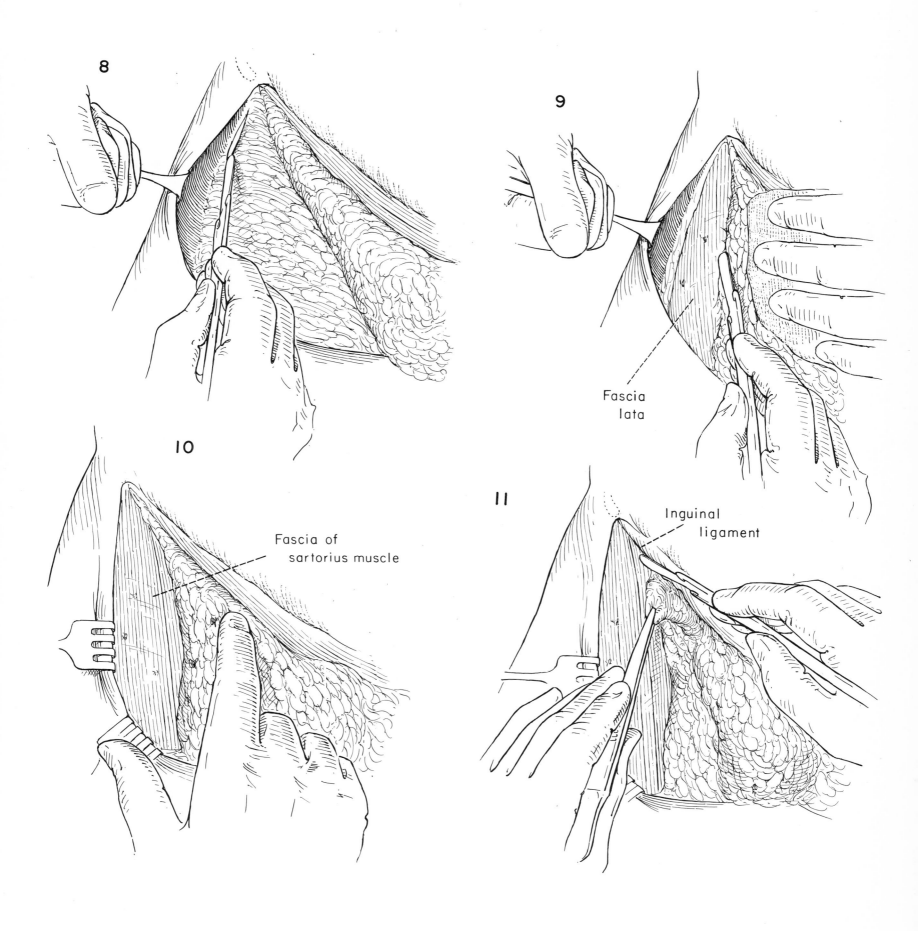

8

9

Fascia
lata

10

Fascia of
sartorius muscle

11

Inguinal
ligament

Figure 12. The overlying fat containing lymphatic channels and nodes has been completely mobilized from the underlying fascia and the position of the femoral vessels identified.

Rake retractors on the lateral edges of the wound provide adequate exposure. The surgeon then draws the mass of fat and nodes medially while he gently incises the femoral sheath on its lateral side. The artery immediately comes in view. The vein lies medial to it and is not visible at this point.

Figure 13. The sheath surrounding the vessels is opened through its full length from the inguinal ligament downward to the top of the adductor canal where the sartorius muscle laterally and the adductor muscle medially come together. With the thighs abducted, as they are for this operation, the course of the vessels will seem somewhat off the axis of the limb.

Figure 14. The surgeon draws the medial edge of the divided femoral sheath toward the midline while he dissects the sheath away from the artery.

As he does so a small arterial branch (the superficial external pudendal artery) comes into view on the medial side. Its position is constant and it is an important landmark in the dissection.

Figure 15. The femoral artery is exposed up to the inguinal ligament. Care must be taken to identify the superficial circumflex artery which appears on the lateral side of the artery just beneath the inguinal ligament. It will usually have to be cut and ligated.

Figure 16. A small, right-angled clamp is placed beneath the superficial external pudendal artery. Tension applied with forceps to the medial edge of the fascial sheath provides adequate exposure.

Figure 17. The vessel is doubly clamped and divided. The stump on the side of the femoral artery is then secured with a silk tie. The clamp on the medial side is removed after the vessel is tied.

Figure 18. The surgeon then draws the femoral artery laterally while the assistant holds the medial edge of the femoral sheath toward him. The surgeon continues the separation of the sheath from the artery on the medial side. As the dissection continues the femoral vein comes into view. The sheath is incised and the vein wall exposed.

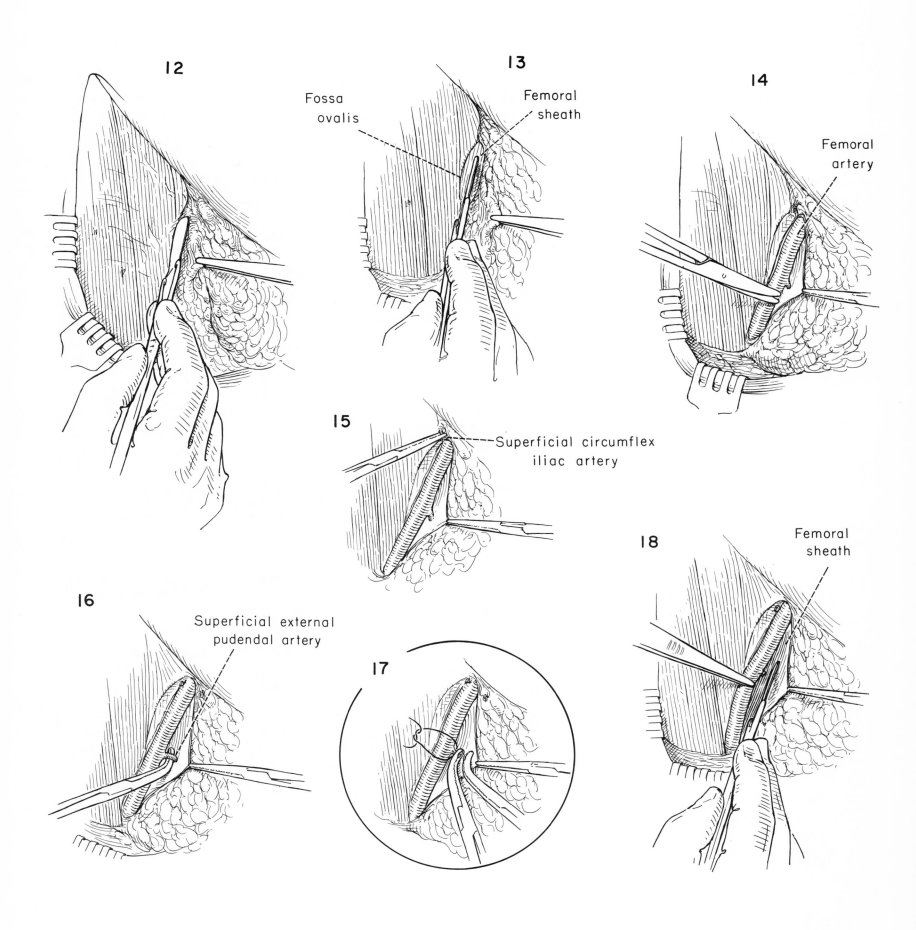

12

13

Fossa ovalis

Femoral sheath

14

Femoral artery

15

Superficial circumflex iliac artery

16

Superficial external pudendal artery

17

18

Femoral sheath

Figure 19. The point of entrance of the saphenous vein into the femoral may be obscure. The small artery noted above always crosses the femoral vein just below this juncture and can be used as a landmark. The surgeon has exposed the femoral vein and has located the probable site of entry of the saphenous into the femoral vein after ligating the superficial external pudendal artery. He now dissects the tissue from the femoral vein which lies deep and medial to the artery. To aid in exposure and to facilitate the dissection, traction is applied to the edges of the wound and to the incised edge of the femoral sheath. The vein is cleaned from the inguinal ligament to the adductor canal.

Figure 20. As the dissection progresses the saphenofemoral junction comes into view. Note the location in relation to the tie on the superficial external pudendal artery. There may be many communicating small veins which empty into the saphenous vein at this location. They must be visualized before the surgeon places a Moynihan clamp across the vessel at the point at which it joins the main femoral trunk.

Figure 21. The saphenous vein is then doubly clamped. At times it may be necessary to clamp and tie individual communicating vessels entering the saphenous.

Figure 22. The vein wall between the two clamps is then divided and secured with a stitch ligature of silk. In placing this suture the surgeon should avoid elevating the clamp to avoid creating a tent-like effect on the femoral vein. If this is done, too much of the side wall of the vein is included in the suture.

Figure 23. The initial stich ligature has been tied. To eliminate the possibility that increase in the venous pressure might dislodge this suture a second ligature is placed in and around the stump of the saphenous vein.

Figure 24. With the saphenofemoral junction divided the surgeon now has a better chance to dissect tissue away from the surface of the vein on the medial side. This is done throughout the length of the exposed femoral vein.

Figure 25. The surgeon then retracts the femoral vein medially and incises the free flap of the femoral sheath that has been created by the dissection along the artery and vein. This will go with the mass of fat and nodes as part of the en bloc dissection. Only by carrying out this dissection with the sheath can one be sure of removing all femoral nodes and lymphatics.

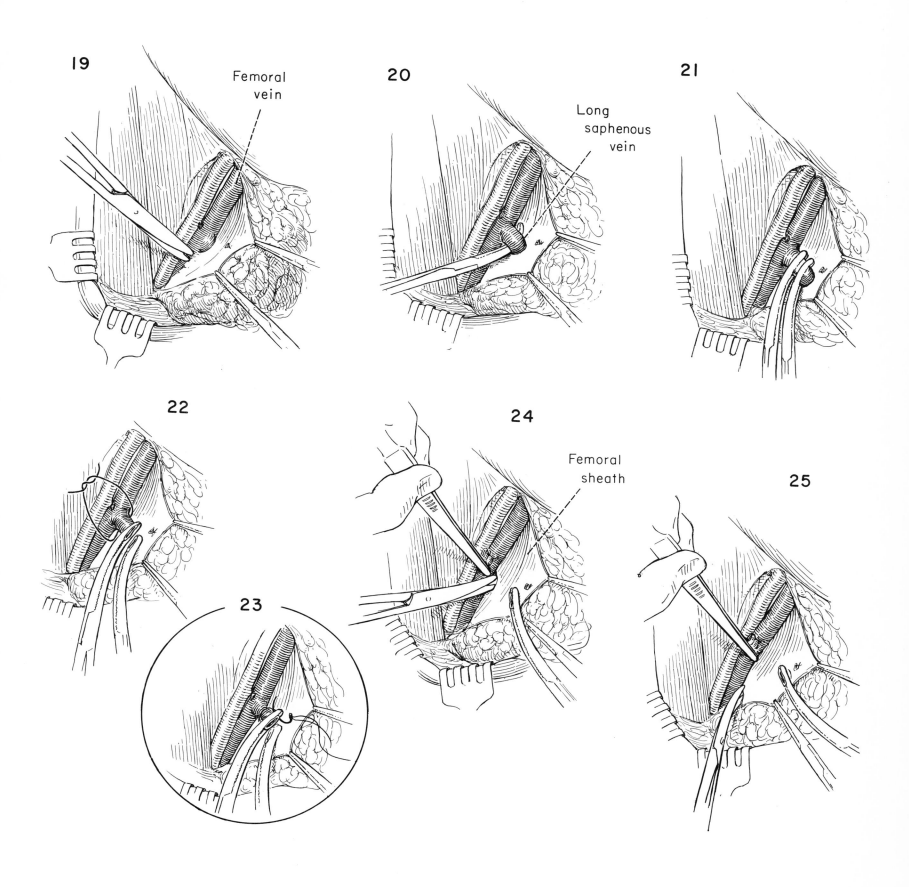

19 Femoral vein

20 Long saphenous vein

21

22

23

24 Femoral sheath

25

Figure 26. Dissection now continues as the surgeon cleans off the tissue from the underlying pectineus fascia.

Figure 27. The mass of connective tissue, lymphatic channels and regional nodes is now entirely free of the vessels except at its two ends. The surgeon first divides the deep tissue on the medial border at the lower pole of the dissection. After division the tissues are secured with a ligature since they contain the main lymphatic channels draining the lower leg.

Figure 28. As the tissue is freed the saphenous vein comes into view at a more superficial level. It is secured with Kelly clamps and divided.

Figure 29. The clamp on the distal portion of the saphenous vein is then tied. This stump is also secured with a stitch ligature as an additional safety factor.

Figure 30. Retraction exposes the lower and medial borders of the wound as the surgeon draws the mass of tissue upward and dissects it free from the fascia and muscles of the medial and upper thigh.

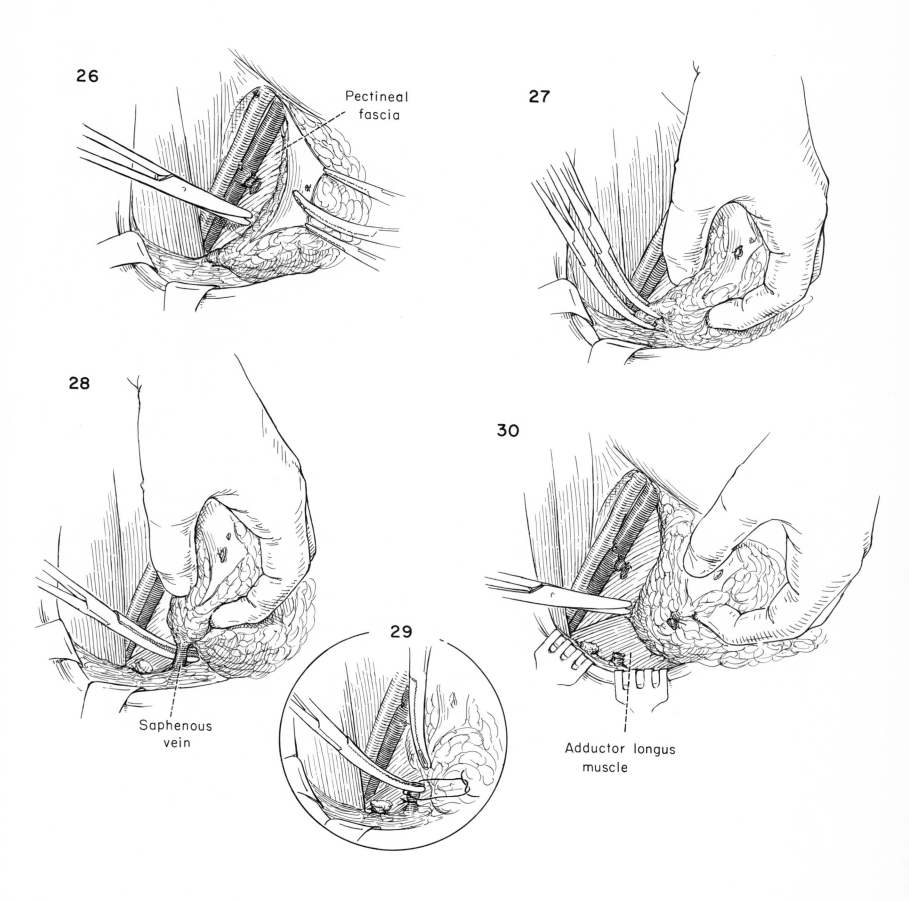

26

Pectineal
fascia

27

28

29

Saphenous
vein

30

Adductor longus
muscle

Figure 31. We have now reached an important area in the dissection. If tumor is going to extend from the superficial inguinal and femoral regional nodes to the deeper channels it will do so at this point.

Just within the femoral canal along the medial side of the femoral vein is the structure designated as Cloquet's node. It can be exposed and brought into the superficial inguinal dissection if the surgeon will exert downward and medial traction on the mass of tissue he has dissected. By gentle dissection along the medial side of the femoral vein Cloquet's node can be included in the mass of tissue that will be excised.

Figure 32. With the vein dissected free the assistant then elevates the inguinal ligament. The surgeon protects the femoral vein with his index finger as he applies a Kelly clamp across the superior attachment of the tissue block just underneath the ligament. This is the only point of transection of the lymphatics within the specimen. It can be obviated only by cutting the inguinal ligament, a step we do not consider desirable or necessary.

Figure 33. Because the tissue is under tension and will retract inside the pelvis when it is released, a ligature secures the tissue held by the clamp. This is left long for subsequent identification.

Figure 34. The surgeon then dissects the mass free from the underlying surface of the inguinal ligament and mobilizes it toward the midline and the spine of the pubis. As he does so the round ligament is exposed.

Figure 35. This illustration shows the superficial inguinal and femoral dissection completed on both sides. The vessels are exposed. The fascia overlying the muscles of the thigh is clean of all tissue.

Above the inguinal ligament the aponeurosis of the external oblique and rectus muscles is shown completely free of all fatty and subcutaneous tissue. The round ligaments emerge from the inguinal canals and are still intact.

The specimen to be removed is shown still attached to the vulva in the midline. When the radical vulvectomy is completed the specimen will include the regional nodes on both sides and the intervening communicating lymphatic channels en bloc with the primary tumor in the vulva.

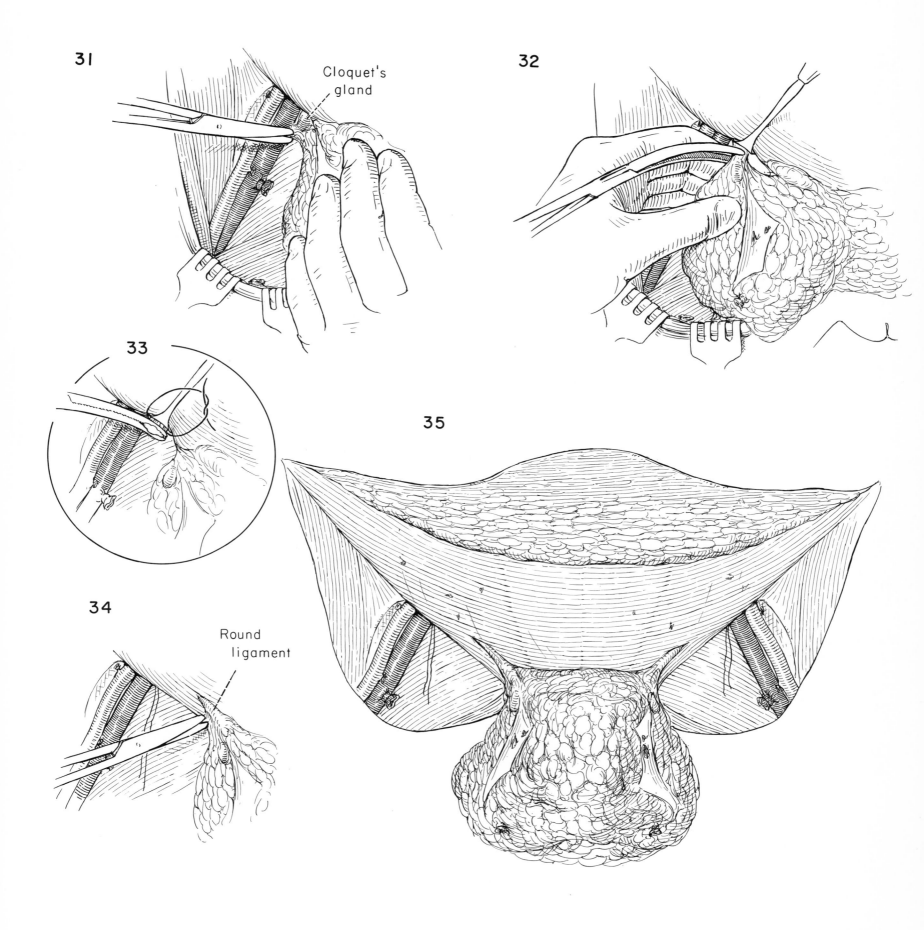

31

Cloquet's gland

32

33

35

34

Round ligament

When metastases occur from a primary tumor in the vulva they invariably lodge first in the superficial inguinal and femoral nodes which have just been dissected. The next area where the surgeon may be expected to encounter them will be in the nodal chain above the inguinal ligament, along the side of the external iliac vein and in the obturator space immediately beneath it.

Ideally, then, a complete operation for cancer of the vulva should include a dissection of nodes in these areas. This is a time-consuming, meticulous operative procedure and a one-stage operation may not be advisable in every patient. The general condition of an older patient may be such that the risks of surgery would outweigh the advantages of including the deep node dissection. If this is the case, the excision of the external iliac and obturator nodes can be postponed until a later date, or even omitted.

In the following illustrations the deep node dissection is being done as a part of a one-stage procedure. The steps would be the same if the extraperitoneal deep node dissection were done at a later date.

Figure 36. With the abdominal skin flap retracted to provide exposure, the surgeon makes a linear incision through the aponeurosis of the external oblique muscle paralleling the inguinal ligament and just above it (see dotted line). The incision extends from the external inguinal ring obliquely upward to the anterior superior spine.

Figure 37. The assistant applies Kelly clamps to both the upper and lower edges of the divided fascia. The assistant then elevates the flap by applying traction to the clamps on the upper edge. This permits the surgeon to dissect it free from the underlying internal oblique muscle. This is done through the full length of the incision.

Figure 38. The internal oblique muscle bundle must be divided. This is best accomplished by having the surgeon introduce the index finger of his left hand into the opening formed by the round ligament as it comes out from under the muscle. The finger is gently advanced in an oblique upward direction, pushing the underlying peritoneum and transversalis away from its undersurface.

Figure 39. With the proper cleavage plane developed by the single index finger it is now possible for the surgeon to introduce both the index and middle fingers into the same space beneath the muscle. The surgeon then incises the muscle lying above them. Any vessels encountered are clamped and the tissue ligated. The muscle is incised to the full length of the incision. Enough muscle is left attached to the inguinal ligament to permit subsequent closure by sutures.

Figure 40. The key to the problem of stripping back the peritoneum to provide exposure of the nodal areas to be dissected lies with the deep epigastric vessels. They must be located, divided and tied off. Any attempt to mobilize the peritoneum without sectioning these vessels will result in the creation of rents in the peritoneum and exposure of the peritoneal cavity.

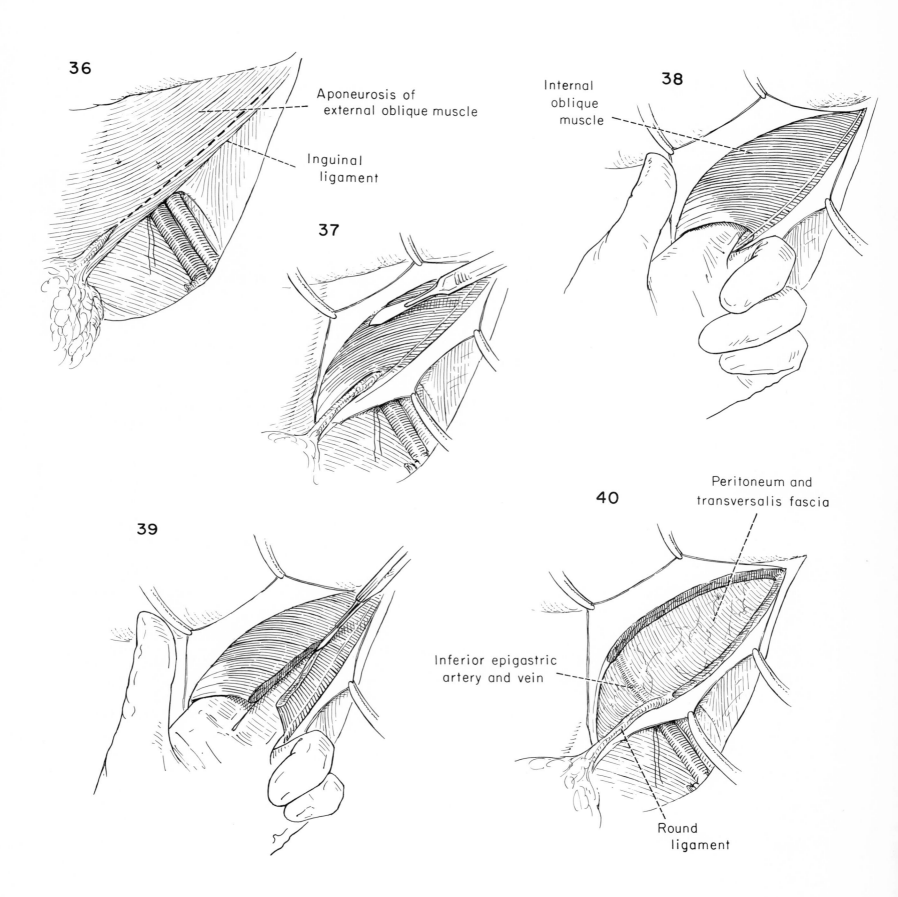

36

Aponeurosis of
external oblique muscle

Inguinal
ligament

37

Internal
oblique
muscle

38

39

40

Peritoneum and
transversalis fascia

Inferior epigastric
artery and vein

Round
ligament

At times the position of the deep epigastric vessels is hard to define, particularly if the patient is obese and there is a large amount of properitoneal fat present. They can always be identified with relative ease if the surgeon will trace the round ligament upward to the point at which it turns to enter the peritoneal cavity. Invariably these vessels can be found lying on the peritoneum just medial to the inner surface of the round ligament.

Figure 41. In this illustration the round ligament has been traced to its entrance into the peritoneal cavity. The inferior epigastric vessels can be seen lying on the peritoneum beneath it. The assistants expose the area by applying traction on the lower fascial edges. The surgeon then grasps the round ligament with Kelly clamps.

Figure 42. The round ligament is divided and both ends are secured with stitch ligatures. The inferior epigastric vessels are now fully exposed.

Figure 43. The surgeon separates the artery from the vein and applies a Kelly clamp across the artery. Another clamp is placed distal to it and the artery is then divided.

Figure 44. The divided ends of the artery included in each clamp are then separately ligated.

Figure 45. The deep epigastric vein is treated in similar fashion.

Figure 46. With the deep epigastric vessels divided the surgeon can now mobilize the peritoneum without incurring the risk of making holes in it and exposing the peritoneal cavity.

The assistants apply traction to the edges of the inguinal ligament as the surgeon, standing on the right side of the table, very gently places the palmar surface of his fingers on the peritoneum and teases it away from the ligament and the psoas muscles lying deep and lateral to it. The direction of the mobilization is upward and inward. Although the transversalis fascia overlies the peritoneum, it is too filmy for separate identification and offers no resistance to this maneuver.

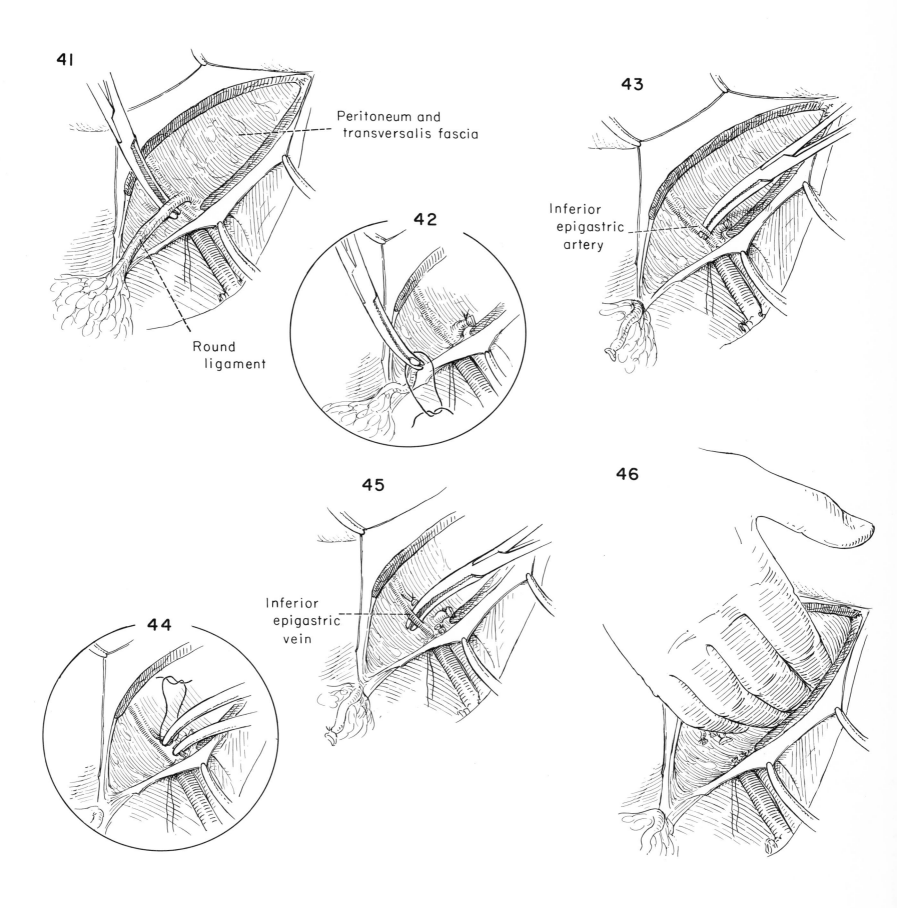

41

Peritoneum and transversalis fascia

Round ligament

42

43

Inferior epigastric artery

44

45

Inferior epigastric vein

46

Figure 47. As the mobilization continues the psoas muscle comes into view, the connective tissue can be seen immediately adjacent, lying on the medial side of the muscle and overlying the external iliac artery.

Figure 48. It is important that the regional nodal chain should be dissected to the bifurcation of the iliac vessels. The peritoneum can easily be mobilized to expose these vessels. The exposure is maintained by a Deaver retractor placed in the upper aspect of the wound.

Medial to the external iliac vessels one can identify the lateral edge of the bladder and the ureter lying on the peritoneum.

The operative field is widened further by placing another Deaver retractor on the bladder to retract it medially.

Figure 49. The assistants put the Deaver retractors on tension to provide adequate exposure. The surgeon then picks up the connective tissue, including the external iliac vessels, at about its midpoint and begins to dissect it away from the pelvic wall with blunt scissors. In almost every respect this dissection is like the lymphadenectomy that is included in the Wertheim (See pp. 342 to 347.)

Figure 50. The surgeon now retracts the artery with forceps and gently dissects the lateral side of the artery away from the medial border of the psoas muscle.

Figure 51. The lateral dissection of the tissue bundle has been completed beginning at the inguinal ligament and extending to the point where the common iliac artery branches to become the internal and external iliac arteries.

If possible, the genitofemoral nerve, lying on the psoas muscle just lateral to the external iliac artery, should be preserved.

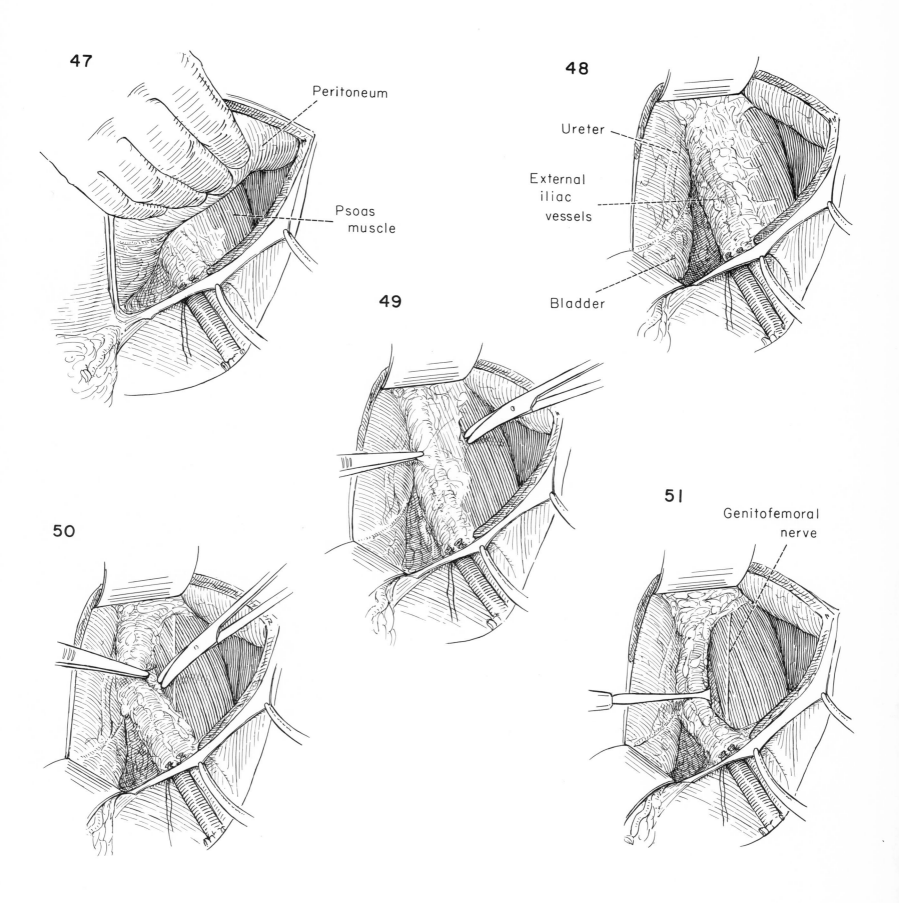

47

Peritoneum

Psoas
muscle

48

Ureter

External
iliac
vessels

Bladder

49

50

51

Genitofemoral
nerve

Figure 52. The medial aspect of the mass is freed from the peritoneum and the ureter, which are retracted. The anterior surface of the common iliac artery is exposed, thus defining the lymphatic bundle at its upper point of transection.

Figure 53. Clamps are applied and the tissues cut across and secured with ties to minimize lymph leakage into the dead space postoperatively.

Figure 54. The overlying tissue is now incised along the course of the external iliac artery and the vessel freed up and out of it.

Figure 55. The vein is similarly unroofed and dissected up and out of the mass, which is allowed to drop back deeper into the obturator fossa.

Figure 56. Any vessels encountered are clamped and then cut and tied off. Venous bleeding from the pelvic wall can be annoying and occasionally terrifying. Often the source proves to be a hole in the side of a larger vessel where a branch was torn off. Pressure will usually control it enough to permit careful clamping and tying, but occasionally it is necessary to temporarily secure the vein above and below and to suture the rent. In this crisis the surgeon should use measures to relieve back pressure along the venous system, such as placing the operating table in Trendelenburg position and removing packs above the field and checking the position of the retractors to be certain they are not resting on the great vessels above the point of bleeding.

Figure 57. The entire mass of fat and nodes now lies free below the iliac vessels. As they are held up it is pushed down and medially.

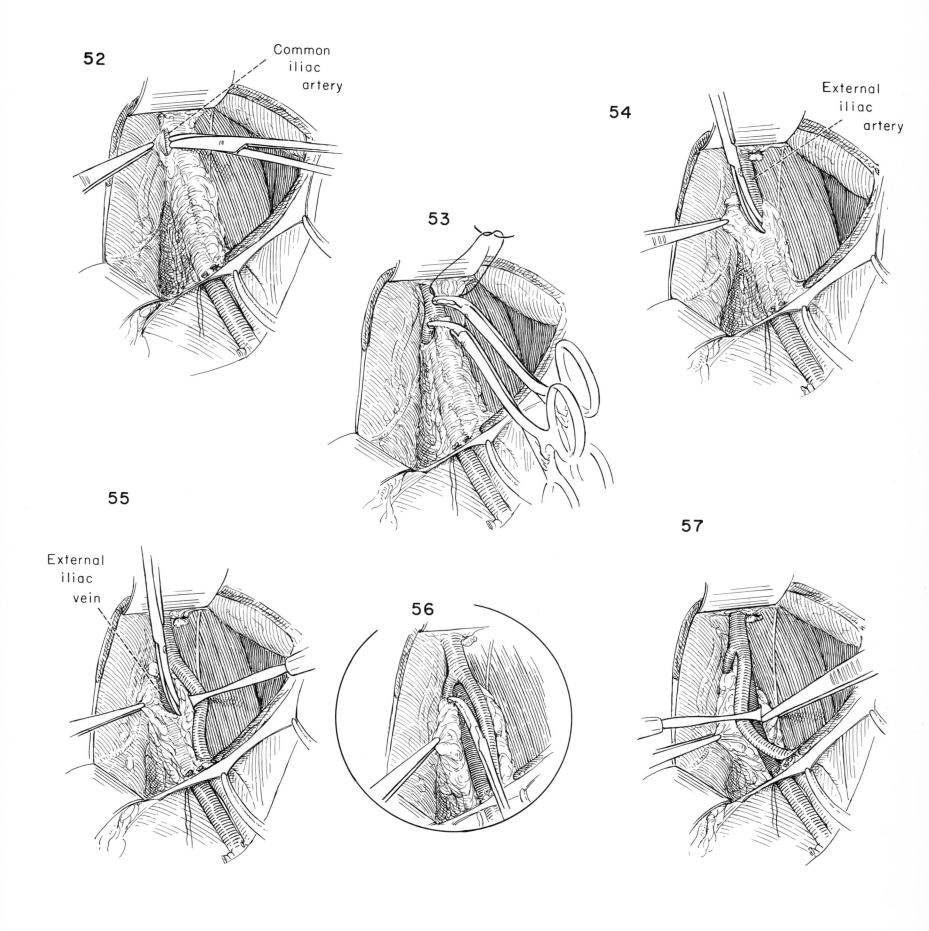

52

Common
iliac
artery

53

54

External
iliac
artery

55

External
iliac
vein

56

57

Figure 58. The surgeon now dissects the node-bearing mass from the lateral side of the internal iliac artery. The assistant provides exposure by applying traction to the Deaver retractors and the Kelly clamps on the inguinal ligament.

Figure 59. This illustration shows the external iliac artery and veins and the internal iliac artery bare of all tissue from the inguinal ligament to the common iliac artery above its bifurcation.

Rarely does the operator find venous branches entering the undersurface of the external iliac vein. The surgeon must be on the lookout and clamp them when he encounters them.

Figure 60. The internal and external iliac portions of the nodal chain have been dissected clean of the vessels. The surgeon is now interested in removing the lymphatic channels and nodes lying beneath and deep to the external iliac vein in the obturator space. The lower border of the space is marked by the obturator nerve.

The surgeon retracts the lateral surface of the bladder toward the midline with the handle end of the forceps. With his right hand he picks up the block of tissue. Gentle traction will free any attachments to the bladder and ureter.

Figure 61. With the mass of tissue free medially the surgeon can now begin the dissection of the obturator space. First, the long tie in the femoral canal is delivered up into the pelvis to be certain that a continuous resection is performed. The assistant draws the mass of tissue toward the midline. The surgeon protects the vein and exposes its undersurface by holding the external iliac vein laterally with the hand forceps as he gently separates the tissue from its undersurface and from the obturator nerve which runs along the lateral aspect.

Figure 62. In this view all the tissue which may reasonably be expected to contain lymph nodes has been excised.

In the upper portion the external iliac artery and vein have been cleaned well up on the common iliac artery. The tissues lying between the internal iliac artery and the external iliac vein are also free. Below it the obturator nerve and vessels can be seen.

Figure 63. Beneath and distal to the inguinal ligament the femoral artery and vein can be seen. The lymphatic pathways beneath the inguinal ligament (the femoral canal) which provide the main link between the superficial inguinal and femoral nodes and the deep nodes above is now clean of all tissue as shown in this illustration.

Figure 64. To close the space between the underborder of the inguinal ligament, the femoral vessels, and the underlying muscle created by the dissection, the surgeon places a few strong sutures into the inguinal and lacunar ligaments. Closure of this space will prevent the later possible development of a femoral hernia.

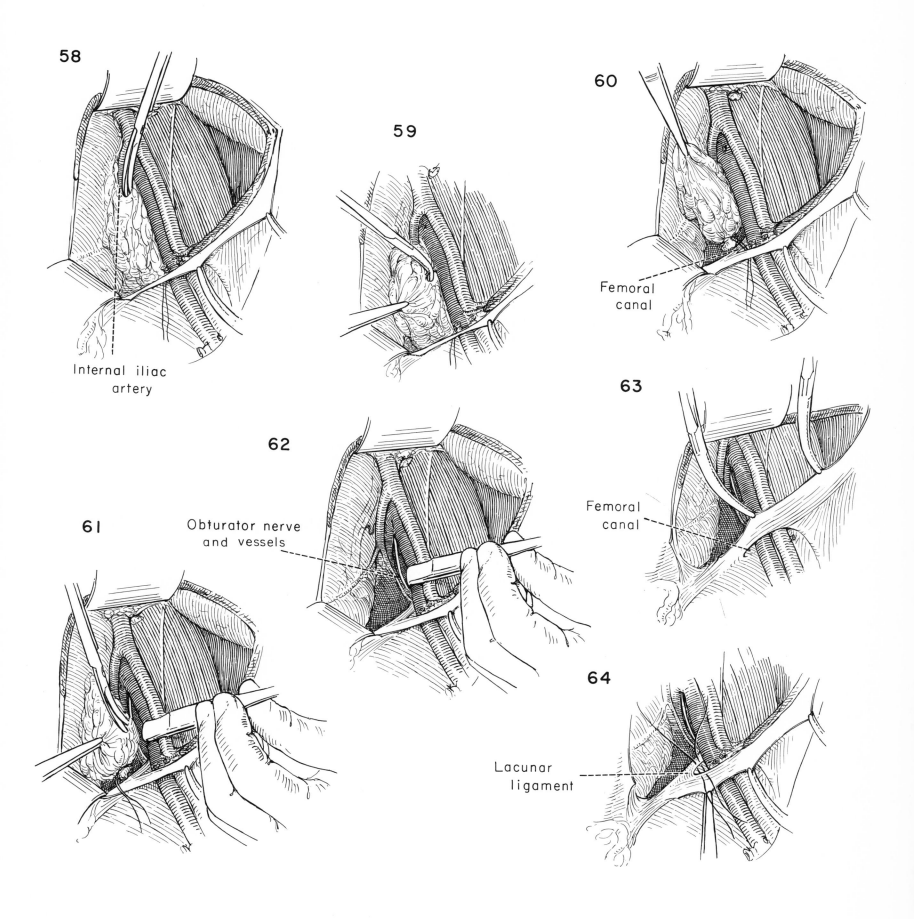

58

Internal iliac
artery

59

60

Femoral
canal

61

62

Obturator nerve
and vessels

63

Femoral
canal

64

Lacunar
ligament

Figure 65. This concludes the procedure on one side. The surgeon now begins to close the wound by placing the first of a series of mattress sutures in the internal oblique muscle at the most lateral point of its division.

Figure 66. A series of these sutures have been placed in the internal oblique muscle and tied. The defect in the muscular wall of the abdomen, left when the round ligament was excised, must now be closed. A series of interrupted sutures are placed which, when tied, will approximate the lower border of the internal oblique muscle to the inguinal ligament as in inguinal hernia repair.

Figure 67. Interrupted sutures are then placed in the aponeurosis of the external oblique muscle, serially tied, and each held on tension to assist in the placement of the next one.

Figure 68. Inasmuch as the dissection must be performed bilaterally, all the steps shown in the preceding illustration are repeated on the opposite side.

With the fascial layers on both sides approximated and tied, the surgeon then dissects the block of tissue containing the vulva and the regional nodes away from the underlying symphysis. Traction in a downward direction helps to establish the cleavage plane.

Figure 69. The lateral wound openings are approximated with interrupted silk on both sides. The area overlying the symphysis pubis is still exposed.

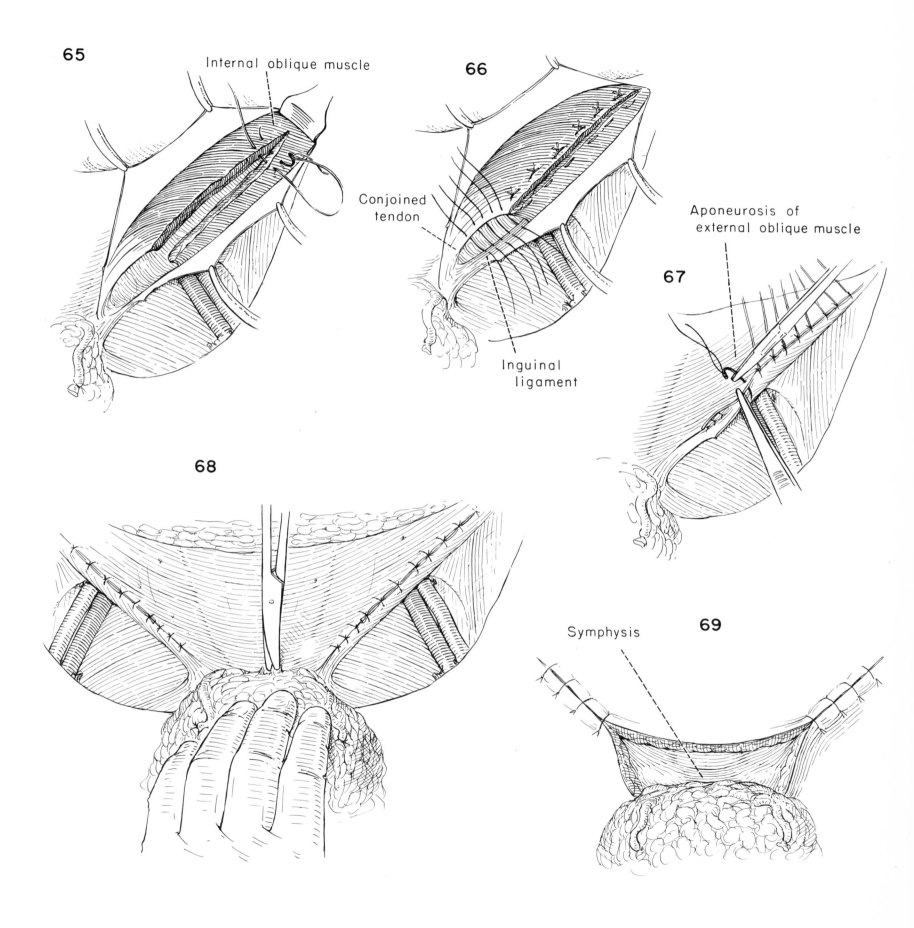

65 Internal oblique muscle

66

Conjoined tendon

Inguinal ligament

67 Aponeurosis of external oblique muscle

68

Symphysis 69

The en bloc superficial dissection to this point has removed the entire lymphatic-bearing area in both groins together with the block of lymphatics intervening between the superficial inguinal nodes and the primary tumor. This tissue remains attached to the specimen.

Figure 70. The patient is now placed in the lithotomy position to permit the removal of the entire vulva. Clamps are placed on the upper skin edges of the specimen within the area of the tissue outlined for removal. The assistant applies upward traction on the clamps as the surgeon grasps the skin opposite and starts the incision along the left side. Note that wide margins are given to the growth despite the fact that the primary tumor is small. Both sides are thus developed.

Figure 71. The inner margin of resection will leave only the urethral and vaginal orifices. To outline it the labia are held apart with Allis forceps for good exposure. The surgeon places the anterior vaginal wall on tension with the palmar surface of the fingers placed over a gauze sponge and incises the epithelium above the urethral orifice.

Figure 72. The labium is held on traction to the right and the anterior vaginal wall to the midline as the operator continues the incision along the lateral wall of the vagina. The same maneuver is repeated on the left side, completely circumscribing the vaginal epithelium except at the fourchette.

Figure 73. The incision lateral to the vulva is deepened to expose the fascia of the underlying muscles. The primary tumor mass is pulled to the midline with the operator's left hand. The use of gauze to provide purchase for the fingers will facilitate this maneuver. Deep rake retractors provide exposure on the lateral side. Individual vessels are clamped as they are encountered.

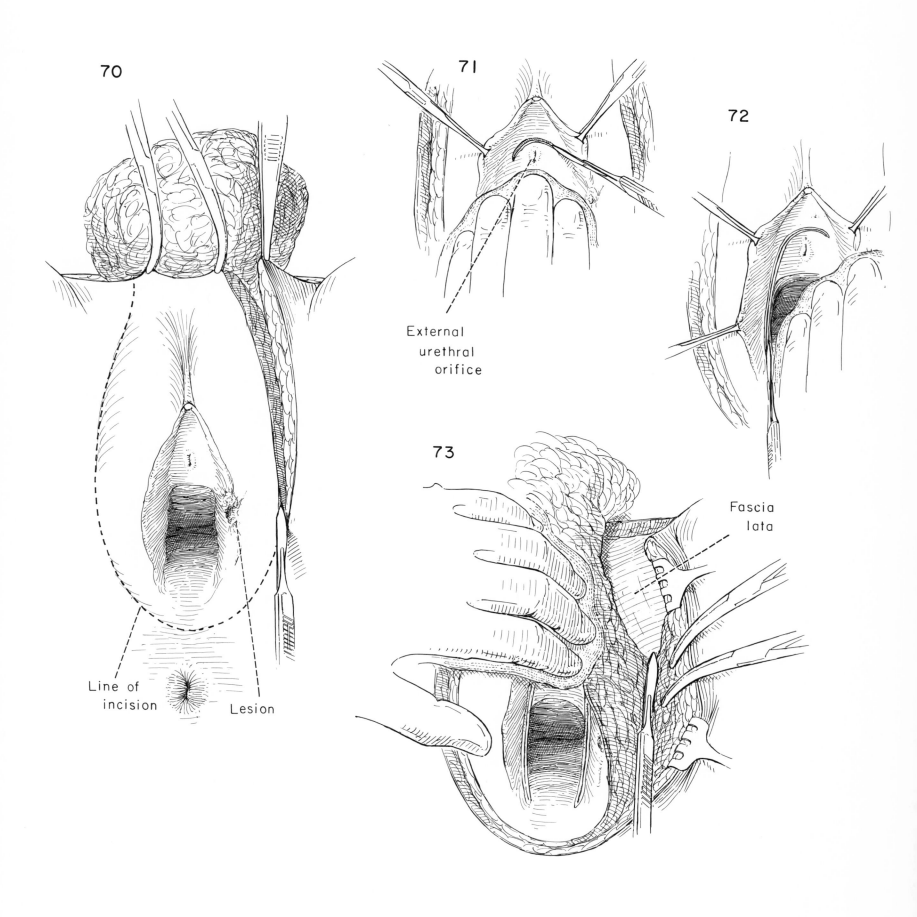

70

71

External
urethral
orifice

72

73

Fascia
lata

Line of
incision

Lesion

Figure 74. The moves are repeated on the opposite side. The entire mass of tissue is drawn downward as it is dissected from the fascia overlying the symphysis and muscles attaching to the pubic rami. The suspensory ligament of the clitoris must be cut across. The mass then falls downward.

Figure 75. By continuing with the dissection in this plane the mass is completely freed from the symphysis, not only on its anterior surface but also underneath the pubic arch. Care must be taken to avoid a plexus of veins in this area. The handle of the knife is useful in making this separation.

Figure 76. The mass of tissue is again drawn sharply to the midline, exposing the perineal vessels appearing just below the level of the midpoint of the lateral dissection. The vessels are being dissected free of the surrounding fat by the tips of a Kelly clamp.

Figure 77. The vessels are doubly clamped as the assistant holds back the lateral border of the skin incision with rake retractors.

Figure 78. The operator then places a ligature around each of the clamps while the assistant maintains the exposure. The same steps are repeated on the opposite side.

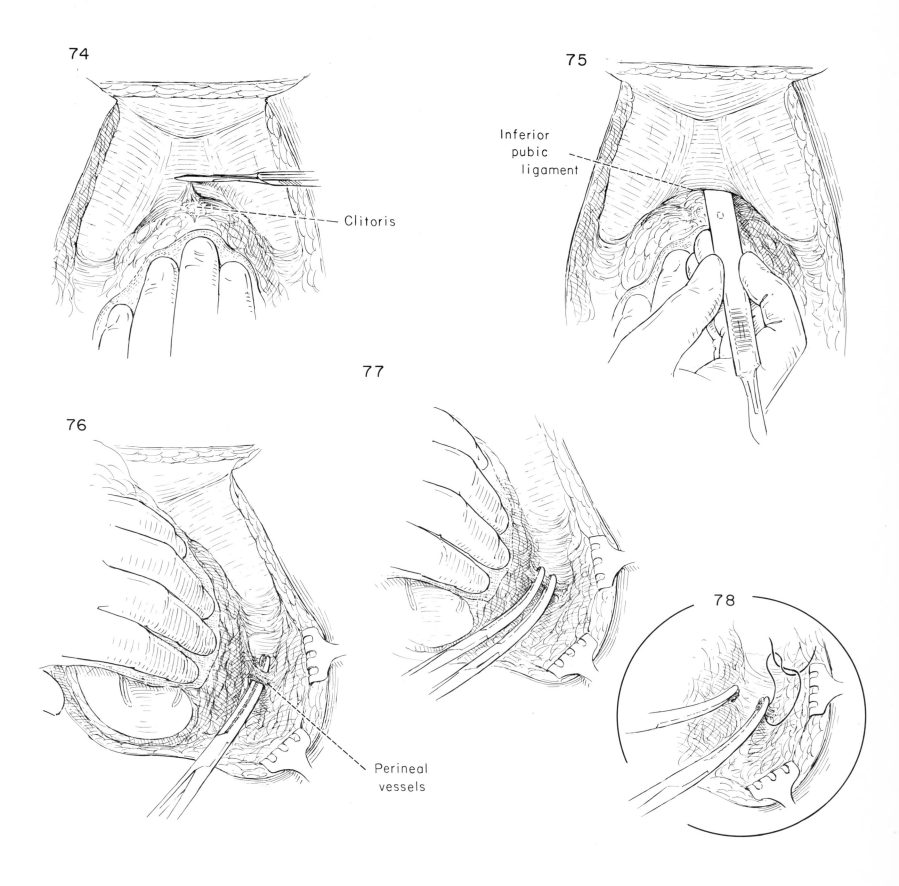

74

Clitoris

75

Inferior
pubic
ligament

76

77

78

Perineal
vessels

Figure 79. The outer aspect of the specimen has now been completely outlined as well as the vaginal aspect on both sides and above; it remains attached in the midline below the fourchette and above the anal opening, which is covered by the drapes.

The perineal incision is now exposed and the plane between vagina and rectum developed.

Figure 80. Upward traction is maintained on the vulva specimen. Two Allis clamps on the edge of the transverse incision below the vagina provide upward traction as the operator separates the vaginal wall from the anterior surface of the underlying rectum. Countertraction with the rake retractors gives additional exposure. This dissection is continued well up between the posterior vagina and the rectal wall to permit approximation of the levators at the time of closure. For this reason the inner incision is not carried across the fourchette.

Figure 81. The specimen is still attached by the tissue between the two areas already dissected. The assistant provides traction to the left as the surgeon divides this fatty connection.

Figure 82. Continuing to hold the specimen upward on tension, the operator connects the lateral dissection with the incision previously made to circumscribe the vaginal epithelium by passing the index finger between the mass, breaking through on the vaginal side.

Figure 83. Before a similar separation over the urethral meatus is accomplished, the canal should be identified by introducing a blunt instrument to demonstrate its course.

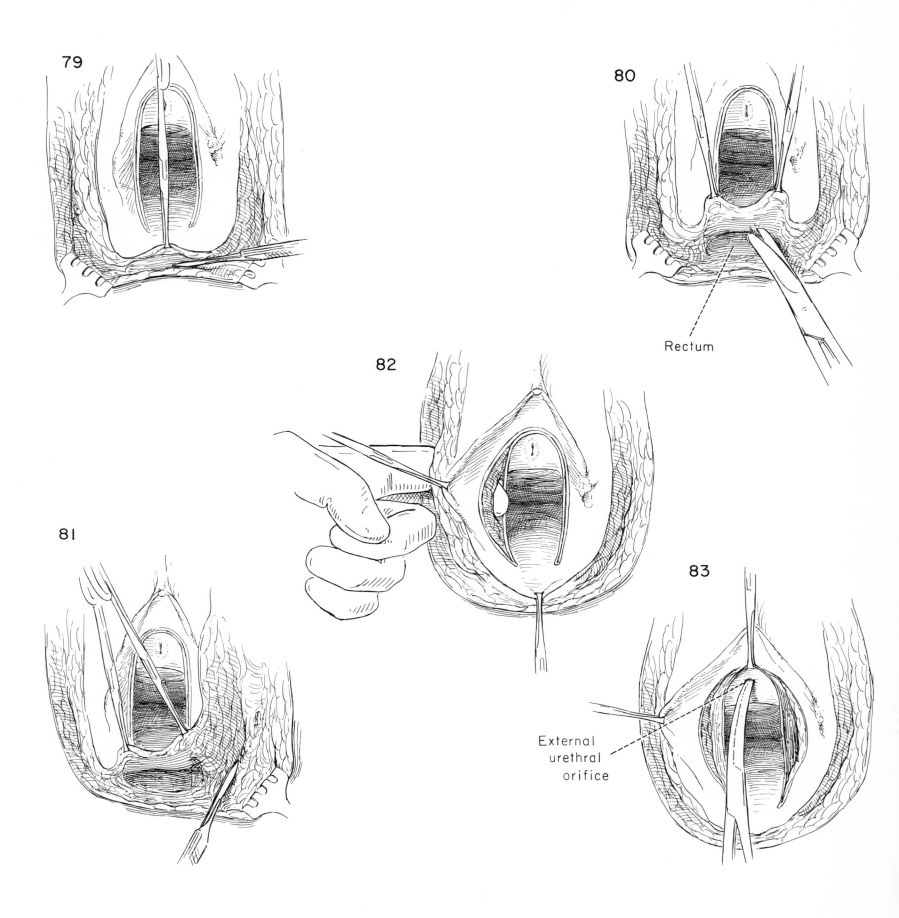

79

80

Rectum

82

81

83

External
urethral
orifice

Figure 84. For the sake of exposure the specimen is again held on tension by lateral clamps. An Allis forceps grasping the upper edge of the incision above the urethra is placed on traction. The surgeon then separates the urethra from the undersurface of the specimen with the knife handle.

Figure 85. This maneuver soon leads into the area of previous dissection from above. The surgeon's left index finger demonstrates this fact.

Figure 86. The specimen is now detached from the symphysis and pubic rami except for the small muscle bundle of the ischiocavernosus which holds it on either side. This muscle is included between two Kelly clamps and the tissue between them divided. The index finger behind the muscle helps to support the weight of the specimen.

Figure 87. The tissue in the lateral clamp is secured with a stitch ligature. The opposite ischiocavernosus muscle is still intact and must be similarly divided, stitched or ligated.

Figure 88. The entire specimen is now held only by the bridge of posterior vaginal wall epithelium. This is now divided and the specimen removed.

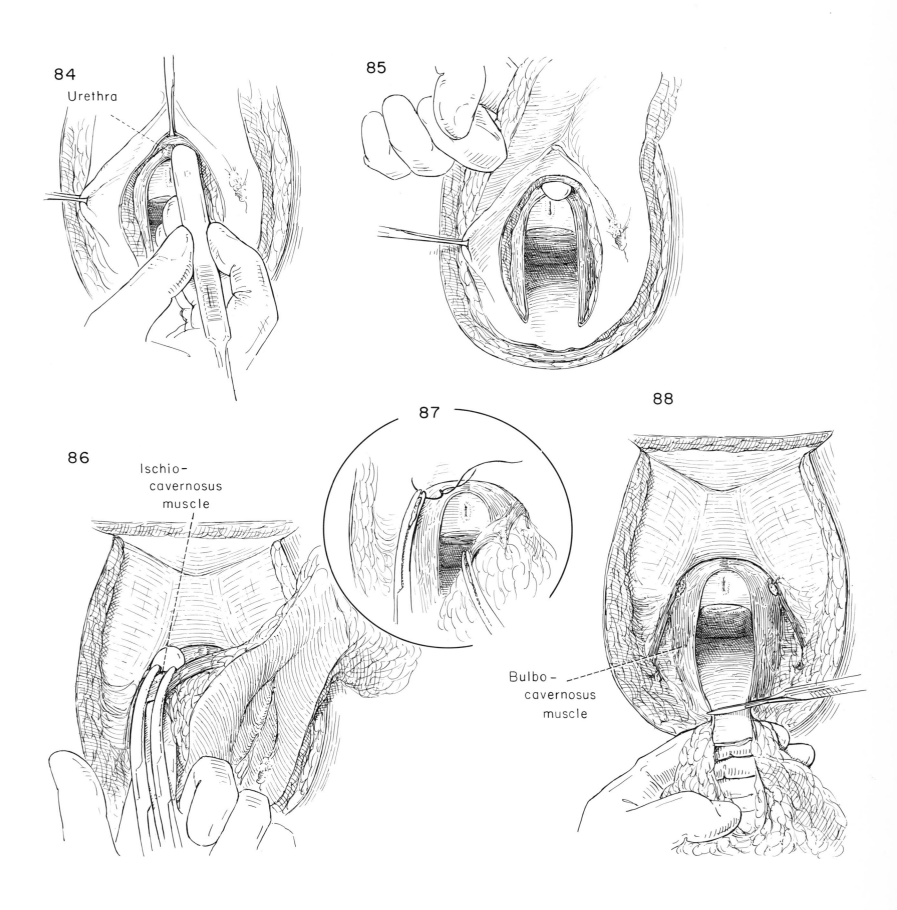

84
Urethra

85

86
Ischio-
cavernosus
muscle

87

88
Bulbo-
cavernosus
muscle

There is a tendency after radical excision of the vulva for a rectocele to later bulge out over the perineal body. This can cause the patient considerable discomfort. To circumvent this the surgeon is advised to reconstruct the levator muscles in front of the rectum.

Figure 89. The lower corners of the vaginal wall are grasped with Kelly clamps and held downward on tension as the operator completes the dissection which separates the vaginal wall from the rectum and exposes the levator muscles on either side.

Figure 90. The rectum is held back by the left index finger, and a series of interrupted catgut sutures is laid into the levator ani muscles in the manner of a perineal repair.

Figure 91. The rectum now lies behind the levator muscles, which are approximated in the midline, and the individual sutures are tied and divided.

Figure 92. So much dead space has been created in this extensive dissection that drainage is an essential part of the wound closure. The surgeon may accomplish this in a variety of ways.

The most effective way today is by the insertion of perforated polyethylene catheters and the establishment of constant suction. There are available small plastic collecting units which maintain constant suction and still permit the patient to be ambulatory.

In this illustration the surgeon is passing a sharp cutting point introducer (to which the catheter is attached) through the abdominal wall above the crescent incision. On the left side the perforated catheter can be seen in the depths of the wound.

Figure 93. The edges of the skin in the upper portion of the dissection are brought together with interrupted silk sutures. The surgeon now approximates the edge of the skin to that of the vaginal wall with interrupted silk sutures throughout the circumference. Because of the extensive dissection the edges will come together with some tension. If they do not fall together easily, one should not hesitate to leave portions of the wound open.

Figure 94. The vaginal wall has been approximated to the skin, and the wound closure is complete. An inlying Foley catheter has been inserted in the bladder. The suction catheters are each fixed to the skin with a suture.

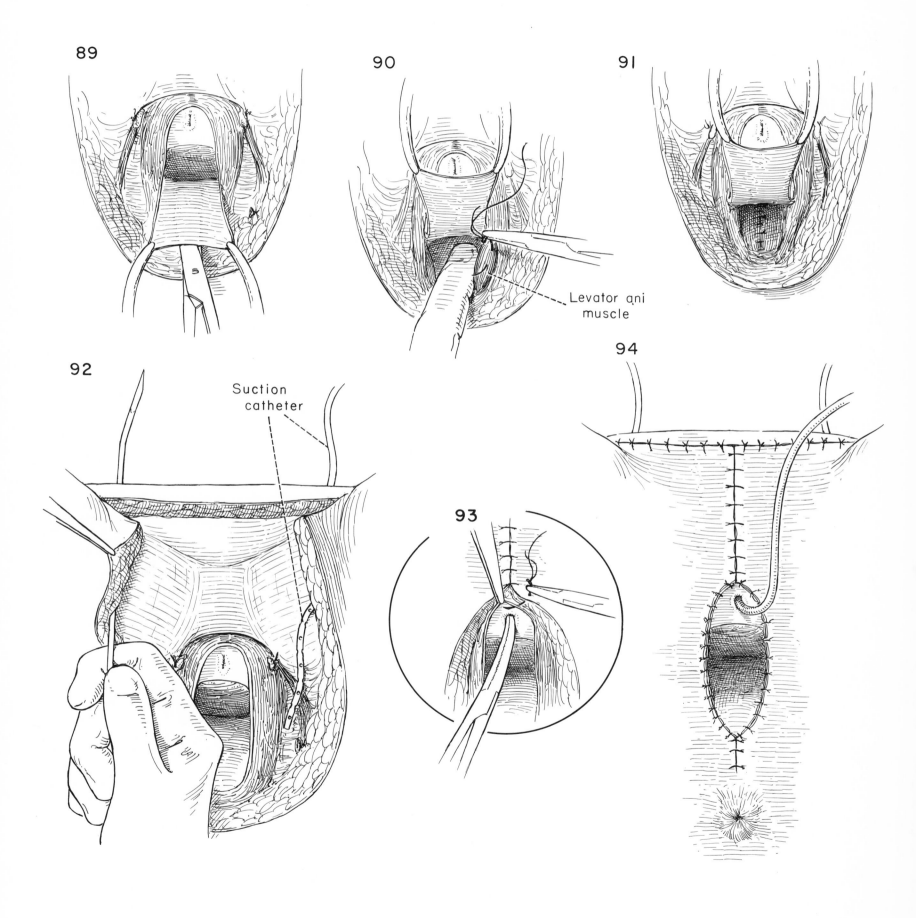

89

90

Levator ani
muscle

91

92

Suction
catheter

93

94

TOTAL PELVIC EXENTERATION

The en bloc removal in one stage of all the pelvic viscera, together with excision of the regional lymph nodes and diversion of the urinary stream and large bowel, is called total exenteration. This term distinguishes it from the anterior or posterior exenteration in which the surgeon elects to spare either the rectum or bladder.

This is a formidable surgical procedure which should never be undertaken lightly. It is usually performed for cancer of the cervix. For the most part it is offered to patients who have failed to respond to a course of radiation therapy. It may on occasion be justified in the patient with far advanced local disease and little hope that radiation will be curative, or again when the surgeon has underestimated the amount of disease when he undertakes to do a Wertheim hysterectomy. The emphasis is always on cure, not palliation.

The procedures have a limited usefulness for other forms of pelvic malignant disease such as carcinoma of the ovary, endometrium, rectum or bladder. Cancer of the vulva and vagina, which have the same sort of life history, may be included with cancer of the cervix, provided bilateral groin dissections are also performed.

This is not an operation that should be performed by the surgeon who deals only occasionally with the problems of cancer in the pelvis. Unless the surgeon has had experience in dealing with pelvic cancer and has at his command a well-trained supporting staff and adequate hospital facilities, the operation should not be offered to the patient. The problems confronting the surgeon are as formidable in the convalescent period as they are in the actual performance of the operation.

INSET A. In this figure the external landmarks are identified. The incision indicated is in the midline. Note that the umbilicus will be excised. This permits an incision of adequate length which can be closed rapidly and securely with full thickness through-and-through wire sutures. The abdominal wall will be opened in one layer.

Figure 1. The midline incision curves around the umbilicus, extending from the symphysis to the midepigastrium.

Figure 2. The ellipse around the naval is completed and excision of the skin begins.

Figure 3. Elliptical excision continues through the umbilicus where all layers, including the peritoneum, come together.

Figure 4. The rounded defect in the peritoneum, following excision of the umbilicus, is identified and held open with forceps.

Figure 5. The assistant and the surgeon elevate the peritoneum away from the underlying intestines and with scissors open the full thickness of abdominal wall in one layer.

Figure 6. After inspecting the lower pelvic cavity and identifying the normal anatomic structures, the surgeon explores the rest of the peritoneal cavity. If no metastasis is found he turns his attention to the bifurcation of the aorta. If nodes are palpable above this point the chances of prolonged survival following total exenteration are remote indeed. Any node found should be excised and presented to the pathologist for frozen section examination.

In this illustration the surgeon has incised the posterior peritoneum and is seen picking up the suspected node in preparation for excision.

A

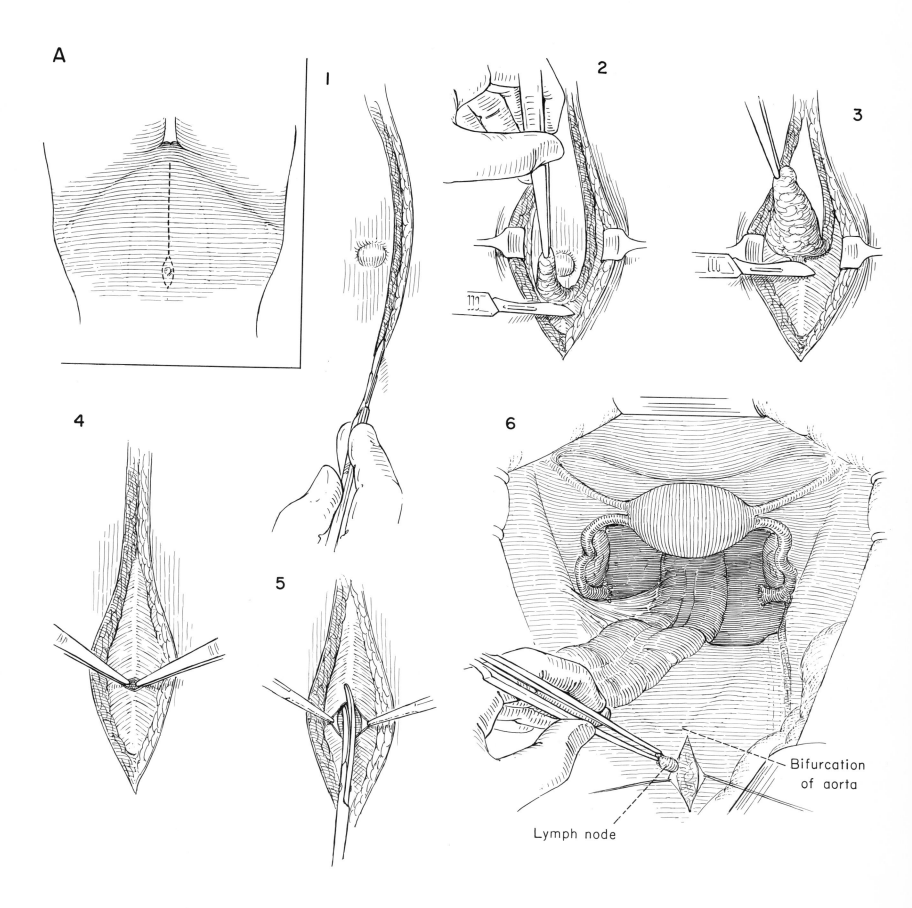

Bifurcation
of aorta

Lymph node

Figure 7. Whether it is wise to continue with the extensive surgery required to complete a total exenteration also depends upon the degree of lateral extension of the tumor. Extensive involvement of the nodal chain in the iliac and obturator areas may influence the surgeon to abandon the procedure, particularly if removal of the metastatic nodes would demand an extensive excision of the iliac vessels. The primary tumor itself may extend laterally into pelvic wall tissues and defy resection.

A quick method of evaluating the extent of lateral excursion of the tumor is to incise the peritoneum lateral to the vessels and parallel to them.

In this view the operative field has been prepared by packing the small intestine out of the pelvis in the usual manner. The surgeon and the assistant then pick up the peritoneum lateral to the external iliac vessels while the surgeon opens it as indicated by the dotted line.

Figure 8. The surgeon then gently inserts the tips of the fingers of the right hand into the space between central mass and pelvic wall and lightly palpates the area to determine the degree of extent and fixation. The left side is explored in the same fashion. Although edema, fibrosis and relative immobility of the central viscera are the rule in these cases, this lateral space on both sides is usually easy to follow to the pelvic floor.

Figure 9. The surgeon has decided that the total exenteration is a reasonable procedure and continues with his exposure and resection. The round ligament is ligated and cut. Stay sutures are then placed on the edges of the incised peritoneum to keep the operative field open. The relationship of the ureter to the ovarian vessels is established. The ureter lies on the medial leaf of the peritoneum. The ovarian vessels are teased away from it and a small Moynihan clamp is placed under the vessels at a point well up under the retracted cecum. A ligature is drawn through and tied.

Figure 10. The ends are left long and held on traction. Another clamp is placed on the uterine side of the ovarian vein. Both the clamp and the stay suture are elevated gently as the surgeon divides the vessels. A stitch ligature is placed on the stump of the ovarian vessels.

Figure 11. The assistant applies traction to the clamp on the distal portion of the ovarian vein and on the traction suture on the medial edge of the peritoneum.

This allows the surgeon to follow the avascular cleavage plane deeper and expose the iliac vessels.

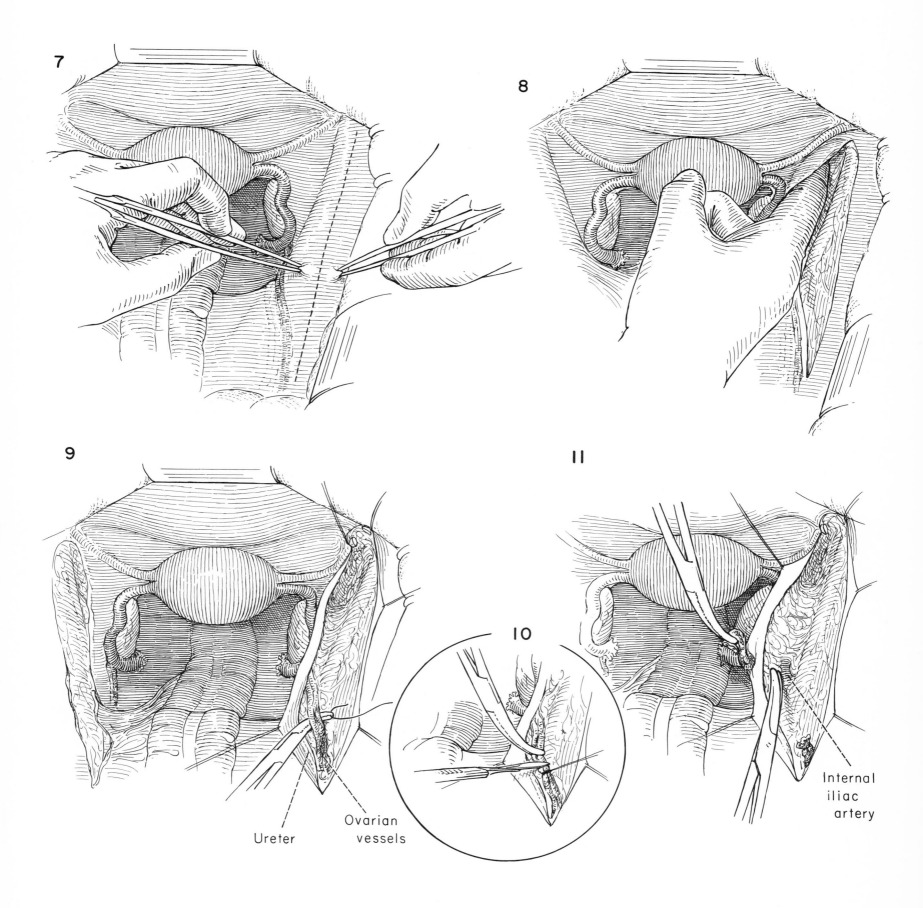

7

8

9

10

11

Ureter

Ovarian
vessels

Internal
iliac
artery

Figure 12. As the dissection continues, the bifurcation of the artery is identified and the internal iliac artery exposed and freed up to enable the surgeon to pass a clamp around it below the point of bifurcation and distal to the major gluteal branch. This must be done carefully to avoid the vein which lies directly beneath. The surgeon then grasps a silk suture fed into the jaws of the open ends of the clamp, draws the suture through and ligates the internal iliac artery. The ends are left long.

Figure 13. Traction is exerted on the stay sutures, on the clamp on the ovarian vessels and on the silk suture just tied around the internal iliac artery. A clamp is then placed across the vessel distal to the point of ligation. The artery is divided with a knife, leaving a cuff of vessel wall distal to the suture previously placed.

Figure 14. The surgeon now secures the stump with a reinforcing stitch ligature. The suture passes through the wall of the arterial cuff.

Figure 15. The stump of the vessel is then elevated and the suture is tied around it.

Figure 16. In the interest of keeping the operative field free of clamps, a tie replaces the clamp on the distal end of the internal iliac artery.

Figure 17. With the distal artery pulled away from its bed, all branches leaving it posteriorly and laterally can be visualized, clamped and cut. All unnecessary clamps are replaced with ties when possible; in this illustration note stump of ovarian vessels above.

Figure 18. Traction on the uterus with clamps or tenacula is of little help when the tissues are unyielding. The reader will note that throughout this series such traction has been omitted and the central mass of organs and supports is not shown displaced until its attachments have been freed.

The internal iliac vein lies directly beneath the internal iliac artery. It must be dealt with by gentle dissection when freeing the lymphatic and fatty tissue from its superior surface. To facilitate this dissection Deaver retractors are placed to hold the uterus and bladder out of the way. They provide a wide open operative field and maintain the tissue planes so essential to a clean dissection. Although the vein can be transected exactly like the artery, it is technically difficult to elevate it from its bed without damage. Our usual practice is to secure all its tributaries as they enter the medial side and to leave the major vessel intact.

Figure 19. With the internal iliac vein retracted gently by the handle of the hand forceps the surgeon then dissects the tissue away from it to find and manage its branches.

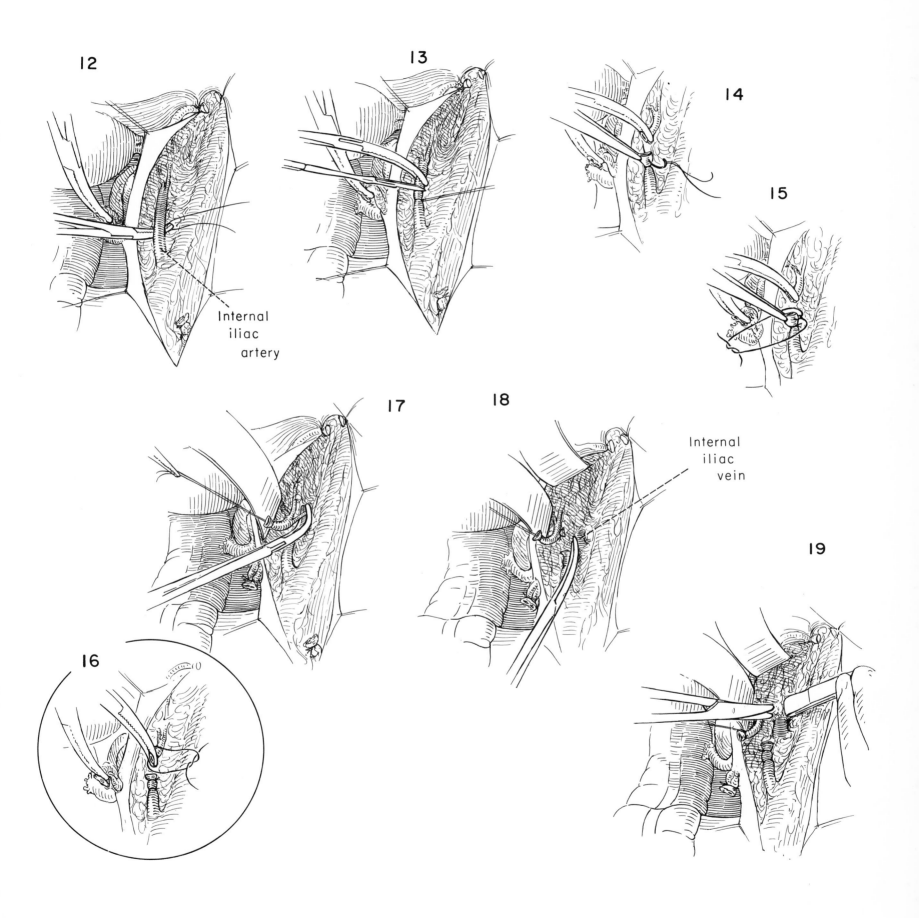

12

13

14

15

Internal
iliac
artery

17

18

Internal
iliac
vein

16

19

Figure 20. Each vessel is meticulously exposed and individually clamped, cut and immediately tied. To leave a clamp on a short branch of the internal iliac vein for any length of time is to risk a tear which may require time, effort and transfusions to control. When this misfortune strikes it may be wise, after one or two failures to reapply the clamp, to pack firmly and to wait. The pack should not compromise the external iliac vein and trap blood in the leg.

Whenever hemorrhage begins to interfere with this operation repeatedly, it is worth stopping, exposing the aortic bifurcation and placing an aortic clamp just above this point. This can be left in place for over an hour, if necessary, while the bleeding sources are visualized and controlled.

Figure 21. The dissection along the internal iliac vein continues until the central mass is completely free from the vessels. Final appraisal of operability is now possible.

Figure 22. The point of no return comes with the division of the ureters. Prior to this time the surgeon could safely abandon the operation without sacrificing any vital structure. The course of the ureter must be traced downward into the pelvis.

Figure 23. The surgeon now identifies the lower end of the ureter as it lies on the medial leaf of the peritoneum. Traction on the stay suture on the peritoneal edge and upon the Deaver retractor placed on the bladder helps to provide exposure. The assistant picks up the periureteral tissue laterally as the surgeon gently separates the ureter from the undersurface of the peritoneum for a short distance.

Figure 24. With the ureter freed, the assistant feeds a suture into the open ends of a clamp introduced into the space beneath it. This suture is then tied and the ends are clamped and left long.

Figure 25. The assistant elevates the stay suture on the peritoneal edge and retracts the bladder medially as the surgeon applies traction on the suture which has ligated the ureter. He then transects the ureter with a knife. Use of a clamp or ligature on the proximal ureter is usually avoided.

Figure 26. The suture on the distal ureter is cut. The surgeon then picks up the peritoneal tissue around the proximal end of the divided ureter and places a suture through the wall. This suture is not tied but is simply clamped and left long. It will help in locating the ureter later when it comes time to begin the diversion of the urinary stream into the bowel.

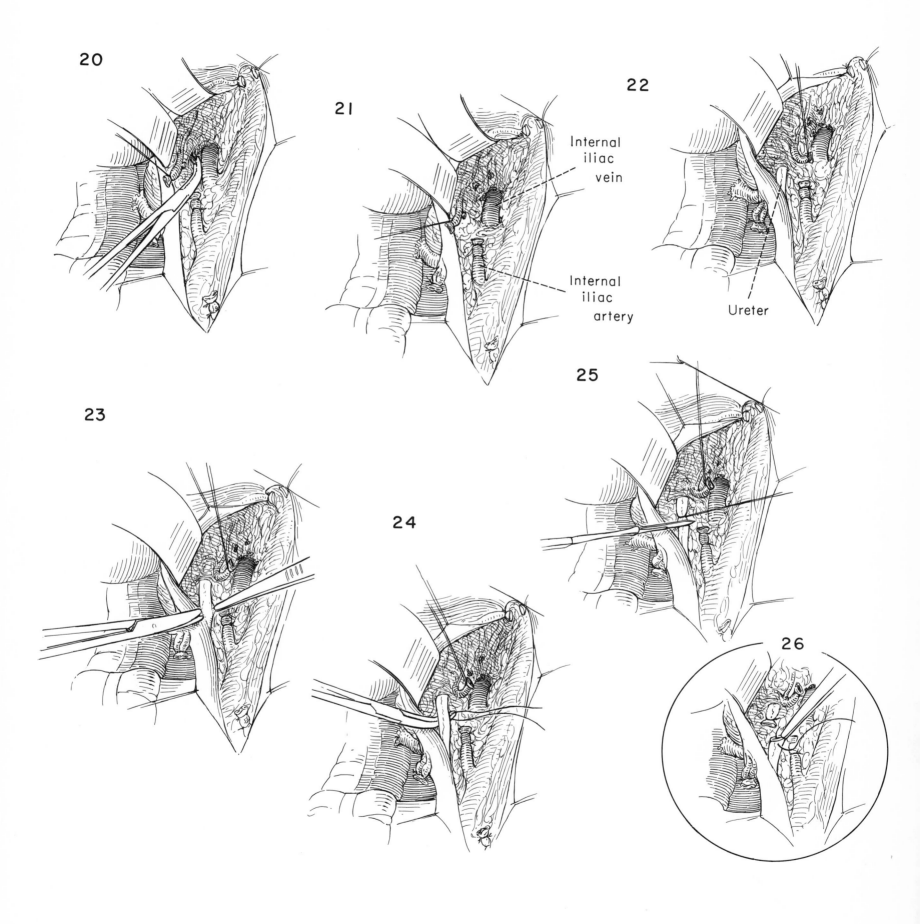

20

21

Internal
iliac
vein

Internal
iliac
artery

22

Ureter

23

24

25

26

Figure 27. This view shows the surgeon outlining a rectangular strip of peritoneum around the right ureter. Note that the flap is longer than the ureter and that the ureter is in contact with its undersurface.

Later on in the operation when the ureter is anastomosed to the bowel any tension upon it can be minimized by simply suturing the edge of the flap to the bowel wall above the point of union. To avoid kinking of the ureter at this point it is necessary that the peritoneum extend beyond the divided end of the ureter.

Figure 28. The other side is now dissected in similar fashion. The asymmetrical origin of the sigmoid mesentery prevents the development of any well-defined peritoneal flap on this side.

With the ureters divided and the peritoneal flaps prepared, the surgeon now turns his attention to the sigmoid which is to be sacrificed. The area to be transected must be carefully selected to ensure having the divided proximal end long enough to pass to and through the abdominal wall, where it should lie comfortably without tension.

The surgeon keeps the bowel on tension and begins to divide the peritoneum of the mesentery on the left side.

Figure 29. The bowel is then drawn to the left side and held on tension as the surgeon incises the peritoneum on the right side of the mesentery.

Figure 30. With traction maintained on the bowel, the individual vessels in the mesentery are identified and doubly clamped. The tissue between them is divided and secured with a stitch ligature. The clamps are then removed.

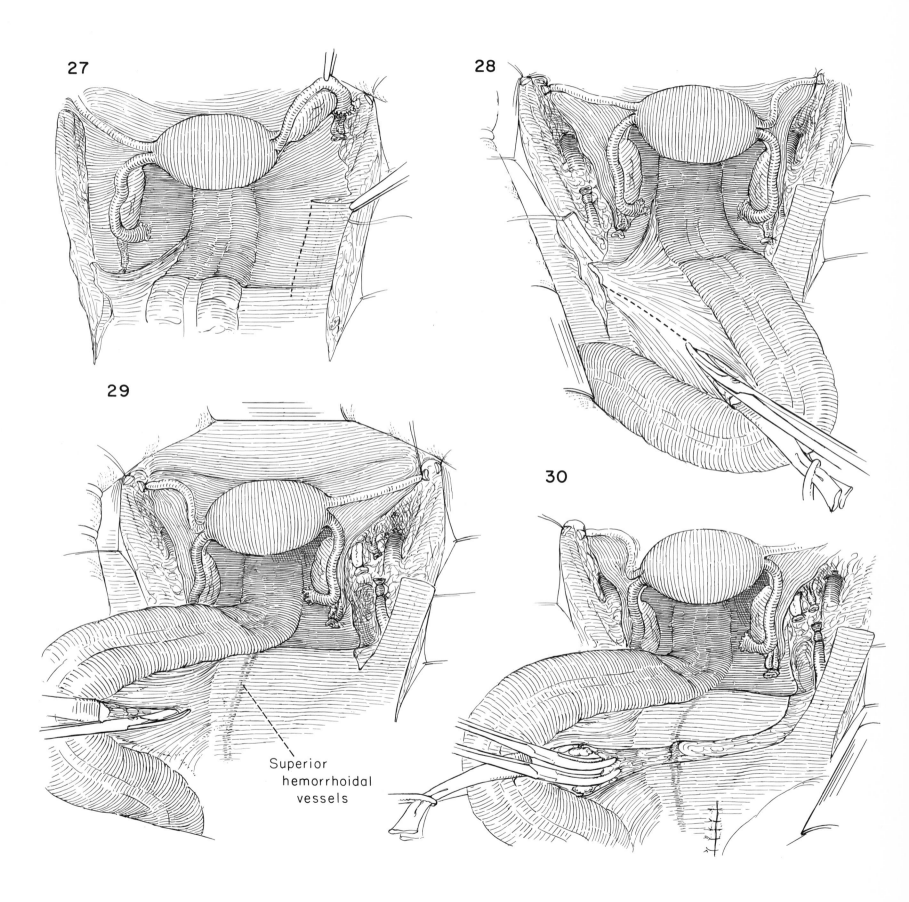

27

28

29

30

Superior
hemorrhoidal
vessels

Figure 31. As the vessels are encountered and sequentially ligated, the space beneath the sigmoid opens up. To assist in traction on the bowel the surgeon then inserts a length of soft rubber drainage tubing beneath the bowel wall. The ends are clamped. When traction is applied to this the mesentery is kept on tension. This is of great help in identifying and isolating the major blood vessels to the distal bowel, the superior hemorrhoidal vessels. When these are sufficiently exposed, a small Moynihan clamp is placed across the vessels.

Figure 32. The vessels are doubly clamped and the surgeon sections the vessel wall. Stitch ligatures are then placed around the vessels and the sutures are tied. The clamps are removed.

Figure 33. Traction on the tape is relaxed as the surgeon selects the area in the sigmoid that he wishes to transect. Troublesome small bleeding vessels are frequently encountered at the point at which the mesentery joins the bowel wall. These should be secured with small clamps and the vessels ligated.

Figure 34. Kocher or narrow blade Allen clamps are then placed across the bowel wall.

Figure 35. The bowel wall is divided between the two clamps. This may be done with a cautery or by sharp knife followed by carbolic acid sterilization and alcohol; the choice of method rests with the surgeon.

Figure 36. To avoid infection through contamination each of the stumps should be covered with gauze. One half of a regular gauze sponge is placed over the clamp.

Figure 37. The assistant holds the clamp and gauze on tension. The surgeon then passes a strand of catgut over the gauze and around the clamp, beginning at the handle end of the clamp. The ends of the suture are brought up and crossed over the top of the sponge. The catgut is held on tension as the surgeon continues the passage over the ends of the clamp. The suture ends are then brought up onto the surface of the gauze, again crossed beneath the clamp on the handle side, brought up and tied on the superior surface. The gauze sponge will have less tendency to slip off and expose the bowel wall edges. The same procedure is carried out on both ends of the bowel.

Figure 38. The assistant then applies traction to the rectosigmoid through the clamp on the divided end while the surgeon introduces his right hand behind the rectum and gently frees the bowel from the wall of the bony pelvis and sacrum.

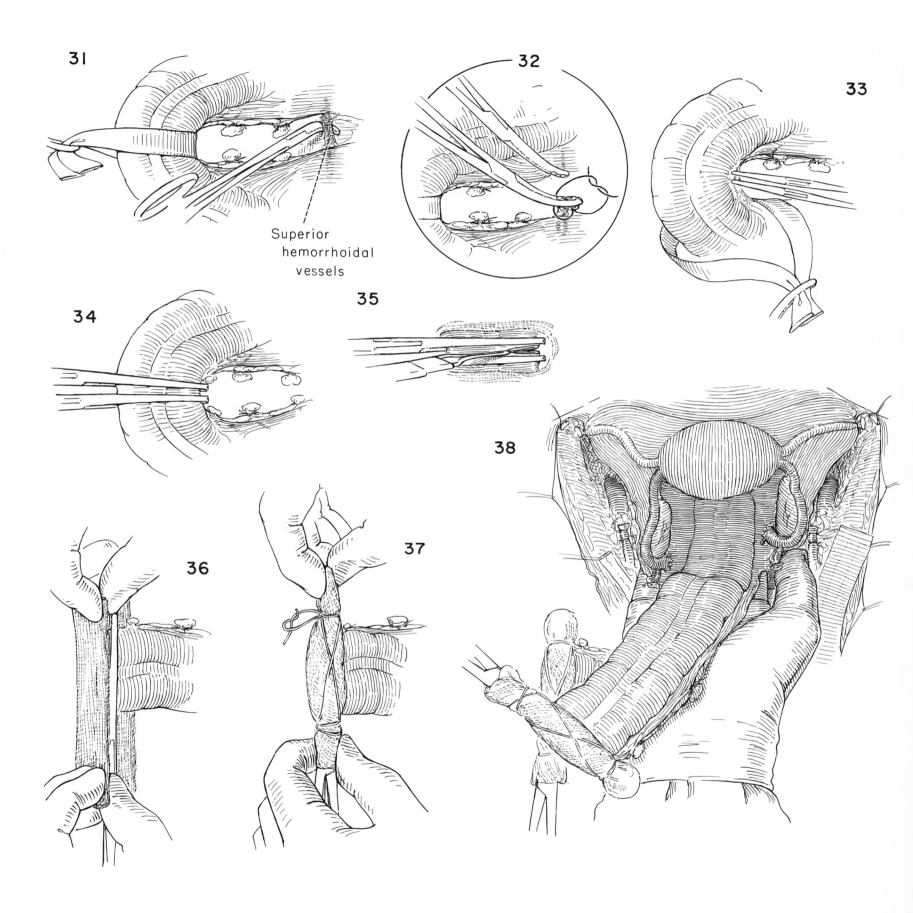

31

32

33

Superior
hemorrhoidal
vessels

34

35

38

36

37

Figure 39. The separation of the rectum from the underlying bony pelvis has made it possible to elevate the entire specimen. To accomplish this the surgeon introduces his left hand into the space behind the rectum. This step allows him easy access to any remaining attachments posteriorly and laterally as the central mass is freed forward off the levator ani muscles.

Figure 40. With the posterior dissection completed the surgeon now turns his attention to the area of the bladder which must be separated from the symphysis and the pubic rami. The lateral peritoneal incisions are extended distally on either side of the bladder until they reach the lower end of the wound.

Figure 41. Dissection is continued deep into the prevesical space. The exposure is markedly improved when the surgeon lays the flat of the left hand on the anterior surface of the bladder and pulls upward and backward with the tips of the extended fingers. This allows him to dissect the attachments of the bladder and urethra from the undersurface of the symphysis. Replacing the retractor over the lower end of the incision increases the exposure.

Figure 42. Maintaining pressure on the bladder in the manner described, the surgeon continues the dissection beneath the symphysis and further detaches the urethra from it. At this point one estimates the extent of the resection necessary below the tumor. Often when the patient has cancer of the cervix it will be found that an adequate distal margin can be resected without recourse to a perineal approach. When this is the case, the distal urethra can be transected at this stage of operation or the vulva entered just above the external urethral meatus.

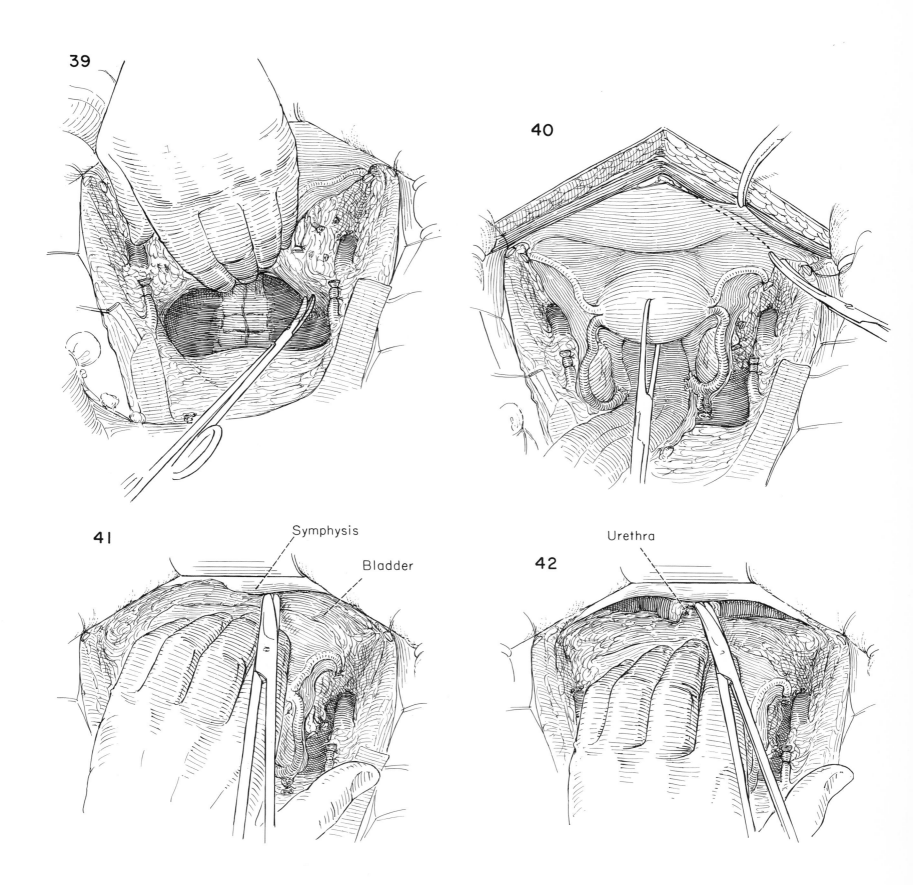

39

40

41   Symphysis   Bladder

42   Urethra

Figure 43. The surgeon then returns to the lateral dissection and begins to separate the lymphatic-bearing nodal tissue off the obturator fascia. The exposure is obtained by having the assistant hold the lower abdominal wall aside with a Deaver retractor while the surgeon draws the specimen upward and medially.

Figure 44. Maintaining the exposure in the same fashion the surgeon now divides the endopelvic fascia, which is clearly visible. Immediately the central mass comes up and forward out of the hollow of the sacrum.

Figure 45. The specimen is now fully mobilized laterally. The lower end of the rectum, anus, vagina and vulva still must be removed en bloc with the main specimen which contains rectum, uterus and bladder, together with all the paracervical, paravaginal and pararectal lymphatic pathways. To get across to the vagina, lower rectum and vulva the surgeon divides the levator ani muscles in circular fashion well lateral to the specimen. It is usually easiest to perforate this layer just below the tip of the coccyx and proceed forward on both sides.

Figure 46. The excision is made under direct vision and with little blood loss when the assistants retract the abdominal wall and the surgeon draws the specimen away from the area to be dissected.

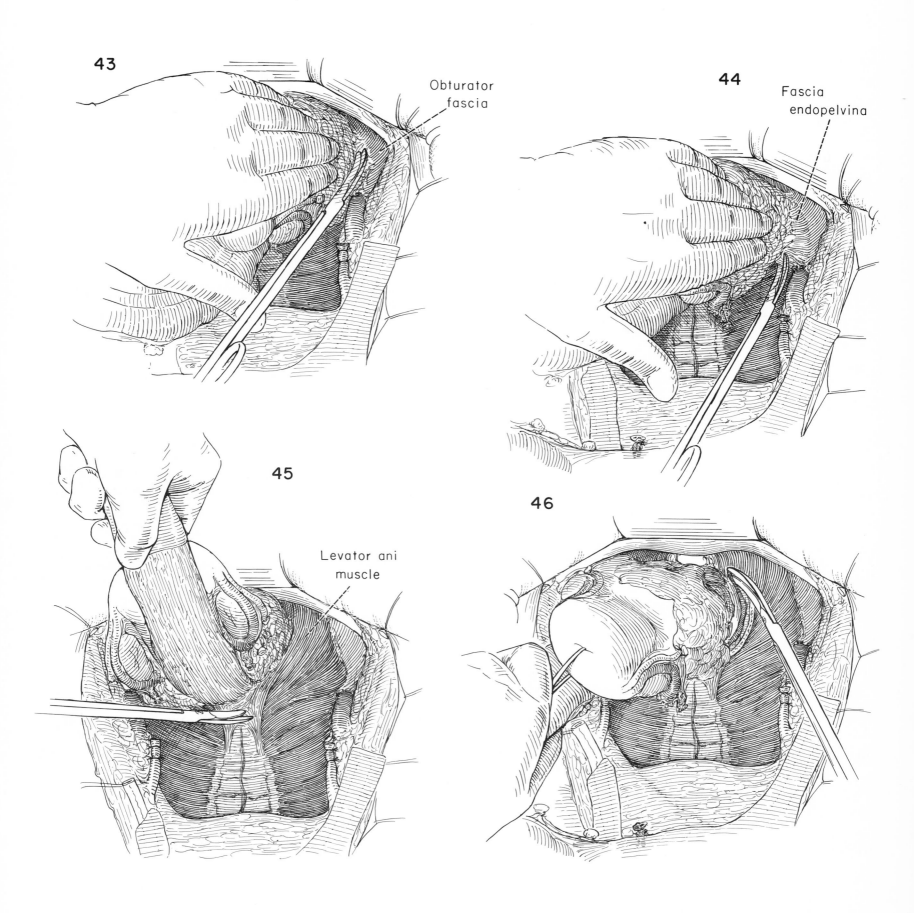

43

Obturator
fascia

44

Fascia
endopelvina

45

Levator ani
muscle

46

Figure 47. After the muscle has been completely divided on both sides, the dissection continues through the fat of the ischiorectal fossa. The assistants provide exposure while the surgeon elevates the entire mass, including the rectum, and dissects the fatty tissue free from the posterior wall of the lower bowel. The excision is carried through the skin behind the anus and extended forward on either side to the opening previously made at the urethra.

Figure 48. The entire specimen has now been removed. This view shows the entire lower pelvis cleared of all tissue, the incised margins of the levator ani and the defect in the skin. To control oozing from the cut edges of muscle and to firm up the pelvic floor somewhat a running lock stitch is placed at the level of the levators.

Figure 49. With the specimen removed there is ample room to examine the field and to secure any persistent bleeding points. It is now planned to excise the presacral nodes. Anatomic landmarks such as the common iliac artery and the left common iliac vein are in direct view as the dissection proceeds. Care must be taken not to damage the presacral vessels which descend longitudinally over the sacrum. They bleed profusely and are hard to control with cautery, suture or dura clip. The best means of stopping the bleeding is by firm packing with gauze.

Figure 50. All tissue is mobilized toward the midline using great care to avoid going laterally beyond the iliac arteries and thereby running the risk of injury to ureteral vessels. The mass of fat is then gently separated from the underlying left common iliac vein. Within this block of tissue lie the presacral nodes.

Figure 51. With the nodal mass free of the vessels beneath, the assistant elevates the tissue by lifting upward on a Kelly clamp applied solely for traction purposes. This allows the surgeon to identify the position of the common iliac vein before he applies clamps to the proximal portion which overlies the bifurcation of the aorta. This pedicle is securely tied in keeping with our feeling about not leaving open lymphatic trunks in the pelvic dissection.

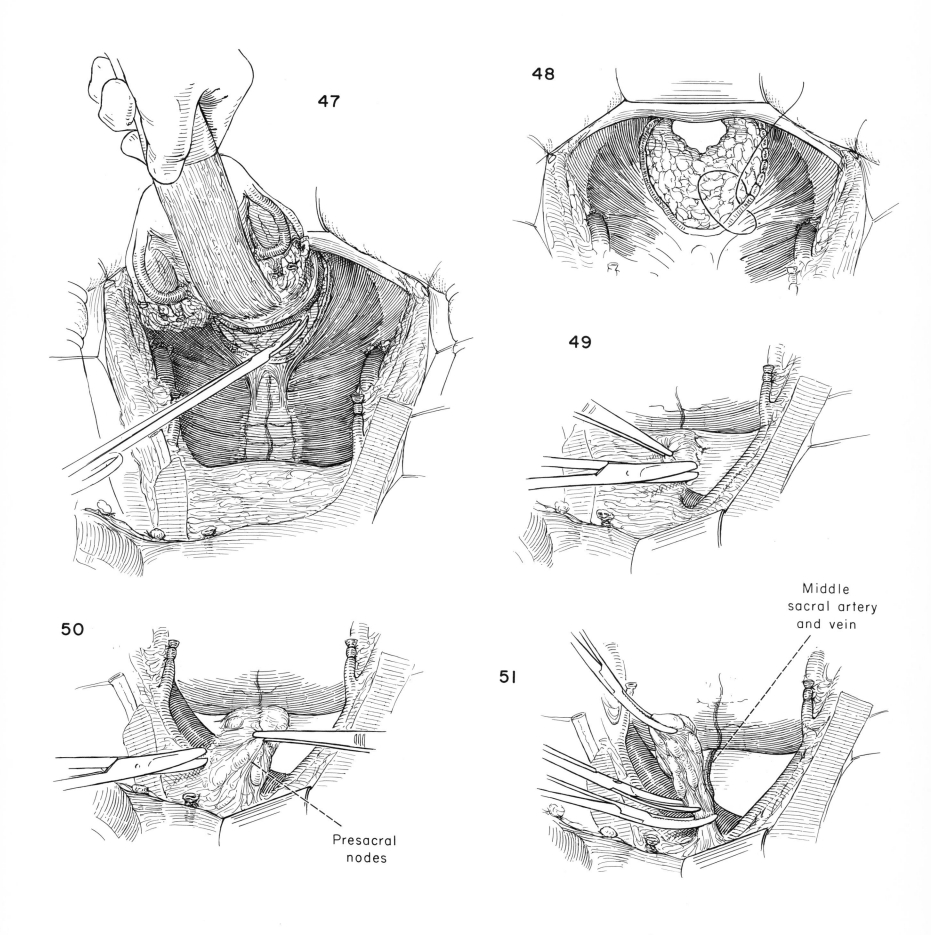

47

48

49

50

Presacral
nodes

51

Middle
sacral artery
and vein

Figure 52. As in the Wertheim procedure (shown in detail on pp. 343 to 347) the pelvic wall nodal dissection begins by freeing of the tissue along the lateral side of the external iliac artery. The tissues are freed from the psoas muscle beneath and mobilized medially until one sees the medial border of the muscle. The tissues are gently freed from it down to the inguinal ligament.

Figure 53. The vessels are cleaned of all lymphatic node-bearing tissue from a point well up on the common iliac artery down to Poupart's ligament. The tissue between artery and vein containing the intermediate chain of nodes is also removed.

The vessels are now retracted laterally and upward with a vein retractor. The surgeon pulls the nodal tissue toward the midline as he dissects it from beneath the external iliac vein and the obturator nerve. This is done bilaterally.

INSET A. Before the surgeon turns his attention from the depths of the pelvis all bleeding points are determined to be secure and drains are placed. Usually a series of cigarette wicks are led out through the perineal skin defect. When excessive oozing causes concern, it is better to lay in gauze packs with their ends at the outlet for removal under light anesthesia five days or so later.

Figure 54. The extirpative portion of the operation is completed when Penrose drains are placed in the posterior defect. The surgeon now faces the problem of diverting the urinary stream. This is usually done in one of two ways: by establishing an ileal conduit or by performing a ureterosigmoid anastomosis. We prefer the former.

A mobile segment of terminal ileum is chosen and the bowel clamped at a point approximately 2 inches from the junction of ileum with cecum. The incision in the mesentery should be extensive enough to allow the distal portion of the isolated segment to be brought through the abdominal wall without tension. The arterial architecture must be closely scrutinized for there is danger of damaging the blood supply by an overenthusiastic attempt to lengthen the incision. The emphasis is on avoiding vessels whenever possible. If any branches are traumatized they should be secured with fine clamps and sutured with silk.

It is important to decide the length of intestine to be used. This will vary, depending on the thickness of the abdominal wall, but the entire segment should be planned to reach from the sacral promontory to the abdominal skin without redundancy.

This view shows the mesentery opened at both ends, the distal small intestine clamped and the proposed line of transection of the proximal portion.

Figure 55. The segment of ileum to be used as the urinary conduit has been isolated by dividing the bowel between the clamps; the two remaining ends have been brought together for anastomosis.

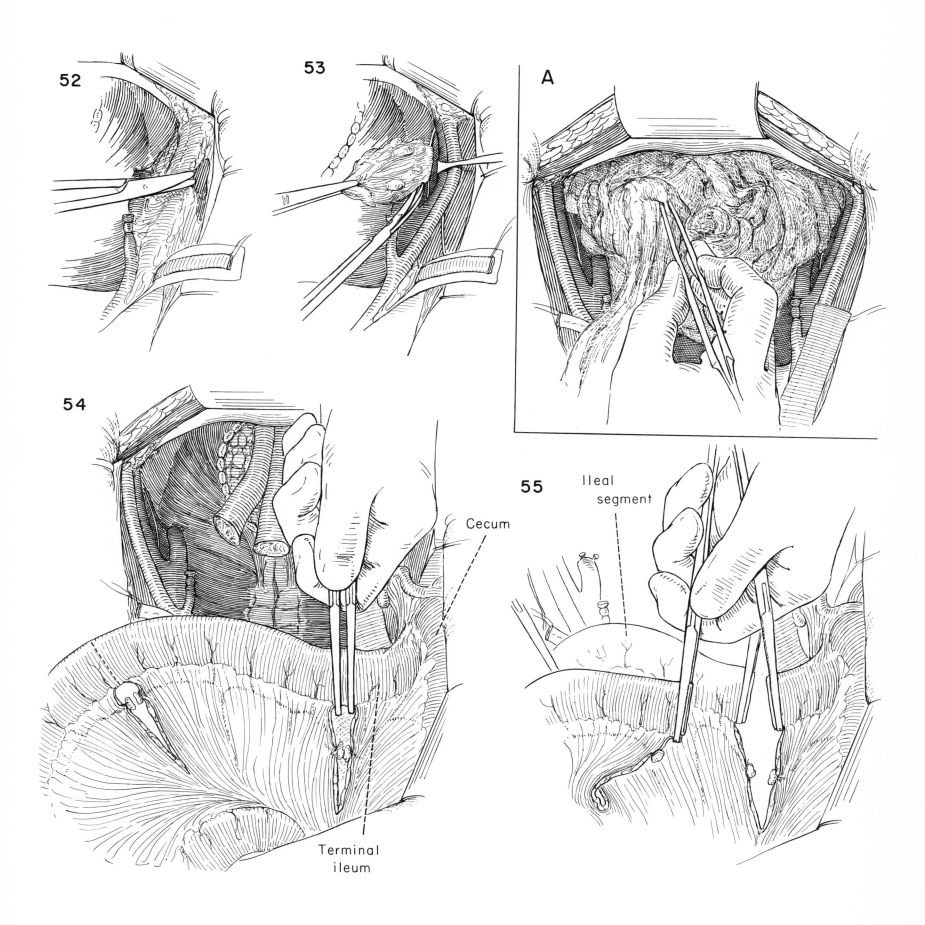

52

53

A

54

Cecum

Terminal
ileum

55

Ileal
segment

Figure 56. Continuity of the small intestine is re-established by end-to-end anastomosis. The assistants approximate the clamps holding the two ends of the bowel as the surgeon places interrupted silk sutures on the serosal surface of the two loops of intestine. When tied, the two ends are approximated.

Figure 57. The surgeon then starts an inner layer of interrupted catgut sutures in the midline. This row of sutures will continue around the full circumference of the bowel. It will be reinforced with a row of interrupted silk sutures placed in the anterior wall of the bowel. (See pp. 113 to 115 for details.)

Figure 58. With the continuity of the small intestine restored the surgeon now prepares to carry out the steps of the uretero-enterostomies. Note the length of the isolated segment and the intact blood supply and mesentery.

Figure 59. The surgeon holds the clamp on the proximal end of the isolated segment and lays in the chromic catgut suture that will close the open end when the clamp is removed. The running suture begins at the end of the clamp and goes from one side of the bowel to the other until the opposite end is reached. Traction is employed on both ends of the suture by the surgeon and the assistant as the surgeon removes the clamp. The continuous suture then returns in similar fashion to the original point at which it is tied. (See p. 111 for details.)

Figure 60. The closure is completed by a series of interrupted silk sutures. Each suture is tied and the ends are left long. The surgeon holds each silk suture as he places the next one.

Figure 61. The silk sutures are not cut but left long to assist in turning the bowel to allow the surgeon to anastomose the ureters on the underside of the bowel.

Figure 62. The surgeon now rotates the ileal loop upward on its long axis by turning the clamp on the distal end and the silk sutures on the closed portion. He selects the areas on the undersurface of the bowel where he wishes to make the two anastomoses. The sites chosen are close to the closed end of the bowel.

56

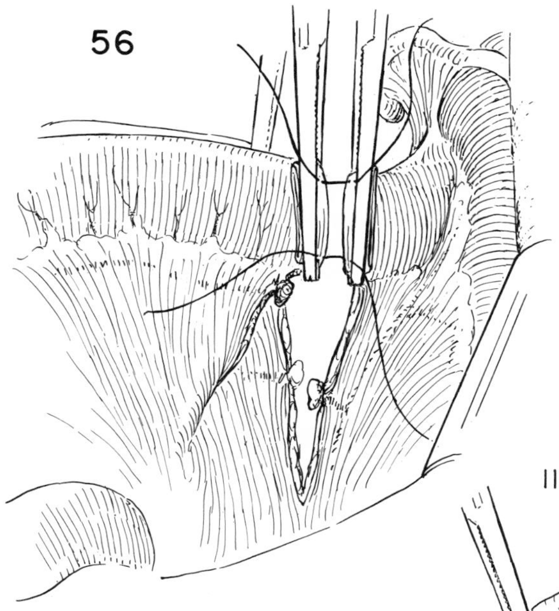

57

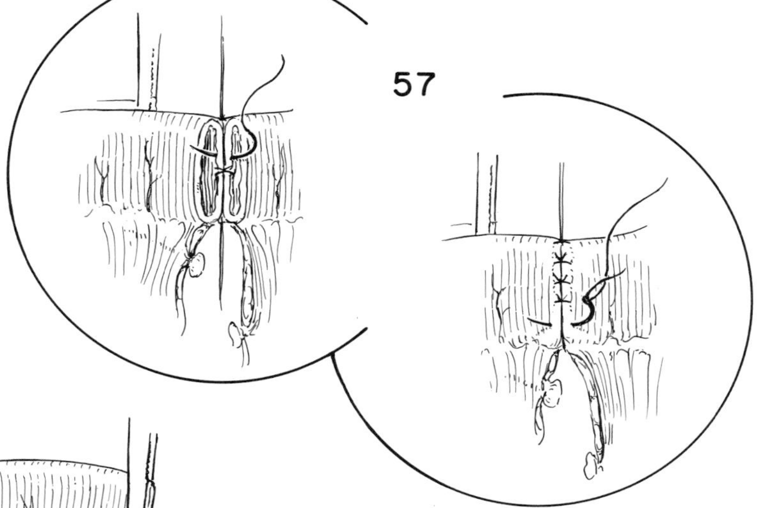

58

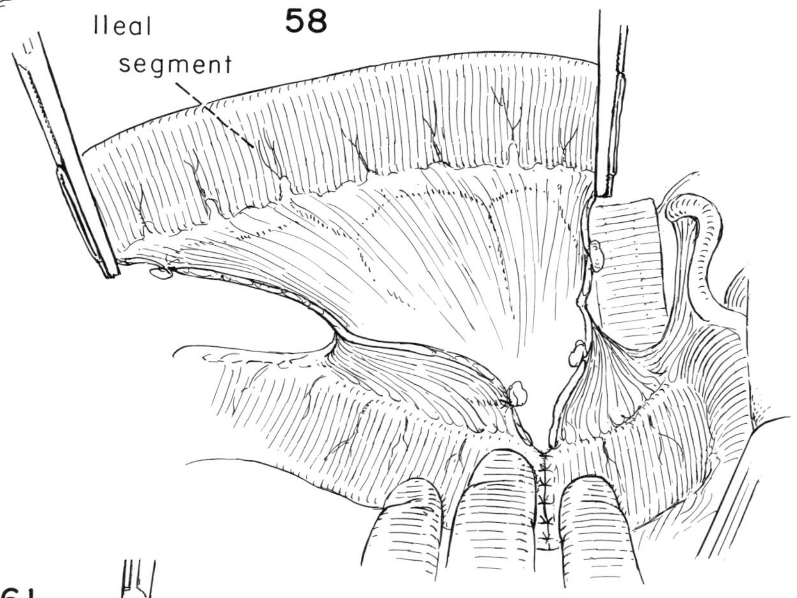
Ileal segment

59

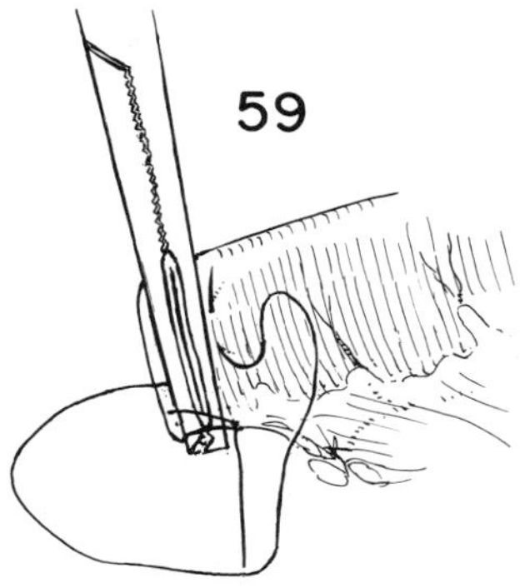

60

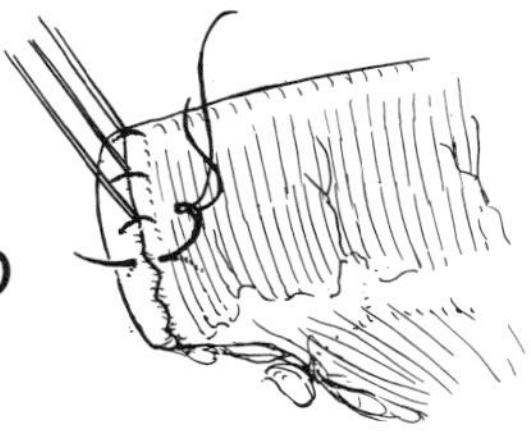

61

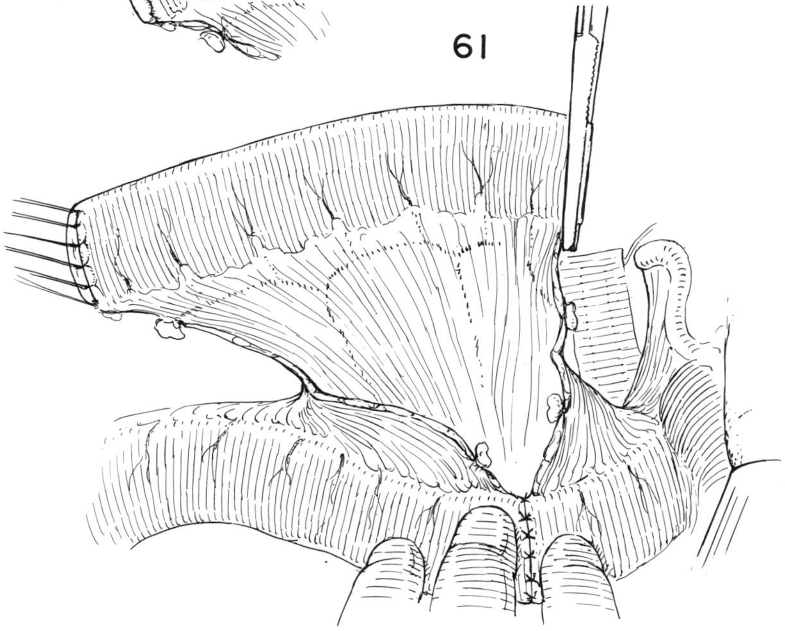

62

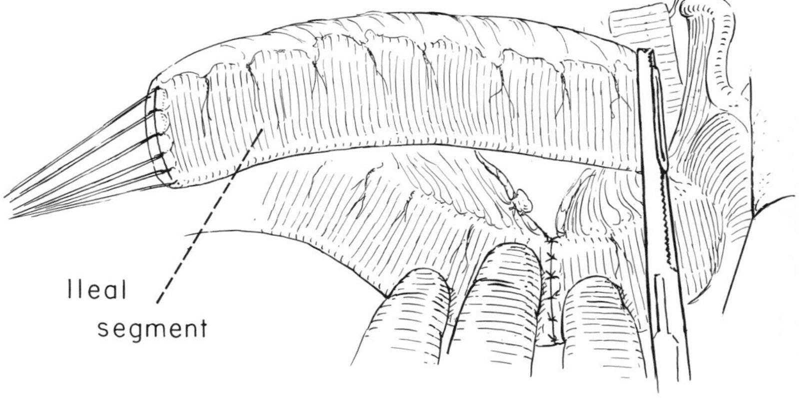
Ileal segment

Figure 63. The assistant holds the loop of bowel on tension as the surgeon incises the serosal and muscular coats of the bowel at the point selected for the anastomosis of the left ureter.

Figure 64. The assistant maintains traction on the silk sutures as the surgeon picks up the edge of the incision and dissects the mucosa of the bowel away from the muscle.

Figure 65. The surgeon grasps the bowel between thumb and forefinger on either side of the incision. This causes the mucosa to pout outward and allows the surgeon to excise with scissors a small circular segment just the right size for the ureter.

Figure 66. The left ureter is drawn toward the opening of the bowel. Interrupted catgut sutures are placed, fixing the periureteral tissues or peritoneum to the bowel wall below the bowel opening. Subsequent tension will then come on this and not on the ureteral anastomosis.

Figure 67. Fine No. 00000 chromic catgut sutures are placed in sequence from the outside into the lumen of the ureter and then from the inside of the bowel to the surface of the bowel. Each suture is then tied and cut. Enough sutures are placed to ensure complete closure, usually five or more. If the ureteral lumen is too small, it may be enlarged by a short axial incision.

Figure 68. The anastomosis has been completed on the left side. The steps are repeated on the right. The ureter is being fixed to the bowel by suturing the peritoneal flap to the bowel wall and the ureter will then be anastomosed to the bowel wall on the right side.

Figure 69. This view shows the anastomoses completed on the underside of the bowel and their relation to the closed end of the ileal loop.

Figure 70. The bowel is rotated back to its original position so that the uretero-intestinal anastomoses are now on the undersurface. In this location there is less danger of kinking of the ureter at the point at which it enters the bowel.

Figure 71. To prevent rotation of the loop the closed end is sutured to the periosteum of the promontory of the sacrum. The ends of suture, previously left long, can be rethreaded and used for this purpose.

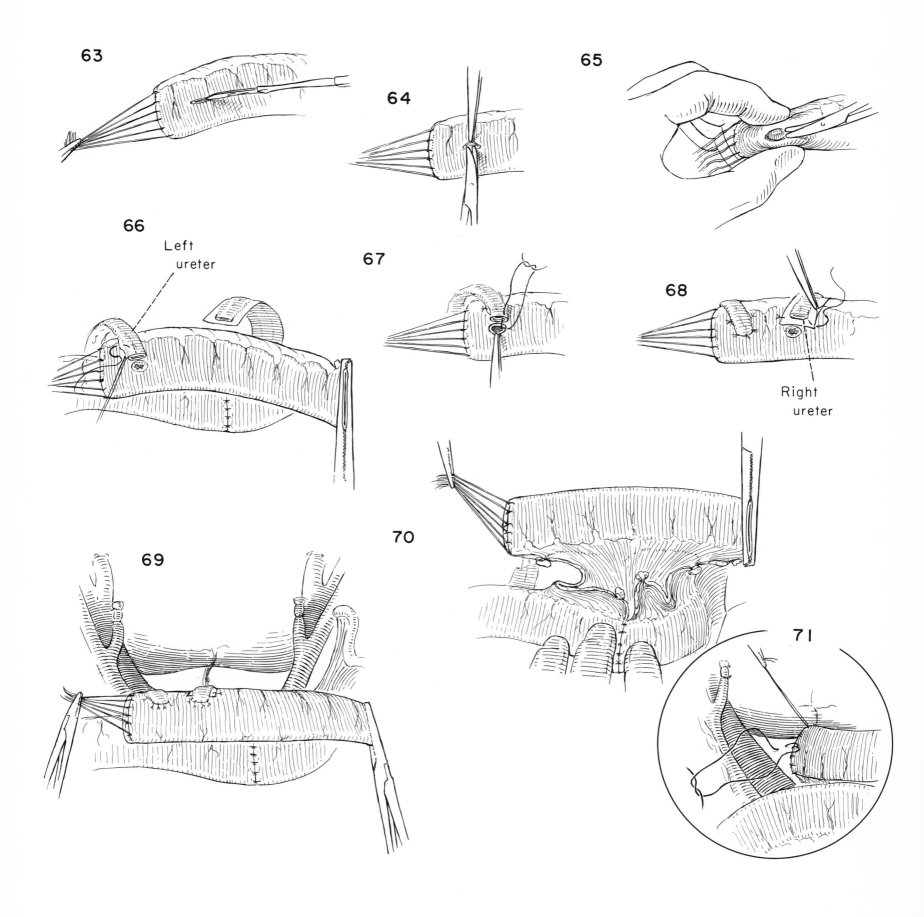

63

64

65

66

Left
ureter

67

68

Right
ureter

69

70

71

Figure 72. This view shows the appearance of the pelvis at this stage. Note that bowel continuity has been re-established and that the rent in the small bowel mesentery has been closed by tacking the edges down to the underlying mesentery of the ileal segment. The pelvis is clean of all structures and the Penrose drains can be seen as they pass out through the perineal skin defect.

All that remains for the surgeon to do is to construct the sigmoid and ileal loop ostia on the abdominal wall before closing the abdominal wall.

Figure 73. The self-retaining and all other retractors are withdrawn from the wound and the drapes are removed. The terminal end of the sigmoid with its gauze cover can be seen in the wound. Figures 73, 74, 75 and 76 demonstrate the technique of formation of the stoma. The formation of the opening in the abdominal wall is the same for both sigmoid colostomy and ileal conduit. The subsequent figures demonstrate only the steps for the ileal loop.

The skin is grasped with a Kocher clamp at a point on the abdominal wall sufficiently far removed from the wound and the anterior superior spine so that the collecting appliance can lie comfortably on a flat surface. The surgeon now excises a disk of skin with the knife held parallel to the surface.

Figure 74. The fat of the abdominal wall is teased away, exposing the underlying external oblique fascia.

Figure 75. Small retractors are placed in the wound to permit the surgeon either to remove a circle of fascia or, as in this illustration, to make relaxing cruciate incisions so that the fascial edges will not constrict the lumen of the bowel as it passes through the abdominal wall.

Figure 76. The surgeon then introduces his hand beneath the abdominal incision and elevates his fingers so that he can continue the dissection through the muscle and the peritoneum.

Figure 77. When the opening has been made the surgeon pushes his index finger through and prepares to introduce a Kocher clamp to grasp the end of the ileal loop by following the finger back through the wound into the peritoneal cavity.

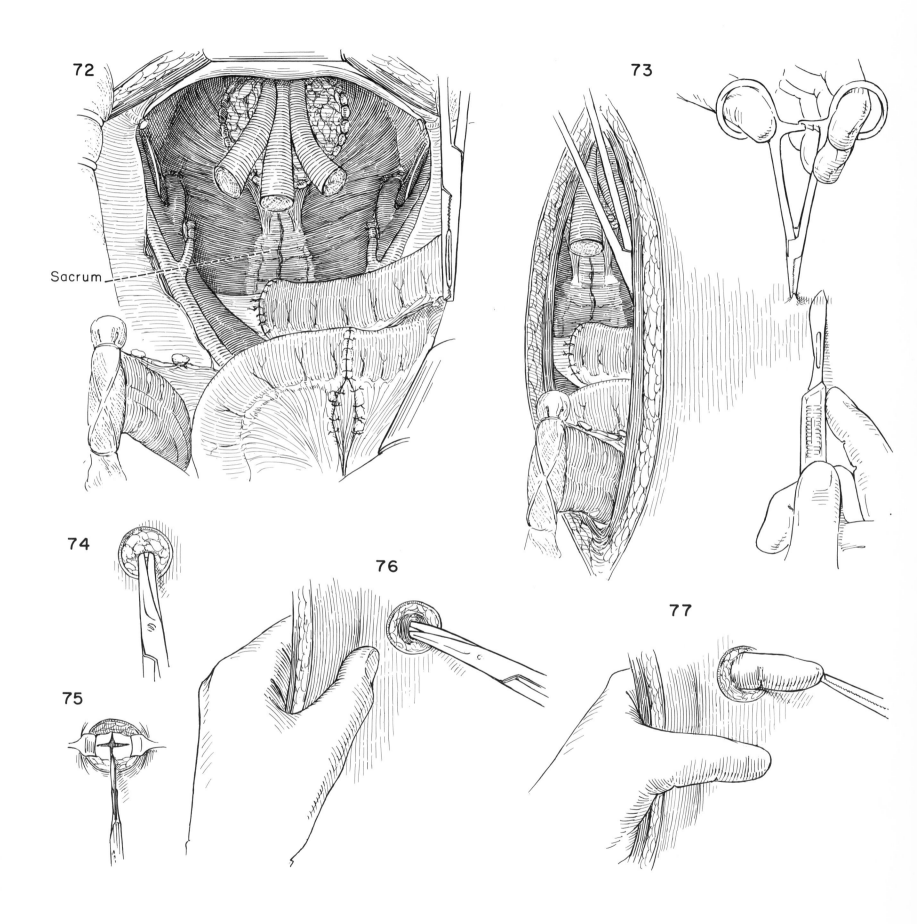

Sacrum

Figure 78. The Kocher clamp has been inserted through the opening and is about to grasp the end of the bowel just below the position of the original clamp. The latter is then removed.

Figure 79. The end of the ileal conduit is drawn through the opening on the abdominal wall. It should lie on the skin without tension.

Figure 80. The Kocher clamp is now removed. The surgeon grasps the edges of the bowel and trims off any excess fat. Great care must be taken not to traumatize any of the blood supply to the terminal end.

Figure 81. The ileostomy will function better if the surgeon can cuff the end. This is done by holding the end on tension and placing a suture which passes first through the skin, continuing on into the bowel wall at the point at which it adjoins the fascia and then again at the terminal end.

Figure 82. A series of these sutures are placed in similar fashion.

Figure 83. When all sutures are tied the mucosa has been everted and is attached to the skin throughout the circumference of the opening. When this maneuver is performed properly there is less danger of retraction of the bowel or stricture of the opening.

Figure 84. The formation of the sigmoid colostomy has not been shown in these illustrations but it must be done in exactly the same way before the abdomen is closed.

Because the operation has been performed for extensive malignant disease, optimum conditions for a solid wound repair do not exist. There is a tendency for these wounds to disrupt. For this reason closure is effected with interrupted sutures of heavy wire which are placed as stay sutures through all layers of the abdominal wall.

Figure 85. The wound is closed in one layer by approximating the wires. They should be loose enough to permit one to pass a finger under the loop. This illustration shows the final closure of the wound with enough additional skin silks to give good coaptation of the edges.

Figure 86. This illustration shows the position of the ostia on both sides in relation to the edges of the wound and to the anterosuperior spines.

78

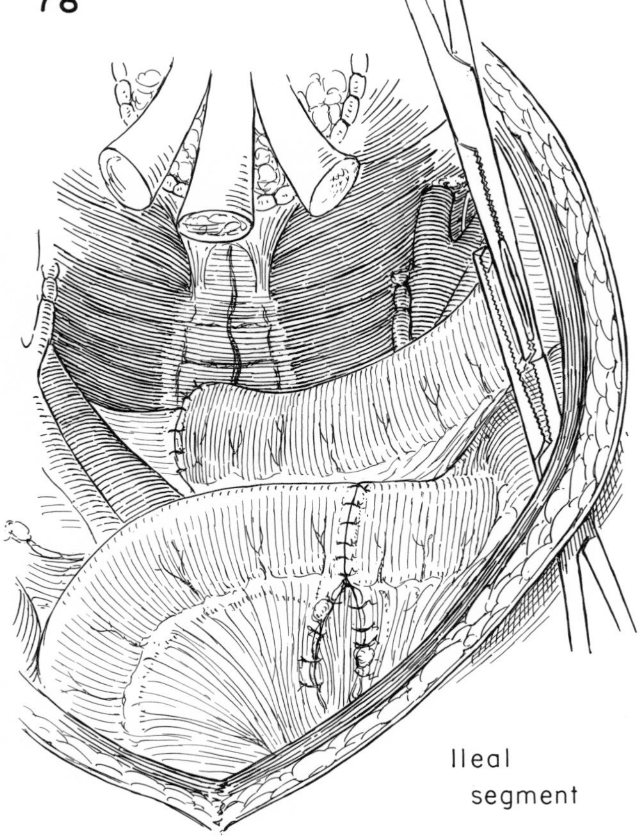
Ileal
segment

79

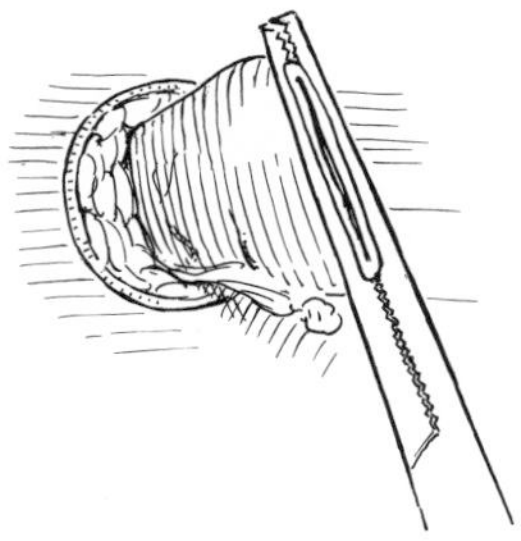

80

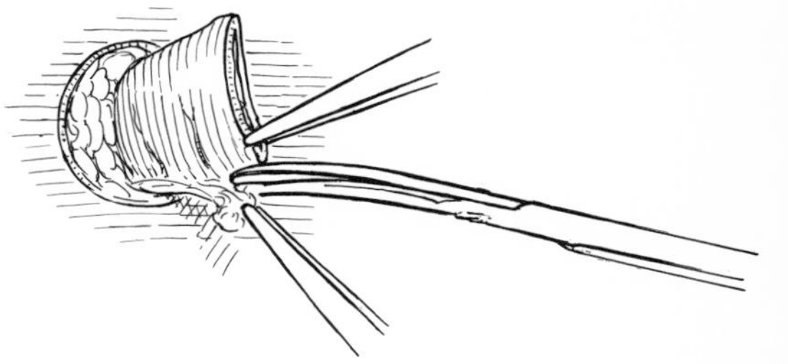

81

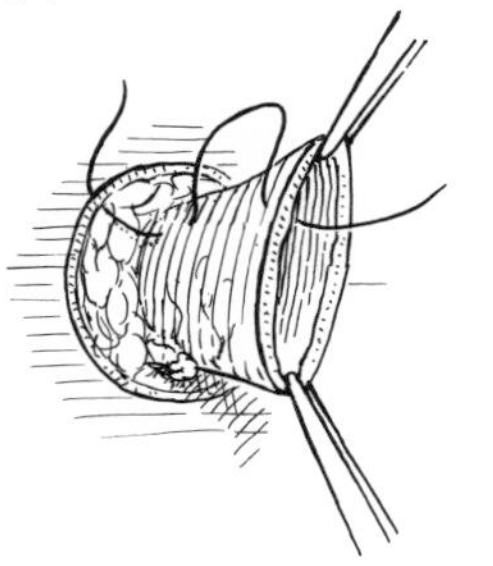

82

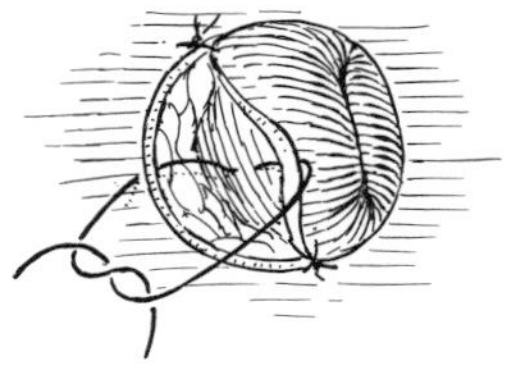

83

84

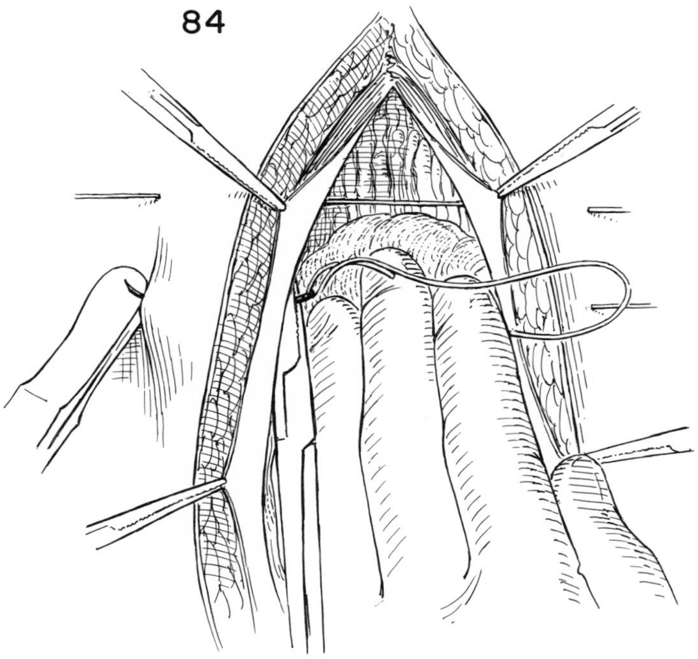

85

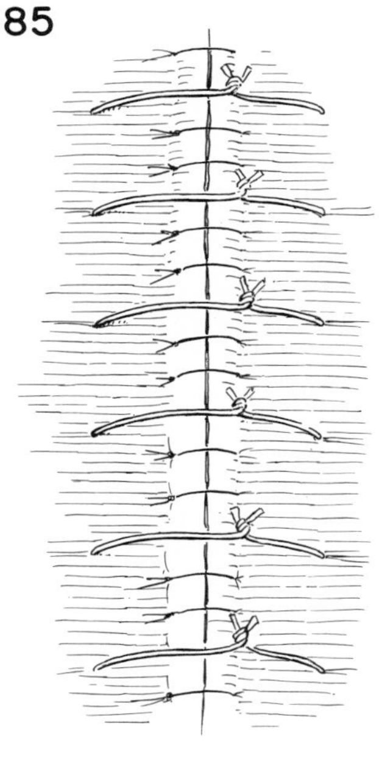

86

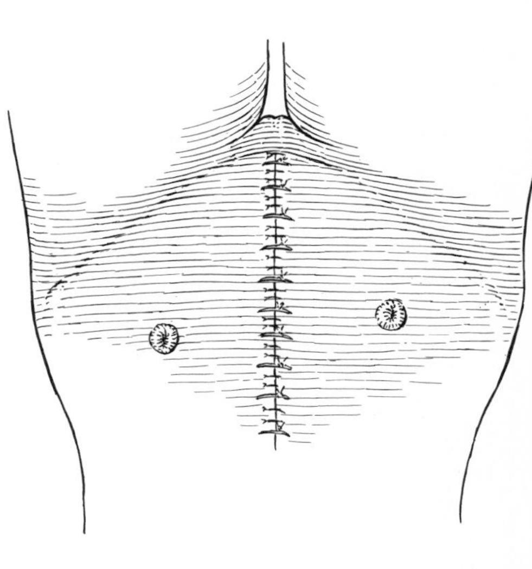

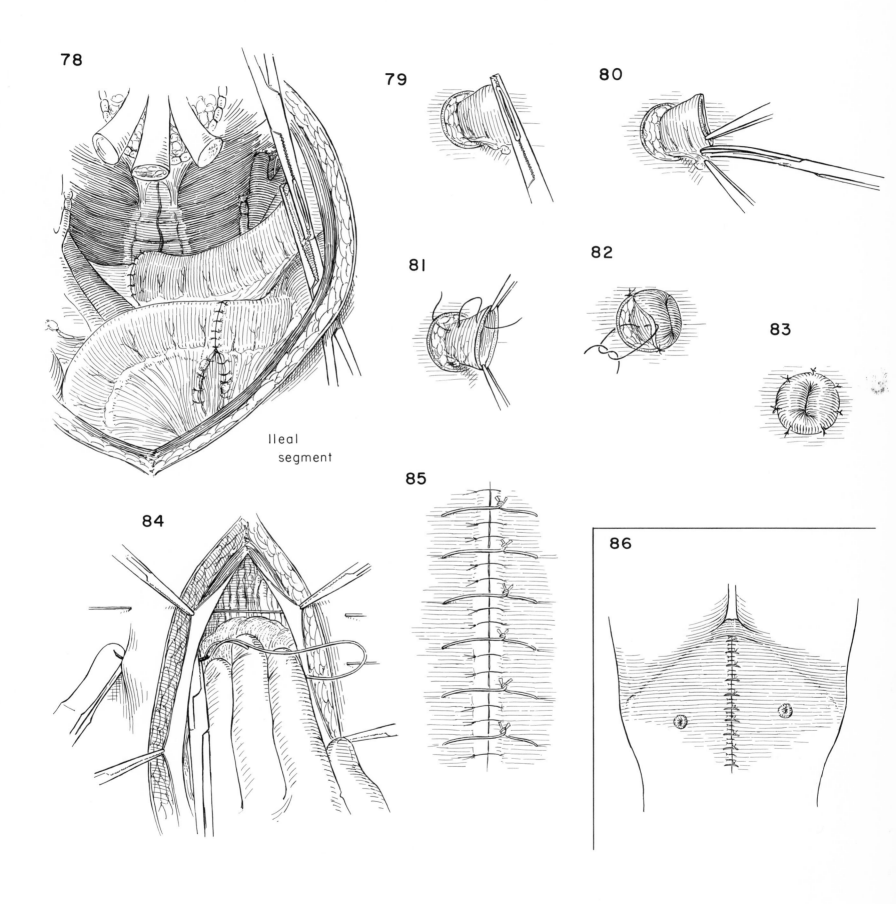

ANTERIOR PELVIC EXENTERATION

Carcinoma of the cervix may grow in an anterior or posterior direction. At times the tumor, while still quite localized, may encroach on or actually invade the bladder wall. When the surgeon finds that a Wertheim type of hysterectomy will be inadequate because of the proximity of tumor to the bladder, he may extend his operation to include the bladder. With the bladder removed it will be necessary to carry out diversion of the urinary stream into either an isolated loop of ileum or into the sigmoid.

The operative steps required to carry out both the anterior and the posterior exenteration frequently duplicate those used in procedures already illustrated in this atlas in great detail. Both procedures therefore will be demonstrated in somewhat abbreviated versions with appropriate reference made when indicated to previous illustrations.

The initial steps follow the pattern outlined for the Wertheim type of hysterectomy (pp. 325 to 329).

Figure 1. The assistant draws the uterus upward and backward by applying traction to a tenaculum placed on the fundus. A Deaver retractor exposes the anterior pelvic cavity. The surgeon has incised the anterior leaf of the peritoneum and developed the space with the index finger on both sides of the cervix lateral to the bladder wall. Kelly clamps are placed on the incised edge of the peritoneum. These clamps are held on tension as the surgeon divides the intervening peritoneum connecting the two spaces.

Figure 2. With the uterus held on tension and the bladder flap on traction the surgeon attempts to strip the bladder from the cervix. When abnormal adherence is found at this point he must decide whether it is wise to continue with this approach or whether removal of the bladder will be necessary. Although partial cystectomy has been performed in patients in whom only one well-localized point of penetration has been found, recurrence in the residual bladder is common and raises some doubt about the wisdom of this compromise.

Figure 3. The surgeon has elected to perform an anterior exenteration and incises the lateral pelvic peritoneum after first identifying the course of the ureter. The ureter lies on the medial leaf and can be seen in close proximity and medial to the ovarian vessels. This relationship must be established before a clamp is placed under the ovarian vessels to isolate them.

Figure 4. A ligature secures the vessels. A clamp is placed distal to the original tie. The surgeon elevates the ends of the suture which have been left long while the assistant does the same thing with the Kelly clamp. He then divides the vessels and secures the pedicle with a second tie.

Figure 5. The uterus is drawn upward and medially as the surgeon places a stitch ligature around the round ligament at two points close to the lateral wall. The surgeon then opens the peritoneum as the assistant lifts the sutures upward to keep the tissues on a flat plane.

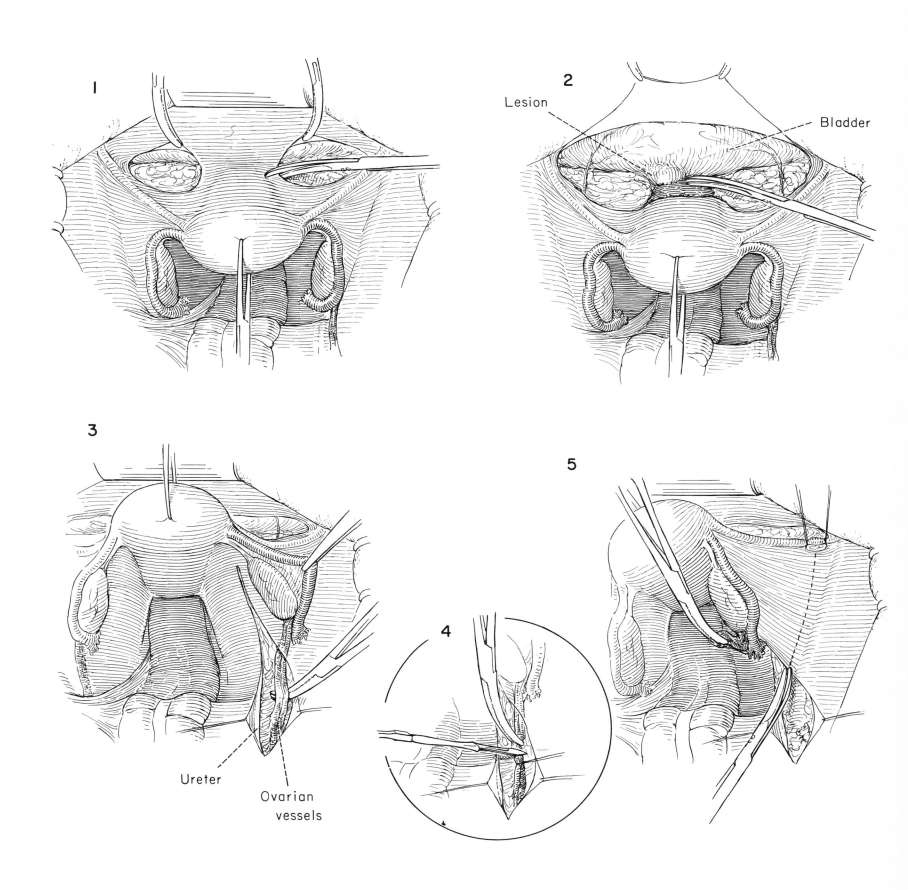

Figure 6. The uterus is drawn sharply to the left to keep the structures on tension. The lymphatic-bearing tissue has been dissected from the anterior surface of the internal iliac artery. The surgeon has identified the terminal uterine and hypogastric branches. A ligature is then placed around the artery at a point just proximal to the area at which the branches are seen. The suture has been tied but the ends left long. A clamp is placed across the vessel distal to the tie. As both the clamp and tie are held on tension the surgeon divides the artery. A second ligature is placed on the stump.

Figure 7. With the uterus held on tension the surgeon dissects the lymphatic tissue from the internal iliac vein, securing all vessels as they are encountered.

Figure 8. The ureter is identified and the surgeon then gently dissects it free from the underside of the medial leaf of the peritoneum well up toward the sacrum.

Figure 9. A ligature is applied distally and the assistant applies traction to elevate the ureter as the surgeon sections it with a knife at a level appropriate for the division procedure.

Figure 10. The cut proximal end of ureter is marked with a fine atraumatic suture which will not be tied but left long for future identification and retrieval.

Figure 11. The same dissection is carried out on the left side in the same sequence. The adnexa are tied up to the tenaculum on the fundus to keep them out of the operative field.

The assistants apply traction on the stay sutures placed on the medial leaf of the peritoneum. The sigmoid has been packed up out of the pelvis. The surgeon now prepares to incise the posterior peritoneum in the manner indicated in this illustration by a dotted line separating the pouch of Douglas from the parietal peritoneum and the rectosigmoid.

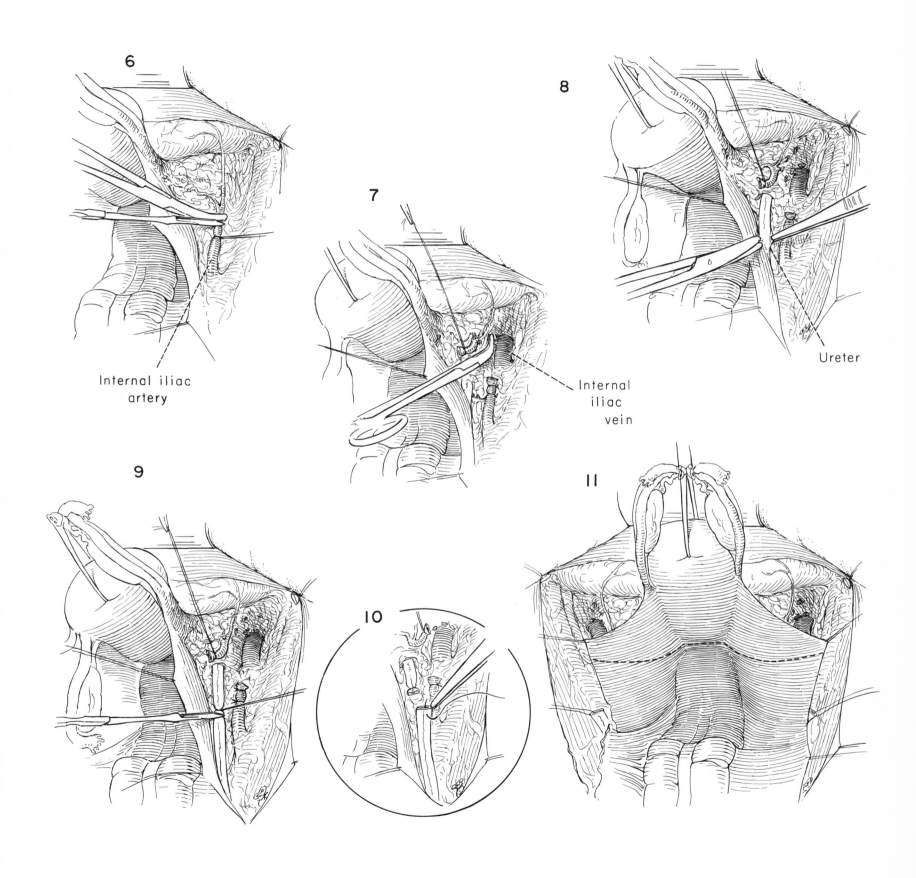

6

Internal iliac
artery

7

Internal
iliac
vein

8

Ureter

9

10

11

Figure 12. With the uterus held on tension upward and against the symphysis the surgeon begins the posterior dissection separating the rectum from the vaginal wall. The left hand placed flat on the sigmoid with the fingers pulling the rectal wall upward and backward helps to establish the proper cleavage plane.

Figure 13. When the cleavage plane is sufficiently developed the assistants elevate the entire specimen while the surgeon inserts his right hand with the palmar surface up into the space developed between rectum and posterior vaginal wall. Manipulation of the fingers will easily separate any remaining adhesions.

Figure 14. The uterus is again held backward and upward while the surgeon begins to divide the peritoneum overlying the bladder and along the anterior ramus of the pubis. The assistant holds the peritoneum upward with a clamp so that the surgeon may stay on a flat plane.

Figure 15. To identify the proper area in separating the bladder from the symphysis the surgeon places the flat surface of his left hand on the anterior surface of the specimen, curls the fingers and draws the mass backward and upward. Scissor dissection separates the bladder and urethra from the undersurface of the symphysis thereby widely opening the prevesical space.

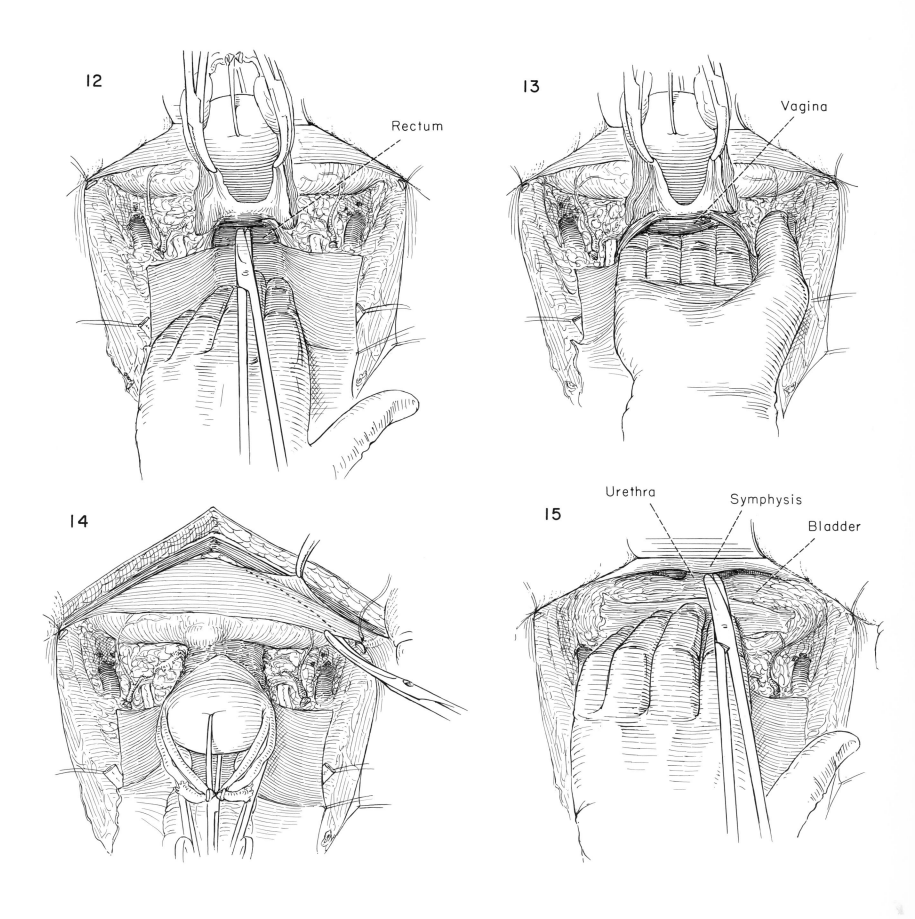

12

Rectum

13

Vagina

14

15

Urethra

Symphysis

Bladder

Figure 16. With the bladder freed anteriorly the surgeon now draws the mass toward the midline with the flat surface of the left hand and gently dissects the space between the specimen and the obturator fascia and the superior surface of the levator muscles on the floor of the pelvis.

Figure 17. The mass is held down by the deep uterosacral ligament on either side of the rectosigmoid. The ligament has been isolated by carrying the dissection down along the side of the rectum. (See p. 337.) This permits the surgeon to place a narrow Deaver retractor along the side of the rectum. The assistant holds the specimen upward and retracts the sigmoid as the surgeon places a large Moynihan clamp at the base of the ligament where it attaches to the posterior bony wall of the pelvis. The tissue within the clamp is cut and secured with a stitch ligature as the clamp is removed.

Figure 18. When the posterior attachments have been sectioned bilaterally, the specimen can easily be drawn upward to provide a better exposure of the lower end of the vaginal canal. A careful dissection is essential and a clear view of the anatomy must be obtained to avoid damaging the anterior wall of the rectum. The secret to the necessary exposure is again traction.

Figure 19. With the posterior dissection completed the specimen is again drawn backward and upward to expose the anterior vaginal wall and the urethra. The separation has been carried out well under the symphysis and its anterior surface. When, as in this case, ample margin below the tumor is apparent, it is permissible to complete excision entirely from above. The urethra is cut across as shown here at the level at which it disappears through the urogenital diaphragm.

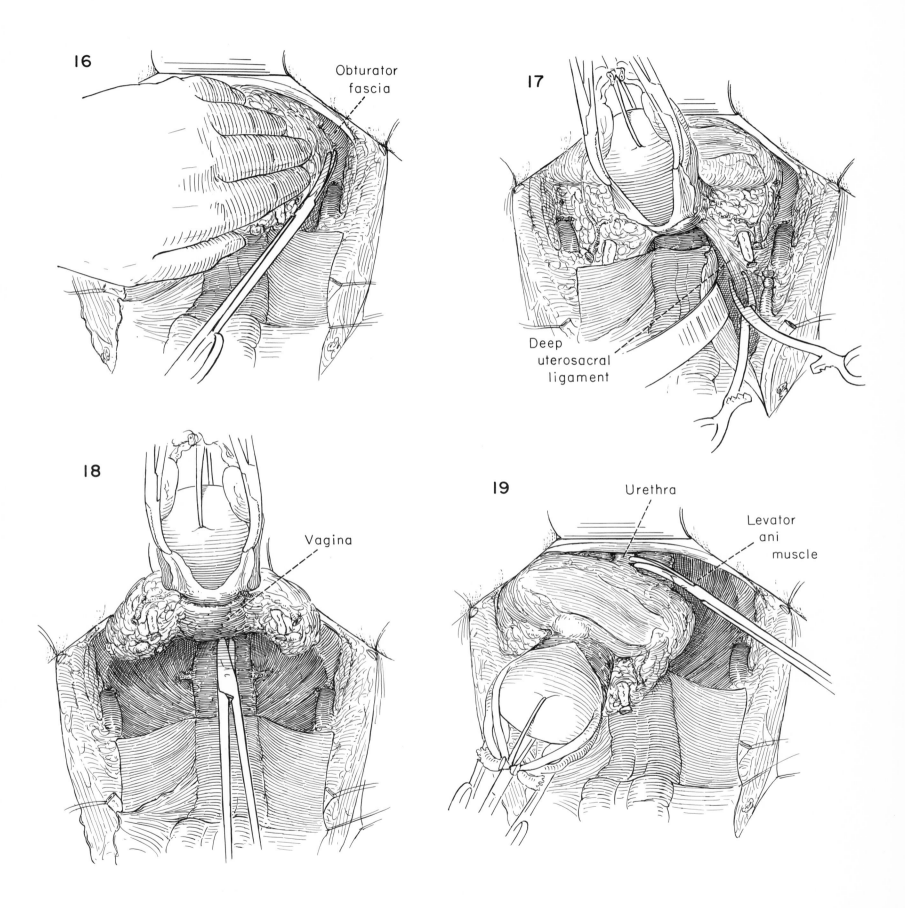

16   Obturator fascia

17   Deep uterosacral ligament

18   Vagina

19   Urethra   Levator ani muscle

Figure 20. The extirpative portion of the dissection has been completed except for the transection of the vagina.

The assistant draws the specimen upward and backward, placing it on tension. Under direct vision the surgeon places Heaney clamps on the edges of the vaginal wall on either side as far down the canal as possible. The vagina is then transected just above the level of the clamps and the specimen is removed.

Figure 21. The tissues included in the clamps on the angles of the vaginal stump are secured with stitch ligatures. The ends of the sutures are left long to provide traction and exposure.

Figure 22. The surgeon now carries out a running, over-and-over lock stitch around the circumference of the vaginal stump for hemostasis. This suture may be placed with ease if the assistant makes extra traction on the Deaver retractor and pulls upward on the long sutures on the lateral margin of the vaginal stump. The vagina is further displayed by traction on a Kocher clamp on its posterior margin.

Figure 23. This illustration shows the appearance of the lower pelvis after the specimen has been removed. Note the cleaned levator ani muscles on the pelvic floor, the vagina, the stumps of the urethra and vessels, the anterior surface of the rectum and the ureters.

Figure 24. With the specimen removed the surgeon now has ample room to carry out pelvic lymphadenectomy under direct vision, which permits him to do this more efficiently with less expenditure of time. (For details see pp. 343 to 347.)

The dissection begins lateral to the external iliac vessels on the surface of the psoas muscle and is carried down over the medial border of psoas. The superior portion of the obturator space is soon entered.

Mobilization of the vessels and development of the obturator space makes the obturator dissection easier and safer. If any bleeding is encountered it can be dealt with from either the lateral side or from beneath the vein.

Figure 25. The lymphatic tissue has been cleaned from the external, common and internal iliac artery, and the intermediate chain between the external artery and vein has been dissected.

With the vessels mobilized a vein retractor is inserted beneath the external iliac vessels to provide more exposure for the surgeon as he dissects the lymph-bearing tissue from the obturator space lying above and medial to the obturator nerve.

Pelvic lymphadenectomy is carried out on both sides.

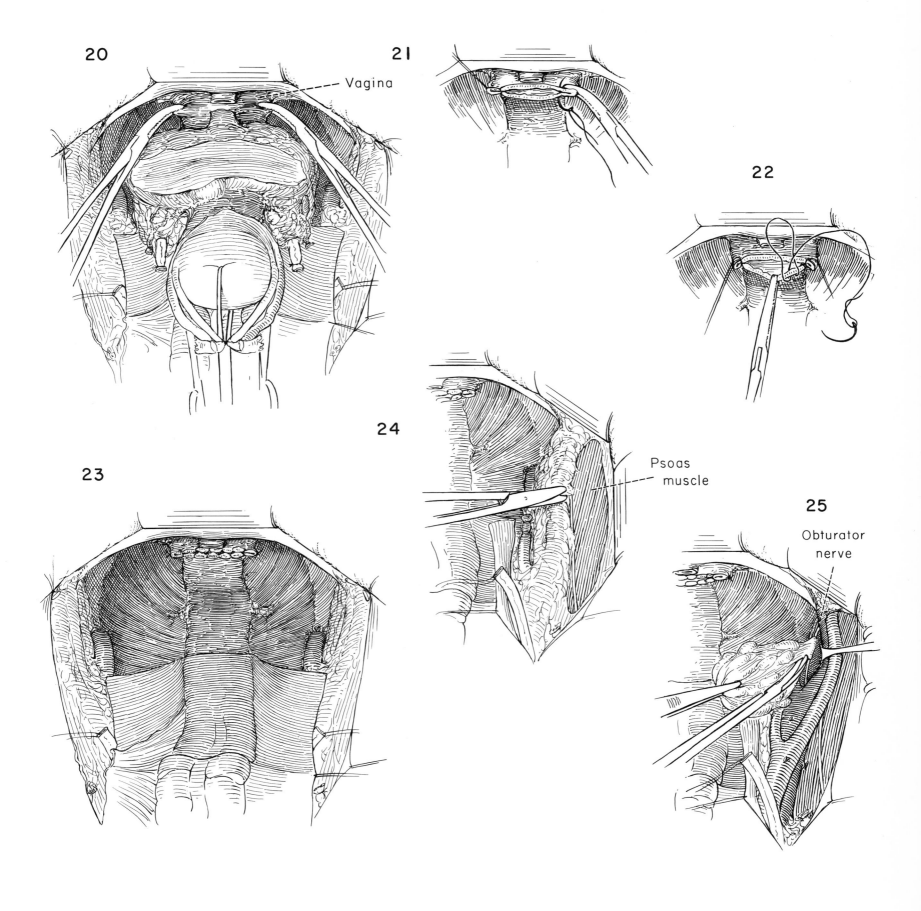

20

21

22

Vagina

23

24

25

Psoas
muscle

Obturator
nerve

The extirpative phase of the operation has been completed. The major problem now is concerned with the diversion of the urinary stream. This may be done by implanting the ureters into the intact colon, or by isolating a loop of ileum and anastomosing the ureters to it. Ureterosigmoidostomy has the distinct advantage of avoiding any ostium on the abdominal wall. There are two major disadvantages: urine tends to collect within the bowel, thereby increasing the tendency toward resorption and hyperchloremic acidosis; and the mucoid secretion from the sigmoid mucosa tends to plug the anastomotic openings and enhance the likelihood of ascending infection and pyelonephritis. For these reasons and others we prefer to use the isolated ileal segment and transplant the ureters into it.

Figure 26. In this illustration the portion of small intestine destined to serve as the ileal conduit has been outlined. Note the length of bowel to be isolated and the distance from the cecum.

To avoid angulation of the ureter an opening is made in the posterior peritoneum and care is taken not to damage the arterial supply to the large bowel. The open ends of the ureters can be seen with stay sutures attached as they are brought to this opening. Note that the left ureter must be led beneath the mesocolon and the inferior mesenteric artery. Avoid stretching or twisting it.

Figure 27. The continuity of the small intestine has been restored. The proximal end of the isolated loop has been closed with catgut and reinforced with interrupted silk sutures which are held long. (For details see pp. 407 to 409.)

Figure 28. The left ureter should be anastomosed to the loop at a point where it will lie easily without angulation or tension. In this instance the ureter is being brought out through the opening in the posterior peritoneum to a point on the lateral aspect of the bowel close to the closed end. There it is anastomosed in the fashion previously described.

Figure 29. The optimum position for the right ureter in this situation is the surface of the bowel opposite to the left ureteral transplant.

The assistant swings the bowel toward the left side by moving the clamp on the distal end in this direction. The right ureter is then transplanted into the bowel lumen in the same manner as the left ureter.

Figure 30. The closed end of the ileal segment is then fixed to the posterior wall by rethreading the silk sutures left long on the stump and attaching them to the presacral fascia.

Figure 31. The peritoneal opening is now loosely attached to the circumference of the bowel above the anastomoses. This takes all tension off them and allows the ureters to remain retroperitoneal in position with a minimum of dislocation.

The opening in the mesentery of the reconstructed segment of ileum is tacked down to the underlying mesentery of the isolated segment to prevent internal hernias, but no effort is made to close the large gutter between the loop and the lateral abdominal wall.

The open end of the loop is brought out in the right lower quadrant and fixed to the skin. The pelvic peritoneum can usually be closed with only moderate tension. The large dead space below it should be drained with cigarette wicks or with suction catheters.

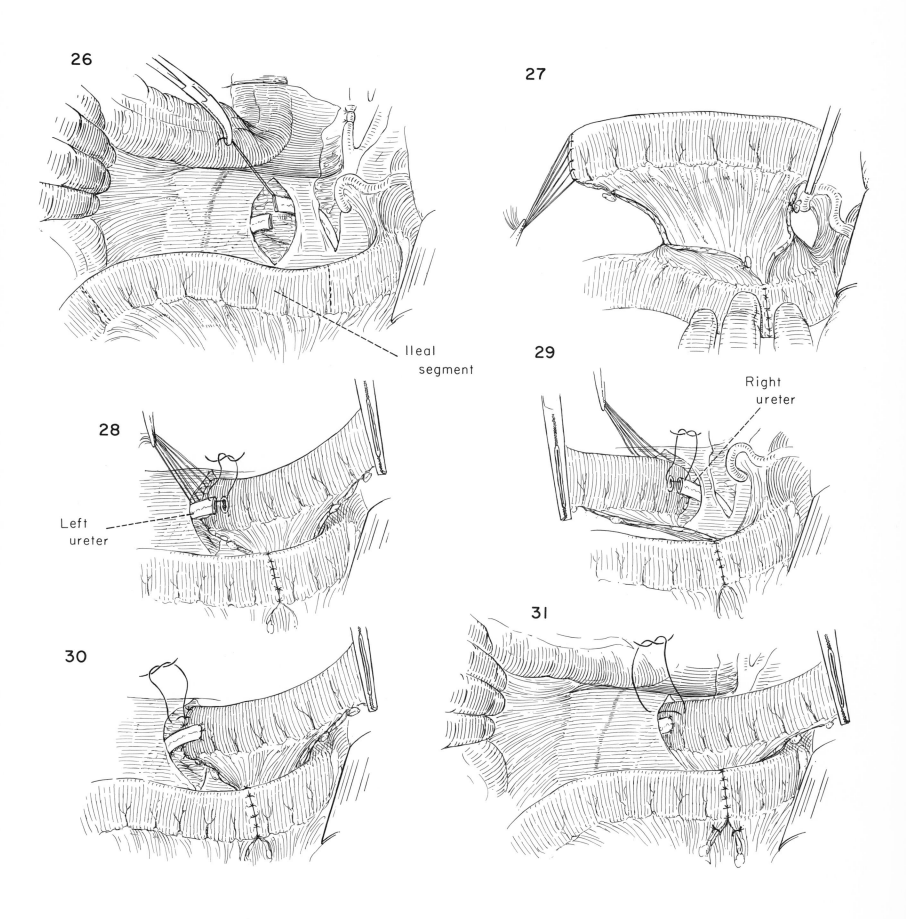

26

27

28   Left
ureter

29   Right
ureter

Ileal
segment

30

31

Perineal Dissection

When the lesion requires more distal resection than has been shown so far, as may be the case in extensive spread of the malignant disease from the cervix to the vagina or when the primary tumor arises in the lower urinary tract, a perineal phase is also performed. In this case the urethra and vagina are not transected from above.

INSET A. The central specimen has been freed completely to a level at or below the levators. It is then pushed deep into the pelvis and the peritoneal floor closed over it. The ileal loop diversion is performed and the abdominal incision closed.

Figure 1. The patient is then placed in lithotomy position and the vulva circumscribed with an elliptical incision which extends only so far laterally as the disease demands. The incision is carried across the perineum between the fourchette and the anus.

Figure 2. The skin incision is deepened to the underlying fascia. Rake retractors maintain wide exposure. The skin and fat are dissected off the fascia. The vessels to the clitoris coming down over the symphysis pubis are clamped, cut and tied.

Figure 3. This is the most important part of the perineal dissection. The vagina must be dissected free from the anterior wall of the anus and rectum. This is best accomplished by placing clamps on the edges of the incision below the fourchette and having the assistant hold them on tension. The assistants keep the operative field open by pulling on the rake retractors.

The surgeon inserts the index finger of his left hand into the anal opening and elevates the bowel as he gently strips the vaginal wall from that of the anus and rectum. This is done in this instance by blunt dissection with the handle of the scalpel.

Figure 4. With the posterior dissection complete the surgeon now continues with the separation of the vulva. Individual vessels are clamped and tied as they are found. The chief vessels encountered are the perineal vessels which run in the fatty tissue in the lower third. The tension provided by the rake retractor helps in making the identification. When found they are clamped, divided and ligated with a chromic catgut stitch.

Figure 5. The surgeon then depresses the mass with the flat surface of the left hand and separates the tissue from beneath the symphysis with the knife handle. When the urogenital diaphragm is reached, he breaks through close to the bone and enters the pelvic cavity and the area of dissection previously developed from above.

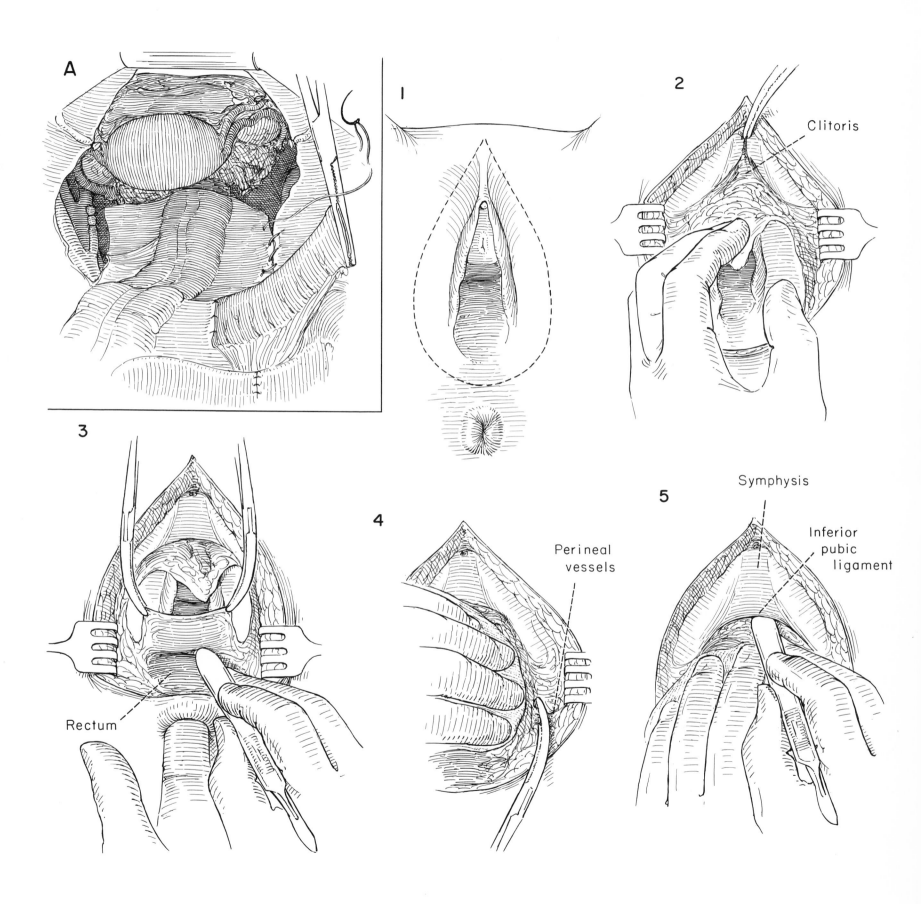

A

1

2

Clitoris

3

Rectum

4

Perineal
vessels

5

Symphysis

Inferior
pubic
ligament

Figure 6. As the surgeon continues to free the central mass from the rami of the pubic bone, he soon encounters the ischiocavernosus muscle on either side. It must be clamped, cut and secured.

Figure 7. As the dissection continues posteriorly the bulbocavernosus muscle is found at the point at which it leaves its circumferential location at the vaginal outlet and joins the transverse perineal band. The bulbocavernosus muscles are both clamped and cut and the dissection then joins with the space previously exposed between vagina and rectum.

Figure 8. With the urogenital diaphragm thus cut free, the true pelvis is entered and the levators visualized. Further dissection along the vaginal wall separates the central mass from levator muscles and frees it completely.

Figure 9. The surgeon then reaches into the prevesical space with the right hand and delivers the specimen. Further separation from the rectum or the levators may be necessary before it can be removed.

Figure 10. With the specimen out of the way the surgeon applies a stitch ligature around any clamps left and ties them as the clamps are removed. Note the levator muscles visible on either side at a deeper level.

Figure 11. Penrose drains are placed in the perineal defect and sutured to the skin. The drains extend upward into the pelvic cavity. The skin edges are then approximated in the midline with interrupted silk sutures. Occasionally, the levators can be loosely approximated at one end or the other to help in the reconstruction of the pelvic floor.

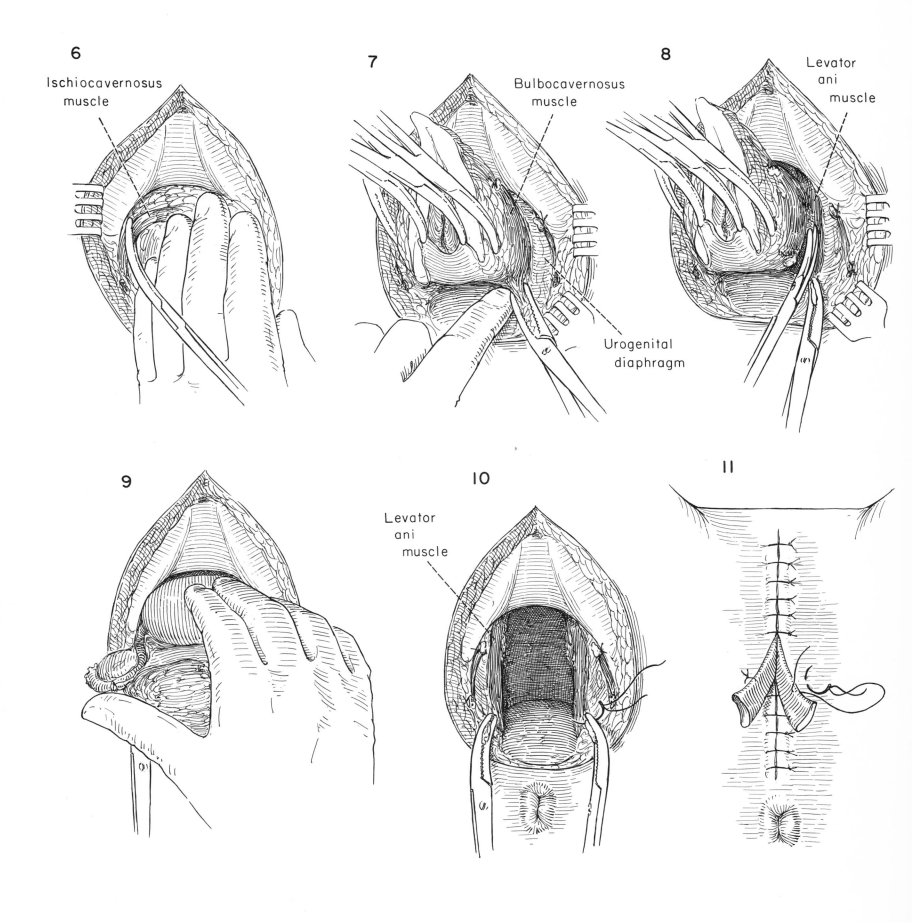

6

Ischiocavernosus
muscle

7

Bulbocavernosus
muscle

Urogenital
diaphragm

8

Levator
ani
muscle

9

10

Levator
ani
muscle

11

POSTERIOR PELVIC EXENTERATION

On rare occasions the surgeon may encounter disease which would make the posterior type of exenteration a reasonable procedure. The difference between an anterior and posterior exenteration focuses on the urological aspects. In contrast to the anterior exenteration the bladder and ureters are not removed. A Wertheim type of hysterectomy is combined with an en bloc resection of the rectum and a pelvic lymphadenectomy.

Figure 1. The initial steps in preparation of an operative field that will permit posterior exenteration follow the same plan outlined for the Wertheim procedure. (See p. 325.)

The fundus of the uterus is held on tension while the surgeon first develops the lateral aspects of the bladder flap and then divides the peritoneum between the two openings as the assistant elevates the peritoneum with Kelly clamps.

Figure 2. The assistant draws the uterus to the midline away from the side to be dissected. The assistant holds the adnexa out of the operative field with forceps. The surgeon identifies the course of the ureter in its upper portion, where the ureter crosses the common iliac artery and where the ovarian vessels and ureter are in close proximity. The peritoneum is opened lateral to the ureter, and stay sutures are placed on the incised medial edge. The surgeon draws the peritoneum medially by traction on these sutures. This permits him to tease the ovarian vessels away from the ureter and allows him to place a right-angled clamp under them and draw a suture through and tie it.

Figure 3. The ends are left long for the purpose of exposure through traction. The surgeon places a clamp on the vessels distal to the tie. Both clamp and tie are elevated as the surgeon divides the vessel, clamps the stump of the vessel distal to the tie and secures it with a second stitch ligature.

Figure 4. The uterus is drawn toward the midline and the round ligament is doubly secured by chromic catgut stitch ligation. The ends are left long after being tied. The surgeon then divides the posterior leaf of the broad ligament and the round ligament.

Figure 5. The anterior and lateral fields of dissection have now been joined and the entire side wall of the pelvis is exposed. All the important anatomic structures can be identified. Note the method of holding round ligament and adnexa up out of the field by tying them to the tenaculum. The uterus is drawn sharply toward the midline. Traction is exerted on the stay sutures on the medial leaf of the peritoneum. The ureter can be seen on its undersurface. The areolar tissue has been dissected from the anterior surface of the internal iliac artery.

Since the bladder is to be left intact it is important to identify the hypogastric and superior vesical arteries. After isolating the uterine artery at its point of origin on the internal iliac artery the surgeon clamps it distal to the point at which the superior vesical and other branches arise.

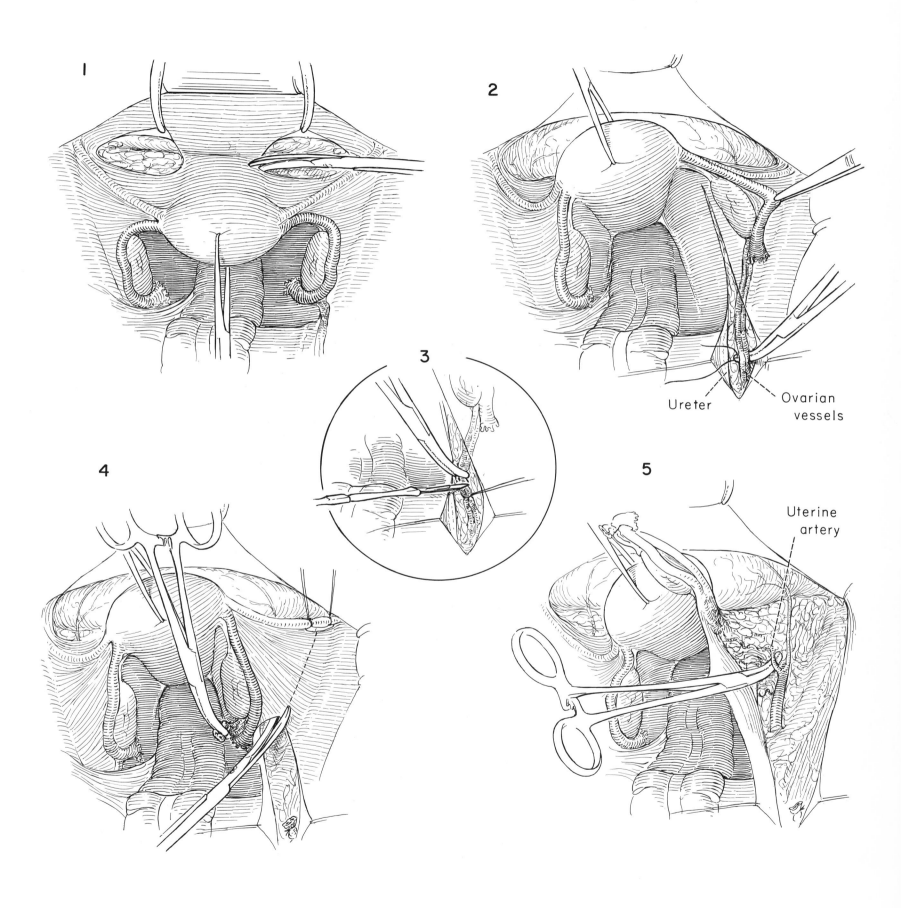

1

2

Ureter   Ovarian
                vessels

3

4

5

Uterine
artery

Figure 6. After dividing and doubly ligating the uterine artery the surgeon gently elevates the hypogastric and superior vesical arteries with round blunt-end forceps and dissects the lymphatic tissue from the underside so that the vessels are lying free. Carrying this dissection deeper along the medial aspect of the iliac vessels, he enters and defines the paravesical space. These steps are repeated on both sides.

Figure 7. The surgeon now moves to dissect the bladder away from the anterior surface of the cervix and the vaginal wall. The assistant draws the uterus upward and backward to provide tension on the tissues. This step helps in identifying the proper cleavage plane. Injury to the bladder is avoided by holding it up gently with ring forceps. The surgeon then dissects the bladder wall from the underlying vagina.

Figure 8. An assistant draws the uterus toward the midline and holds the stay suture on the medial peritoneal edge on tension. The surgeon then gently separates the ureter from the undersurface of the peritoneum. The arterial branch to the ureter which takes origin on the internal iliac should be identified and preserved and the periureteral vascular plexus carefully handled. This plane of dissection is followed until the pararectal space has been developed.

Figure 9. The uterus is drawn firmly toward the midline. The bladder wall is elevated with forceps and the ureter identified at the point along the lateral vaginal wall at which it emerges from below the canal made up of the uterine artery and vein and their branches. This can be a very bloody area. After establishment of the anatomic relationships a small Moynihan clamp is introduced into the canal above the ureter which lies beneath the vessels. Traction on a vein retractor placed beneath the ureter will help the surgeon to place two clamps safely across the vascular bridge and divide it. This step unroofs the canal.

Figure 10. The vessels included in the clamps are secured with chromic catgut stitch ligatures. The sutures are tied and the clamps are removed.

Figure 11. The assistant continues to apply tension on the vein retractor so that the ureter maintains a straight course and does not kink. The surgeon elevates the overhanging edge of the bladder wall and divides the bloodless areolar tissue above the ureter to complete unroofing of the canal.

These steps are carried out on both sides.

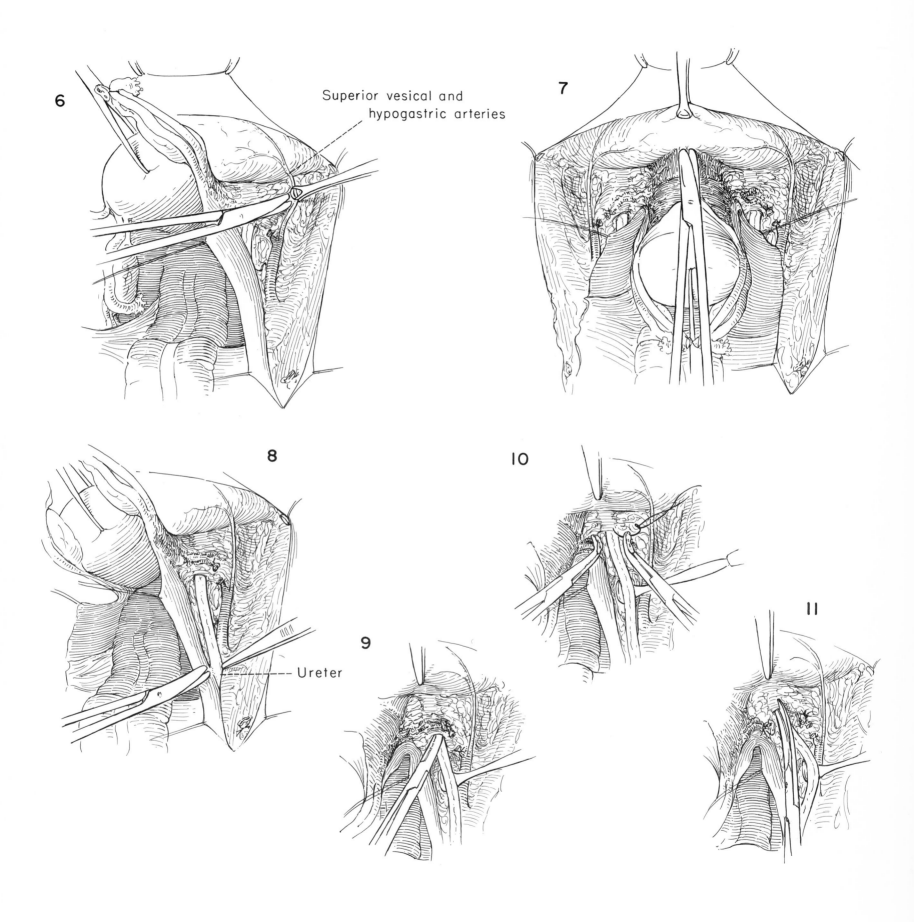

6

Superior vesical and
hypogastric arteries

7

8

Ureter

10

9

11

Figure 12. The course of the ureter into the bladder wall is outlined and freed from all tissue by having the assistant elevate the ureter as the surgeon picks up the adjacent bladder wall and gently dissects the ureter free from its bed. This dissection continues well below the point where the ureter disappears into the bladder wall.

Figure 13. The lateral bladder extension is now freed from the parametrial tissues. To provide exposure the assistant pulls on a vein retractor placed beneath the superior vesical and hypogastric vessels. This must be done gently for they can be very easily divided if the traction is too forceful.

Figure 14. With the dissection in and around the ureters and bladder completed the surgeon now selects the point on the sigmoid wall where he wishes to divide the bowel. The uterus is drawn toward the symphysis and the sigmoid back toward the patient's head. With the mesentery on tension its peritoneum is divided on both sides. An effort is made to preserve as much of the peritoneal covering of the two ureters as possible.

Figure 15. The individual vessels in the mesocolon are doubly clamped, divided and secured with a stitch ligature until the entire mesentery has been sectioned.

Figure 16. The bowel is then transected between clamps. The clamp on the proximal end which will serve as the terminal colostomy is covered with gauze in the manner previously described in the technique of total exenteration. (See p. 397.) The distant portion of the bowel is treated differently. Since the final extirpative steps are to be carried out from below, the clamp on the open end of the distal colon must be removed. A piece of rubber drain or glove is firmly tied around the open end as the clamp is removed.

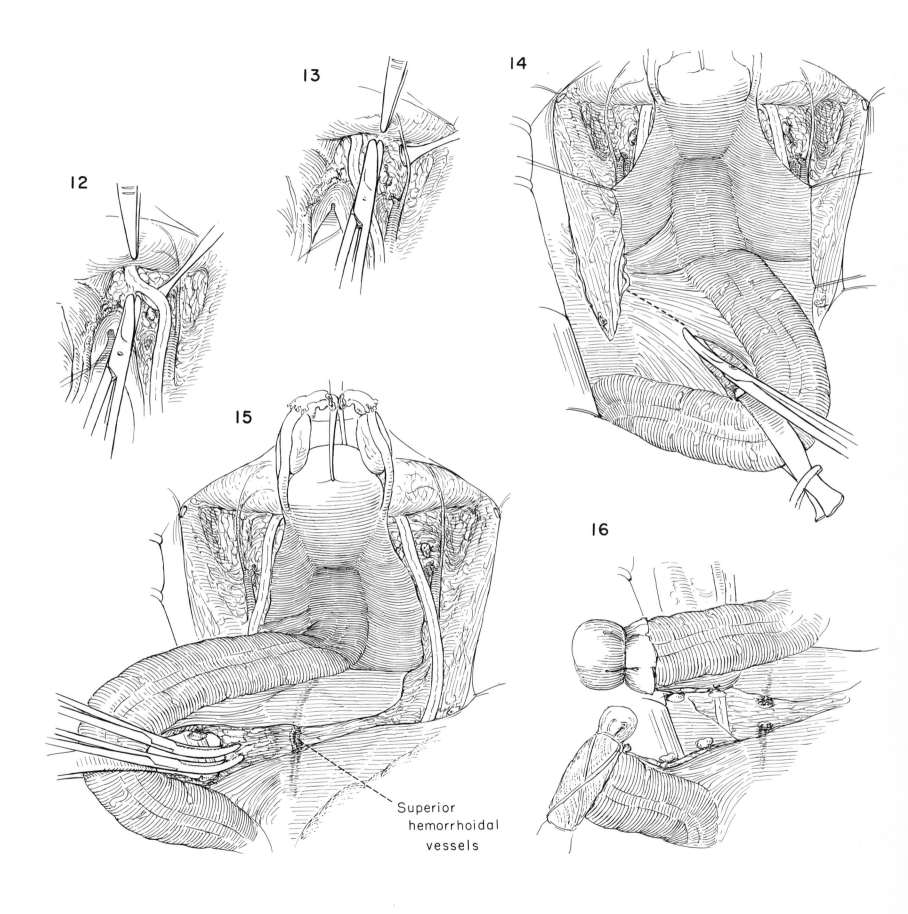

12

13

14

15

16

Superior
hemorrhoidal
vessels

Figure 17. The sigmoid has been transected and the open ends covered. The mesentery of the sigmoid has been developed by incising it and applying individual stitch ligatures to the vessels as they are identified. The assistant places the uterus on traction as the surgeon inserts his right hand behind the rectosigmoid and gently separates the attachments of the bowel to the posterior bony wall of the pelvis.

Figure 18. The surgeon then elevates the specimen which contains the uterus and rectum toward the midline while the assistant retracts the ureter.

The deep uterosacral and cardinal ligament pedicles are then secured with long-handled Moynihan clamps in pairs. These are immediately replaced with suture ligatures. The surgeon will be well advised to apply the initial stitch ligature on the medial clamp. When it is tied and the clamp removed, more room is provided for applying and tying the tissue within the lateral clamp. These clamps are deep in the pelvis, the lateral clamp containing the blood vessels at their point of origin. There is a tendency for these ties to slip out of the clamp as they are ligated. They can be more readily grasped and the bleeding controlled if the surgeon has a free space in which to work.

Figure 19. The surgeon continues to place the tissues on tension by drawing the mass upward and toward the midline as he applies clamps in sequential fashion across the "web." The tissue between them is divided.

In this illustration the Moynihan clamp is being placed across the middle hemorrhoidal vessels. The clamps will continue to be applied and the tissue divided and sutured until the specimen is freed of all attachments to the side wall of the pelvis.

Figure 20. The steps previously outlined are duplicated for the opposite side.

The assistant then draws the specimen backward and upward toward the head of the patient. The surgeon places clamps on the lateral edges of the vaginal wall on both sides. The tissue between the clamps is divided and each clamp is replaced with a stitch ligature. After being tied the ends of the ligatures are left long and clamped.

Traction is placed on them as the surgeon holds the bladder wall back with the forceps handle and completes the transection of the anterior vaginal wall. This is usually at the level of the bladder neck.

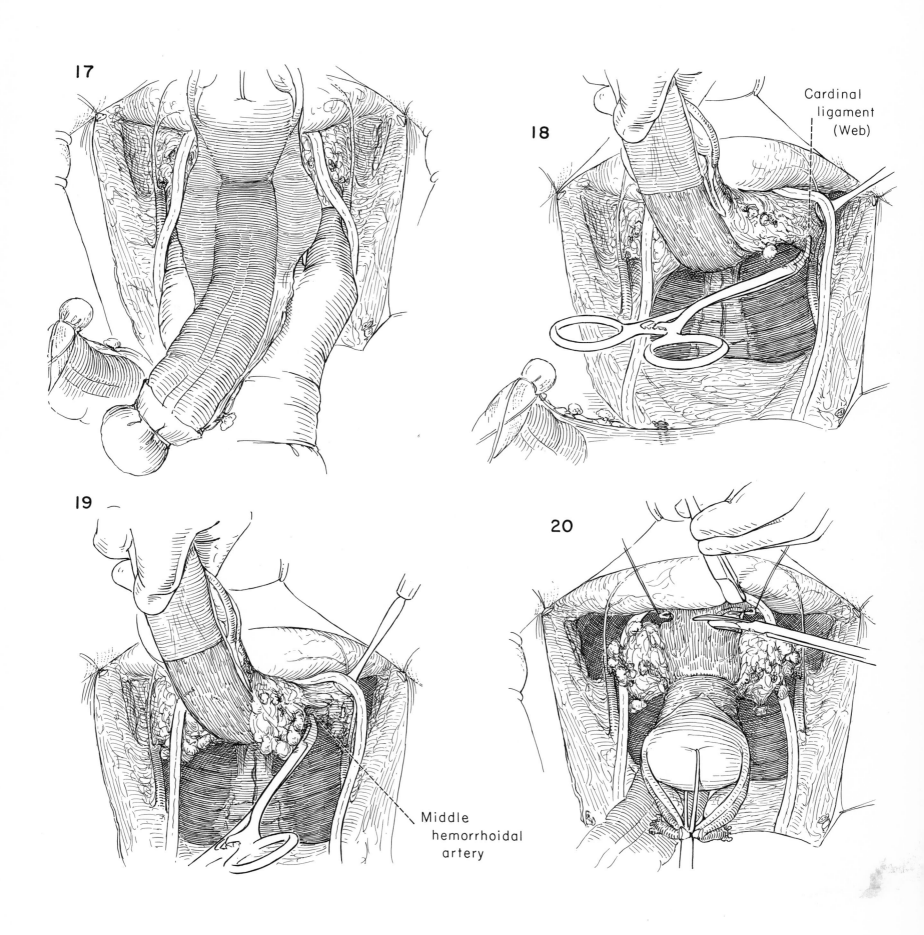

17

18

Cardinal
ligament
(Web)

19

20

Middle
hemorrhoidal
artery

Figure 21. The surgeon now turns his attention to the dissection of the regional nodes.

The tissue lying over the bony promontory of the sacrum is cleaned from it and from the posterior surface of the left common iliac vein which crosses the midline to join the inferior vena cava lying on the right side of the aorta. In making this dissection the surgeon should take care not to damage the middle sacral vessels which run longitudinally over the sacrum in the midline.

Figure 22. The mass of tissue containing the presacral nodes is freed from the underlying iliac vein and elevated and the pedicle is clamped at the level of the bifurcation of the aorta. The tissues included in the clamp are secured with a stitch ligature and the clamp is removed. As a general policy, all terminal pedicles containing lymphatics are clamped and ligated whether proximal or distal to the field of operation. Lymph drainage can sometimes be profuse and lymphoceles troublesome. Our incidence of this complication is very low, and we give credit for this to our invariable rule of ligating all pedicles.

Figure 23. The pelvic lymphadenectomy begins by separation of the tissues from the surface and the inner border of the psoas muscle.

Figure 24. The steps follow the same pattern previously outlined for the Wertheim and other exenteration procedures. (See pp. 343 to 347.) The external iliac artery and vein as well as the area between the two are cleared of all lymphatic tissue. The dissection continues upward along the common iliac artery and vein. The tissue is elevated as the surgeon places a clamp on the proximal portion. The level chosen is approximately that of the aortic bifurcation. The tissues are divided and secured with a stitch ligature. The clamp is them removed.

Figure 25. With the external, common and internal iliac arteries free of all lymphatic tissue, the assistant places a vein retractor beneath the external iliac vein and elevates it to provide better exposure for the surgeon as he cleans the nodal mass from beneath. The obturator nerve runs through the tissue and must be freed from the mass. The entire obturator space is cleaned as the surgeon draws the mass of tissue containing the nodes toward the midline and gently dissects the tissue from the nerve and the anterior surface of the internal iliac vein.

Figure 26. This illustration shows the vessels cleared of all node-bearing tissue, the ureters lying free and the bladder intact. The specimen, including the rectum with the rubber drain tied over its open end, lies deep in the pelvis. The proximal end of the sigmoid colon is brought out, as a colostomy, through a separate opening in the abdominal wall on the left side.

The final steps of actual removal will be carried out from below. The pelvic peritoneum is reconstructed, usually without difficulty, and the abdomen is then closed. Braided wire sutures may be used on the fascia and supplemented by wire stay sutures.

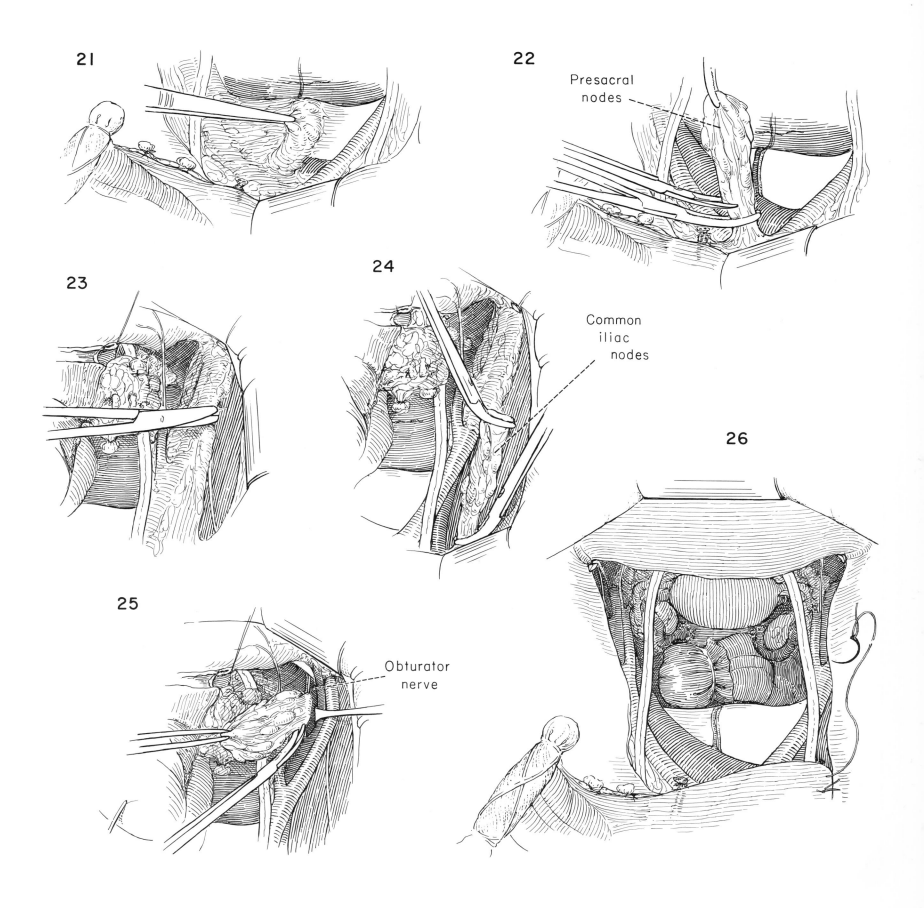

Figure 27. The patient's legs have been placed in stirrups in the lithotomy position. The operative field has been suitably prepared and draped. The surgeon now outlines the portion of the vulva and vagina he wishes to remove.

Figure 28. The skin incisions are deepened as the dissection is carried around and below the anal opening. The anal opening is sealed off by oversewing the edges of skin with a running silk suture. The ends of the sutures are left long after tying. Traction on them will help the surgeon to carry out his dissection in tissue planes.

Figure 29. The assistant holds the skin edges back with Allis clamps as the surgeon draws the anal mass laterally to expose the vessels as they are encountered. They are doubly clamped and the tissues divided and sutured with chromic catgut stitch ligatures.

Figure 30. The turned-in stump of the bowel is elevated as the surgeon follows the posterior wall of the anal canal and lower rectum to the firm ligamentous attachment at the tip of the coccyx. This is cut across and the presacral cavity entered.

Figure 31. The levator muscles are exposed. The specimen is drawn to the opposite side as the surgeon places the index finger in the space behind and sections the muscles, with the finger acting as a guide. All bleeding vessels are clamped and tied as they are confronted. The steps are repeated on the opposite side. Note that the posterior wall of the vagina is still intact.

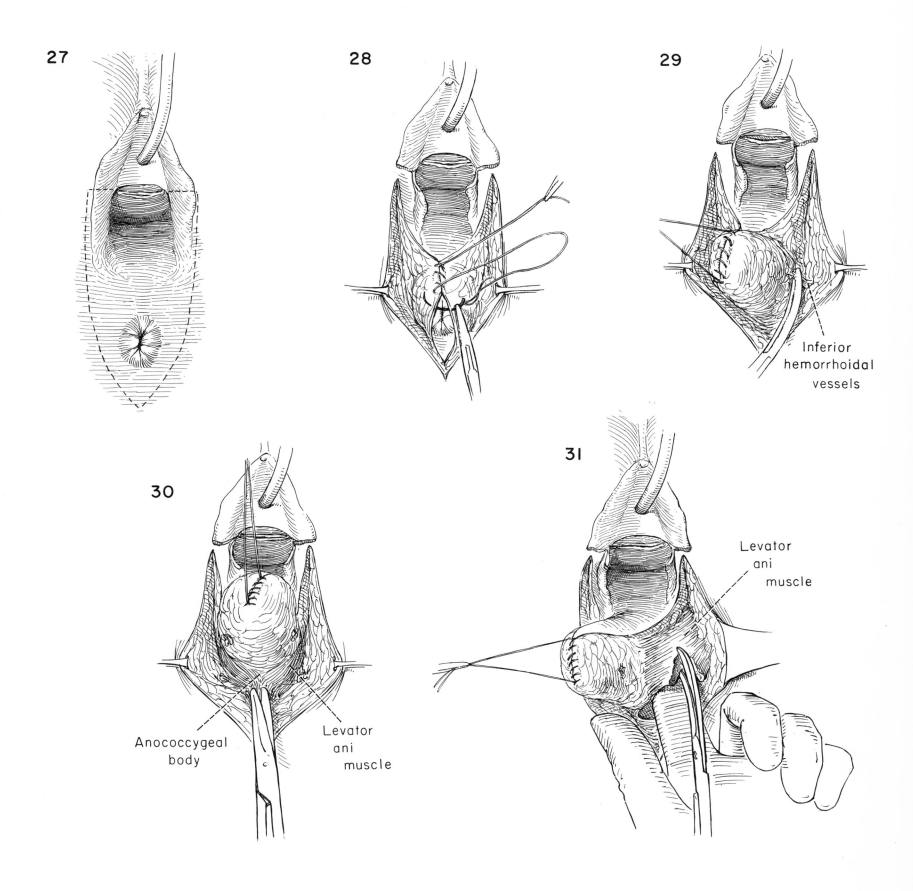

27

28

29

Inferior
hemorrhoidal
vessels

30

Anococcygeal
body

Levator
ani
muscle

31

Levator
ani
muscle

Figure 32. The transverse septum, consisting of the conjoint bulbocavernosus and transverse perineal muscles, is clamped at both ends and divided and the stumps ligated. Frequently, several steps like the one shown here are required before the specimen is freed completely.

Figure 33. With all muscle attachments divided, the intra-abdominal mass is now drawn through the opening in the pelvic floor. The only remaining point of fixation is the lateral vaginal walls on both sides.

The surgeon now introduces the index finger of the left hand into the opening created by the transverse section of the anterior vaginal wall. The bladder wall is gently pushed backward and upward as the finger is introduced. The surgeon, using his index finger as a guide, now divides the vaginal wall with scissors. The steps are repeated on the opposite side and the entire specimen is removed.

Figure 34. This illustration shows the area after the vulvar dissection and the removal of the specimen. Note the catheter in the bladder.

Perineal support is often obtained by bringing the muscle partially together in the midline with interrupted catgut sutures.

Figure 35. After several drains have been placed through the lower portion of the incision into the lower pelvic cavity, the skin and fat are loosely approximated with heavy silk sutures.

Alternate Method of Closure

When the extent of excision of pelvic floor supports does not permit any form of reconstruction, and particularly when the peritoneum was inadequate for closure, it is desirable to use a combination of pack and drain that will allow the abdominal contents to agglutinate inferiorly and seal themselves off from the raw pelvic cavity during the early phases of healing. One method of achieving this goal is shown in the inset. A large square of rubber dam with holes cut in it for drainage is gently pushed up into the pelvis from below by packing several large gauze strips into its concavity. Starting on the fifth postoperative day, the bulk is gradually diminished by withdrawal of sections of the pack. It is usually all out by the ninth or tenth day.

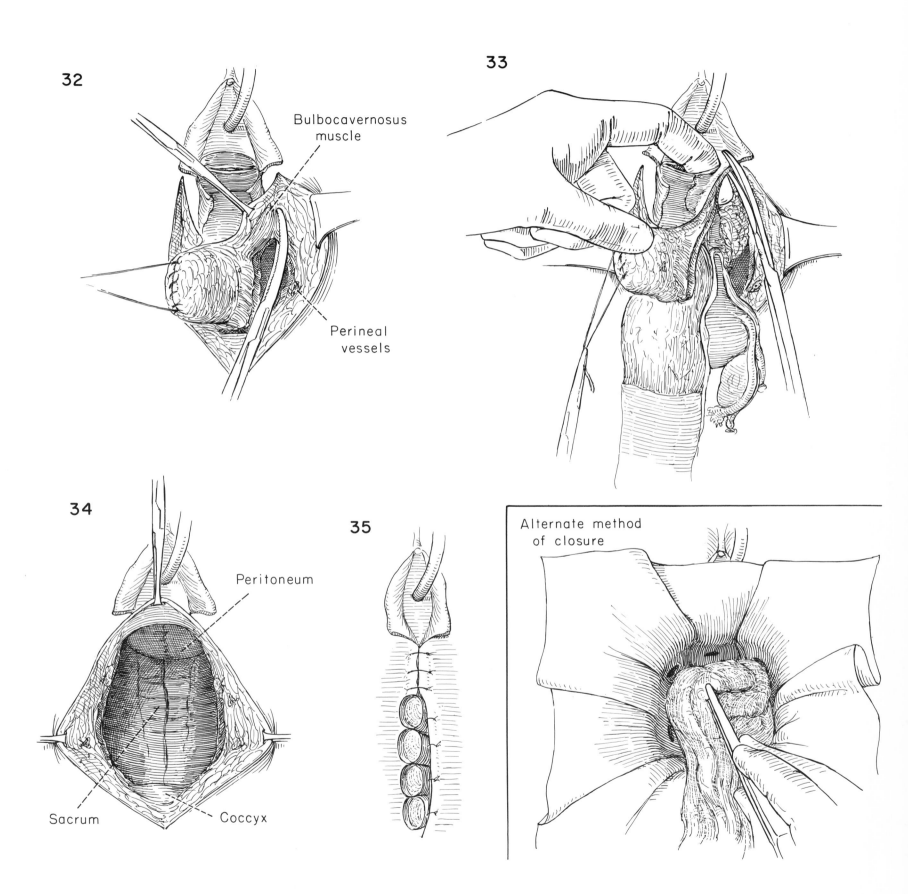

32

Bulbocavernosus muscle

Perineal vessels

33

34

Peritoneum

Sacrum

Coccyx

35

Alternate method of closure

Index